State of the Art in Biomaterials for Drug Delivery

State of the Art in Biomaterials for Drug Delivery

Guest Editor

Chengzhen Liu

MDPI

Basel • Beijing • Wuhan • Barcelona • Belgrade • Novi Sad • Cluj • Manchester

Guest Editor
Chengzhen Liu
College of Life Sciences
Qingdao University
Qingdao
China

Editorial Office
MDPI AG
Grosspeteranlage 5
4052 Basel, Switzerland

This is a reprint of the Special Issue, published open access by the journal *Journal of Functional Biomaterials* (ISSN 2079-4983), freely accessible at: https://www.mdpi.com/journal/jfb/special_issues/bio_drug_delivery.

For citation purposes, cite each article independently as indicated on the article page online and as indicated below:

Lastname, A.A.; Lastname, B.B. Article Title. *Journal Name* **Year**, *Volume Number*, Page Range.

ISBN 978-3-7258-4955-0 (Hbk)
ISBN 978-3-7258-4956-7 (PDF)
https://doi.org/10.3390/books978-3-7258-4956-7

Contents

About the Editor

Chengzhen Liu

Doctor, Assistant to the Dean of the College of Life Sciences, Associate Professor, Master's Supervisor.

I am currently an associate professor in the School of Life Sciences, Qingdao University. My research interests include the intensive processing and design of nano-enzymes, the stabilization of functional components, and the development of functional foods, with publications in AM, Nano Lett., JCIS, JAFC, and Food Hydrocolloids. And other internationally renowned journals published more than 40 SCI papers, with an h index of 26, and have been cited nearly 2600 times. I applied for more than 10 invention patents and participated in two works (one national high-quality teaching material). I am currently a visiting editor of the Journal of Functional Biomaterials. I am in charge of the National Natural Science Foundation project, the youth innovation team of colleges and universities in Shandong Province, the industry-school contract coordination education project of the Ministry of Education, the "Golden seed" talent project of Qingdao City, and the introduction of the scientific research startup project of Qingdao University, etc. As the backbone of scientific research, I participate in the national key R&D program, the Qingdao Huimin special project, and so on. I have made achievements recognized by my counterparts at home and abroad in my field and have been invited to give a report at international and domestic conferences. "Early screening and rehabilitation team for major diseases"—the core member of the 2023 excellent graduate guidance team of Qingdao University, was awarded as "Elsevier Young Scientist Award", "Outstanding Instructor of National College Student Life Science Competition", "Outstanding Instructor of the 14th Shandong University Student Science and Technology Festival", "Excellent Head Teacher of Qingdao University".

Journal of
Functional
Biomaterials

MDPI

Article

Development of Multilayer Ciprofloxacin Hydrochloride Electrospun Patches for Buccal Drug Delivery

Jorge Teno [1,†], Maria Pardo-Figuerez [2,†], Kelly J. Figueroa-Lopez [2], Cristina Prieto [2] and Jose M. Lagaron [2,*]

1 R&D Department, Bioinicia S.L., Calle Algepser 65 nave 3, Paterna, 46980 Valencia, Spain
2 Novel Materials and Nanotechnology Group, Institute of Agrochemistry and Food Technology (IATA), Spanish Council for Scientific Research (CSIC), Calle Catedrático Agustín Escardino Benlloch 7, Paterna, 46980 Valencia, Spain
* Correspondence: lagaron@iata.csic.es
† These authors contributed equally to this work.

Abstract: Bacterial infections in the oral cavity can become a serious problem causing pain, sores and swelling for several weeks. This type of infection could be alleviated using mucoadhesive delivery systems, allowing local administration of the antibiotic to inhibit bacterial spreading. This work reports the development of a multilayer antibiotic patch containing ciprofloxacin hydrochloride (CPX)-loaded electrospun fibers for the treatment of such infections. For this, the release kinetics of the CPX-loaded fibers was modulated using different ratios of polyester blends. The selected reservoir layer was analyzed by scanning electron microscopy (SEM), Fourier transform infrared spectroscopy (FTIR), wide angle x-ray scattering (WAXS) and differential scanning calorimetry (DSC). These analyses confirmed the presence and good distribution of the drug in the fibers and that the drug is in an amorphous state within the reservoir layer. To enhance mucoadhesion whilst ensuring drug directionality, the reservoir layer was assembled to a backing and an adhesive layer. This multilayer patch was assessed in terms of in vitro drug release, adhesion and antimicrobial properties. The multilayer strategy showed excellent antimicrobial properties over time and also a strong adhesion patch time in the volunteers for an average of 7 h. These results highlight the capabilities of multilayer electrospun patches as platforms to treat oral infections.

Keywords: ciprofloxacin hydrochloride; electrospinning; transmucosal patch; biopolyester; antimicrobial

1. Introduction

Infections are illnesses caused by certain organisms such as bacteria, fungi, viruses and parasites [1]. Among them, bacterial infections are the most commonly reported, and although some of them may result in minor symptoms that usually resolve themselves, some others may cause serious life-threatening conditions, such as pneumonia or sepsis [2–4]. Bacterial infections can also be a serious problem in the oral cavity, with a particular worst-case scenario for immuno-suppressed patients, where the microorganisms present in the mouth can cause ulcers and wounds that can last for weeks [5–10]. These infections are commonly treated with formulations based on gels, sprays, tablets and mucoadhesive systems, with the latter presenting the most promising effects [6,7,11]. Mucoadhesive delivery systems present numerous advantages such as easy administration, sustained delivery to prevent bacteria spreading, rapid onset of action and avoidance of first-pass effect for certain drug types [1,12,13]. Additionally, these systems are often preferred to conventional dosage forms for the patients since they protect the site of action and are more comfortable to use [1,5].

Although mucoadhesive drug delivery presents many advantages, the vast majority of drugs, such as antibiotics, are most popularly administered through oral delivery and subsequent gastrointestinal tract absorption [1,14]. However, this route of delivery is quite limited, not only for the reported side effects but also for the low solubility and permeability of commonly used antibiotics, which are mainly classified as class II (low solubility) or IV (low solubility and low permeability) according to the biopharmaceutical classification system (BCS) [2,15]. In an attempt to increase the bioavailability of such active ingredients, the technique of electrospinning has been frequently used. This technique can be used to generate solid dispersions of an API within a polymer matrix, generating solid pharmaceutical formulations that can adhere to the mucosa membrane. Electrospinning is based on the application of a high electric field to a polymeric solution to generate ultrathin fibrous structures. The rapid evaporation rate of the solvent during the process leads to rapid entrapment of the drug within the polymeric matrix, leaving little possibility for the API to reorganize itself and crystalize [16,17]. Furthermore, the resultant fibrous materials have a high specific area, tunable pore size and controlled mechanical properties, making them attractive in drug delivery applications [18].

Different electrospinning methods such as blending [19], coaxial [20] or emulsion electrospinning [21] are used to efficiently encapsulate active ingredients. It is known that API release kinetics can be tuned with the right selection of the polymer matrix, the morphology, as well as the compatibility of the drug–polymer matrix [19,22]. With an appropriate selection of these parameters, the electrospun fibers can provide a controlled release of antibiotics at the local site, thus actively preventing infection.

Herein we present the development of a multilayer system for the release of ciprofloxacin hydrochloride (CPX) by means of blend electrospinning. CPX is an antibiotic belonging to the fluoroquinolones family, with broad antibacterial activity against Gram-negative and Gram-positive bacteria [7]. Such antimicrobial effects make CPX attractive for treating infections in the urinary tract, skin [23,24], sexually transmitted diseases such as HIV [25] and oral diseases [5–7]. Being considered a class IV drug by the BCS, CPX has limited water solubility at physiological pH as well as a heavy first-pass effect, which makes it an ideal candidate to be administered in a mucoadhesive drug delivery system [7,15].

Some studies have presented the vehiculation of CPX in electrospun fibers. In a study presented by Yarin et al. (2016), the release of CPX was modulated by electrospinning a blend of Poly(methyl methacrylate) (PMMA) with hydrophilic polymers [19]. The different hydrophilic polymers used in the blend (chitosan, polyethylene oxide (PEO) or polyvinyl alcohol (PVA)) dramatically altered the CPX release profiles, with chitosan revealing a slow, gradual release and PEO delivering a burst effect, while PVA yielded a two-stage release. Similarly, Moydeen et al. (2018) utilized core–shell nanofibers of PVA/dextran prepared by emulsion electrospinning to encapsulate CPX. In vitro drug release studies showed that the PVA/Dextran nanofibers could modulate a sustained drug release of CPX, and this could be further tuned by altering the concentration of dextran in the mixture [26]. Another study reported by Wu et al. (2020) presented the delivery of CPX with polymeric blends, in which the second polymeric component modulated the release of CPX [27]. These studies efficiently analyzed the release kinetics of CPX; however, they were based on monolayer systems and did not specify the end application, making it difficult to correlate the release kinetics data with the application time of the delivery system at the site of action.

In the case of mucoadhesive systems for drug delivery, a study based on a buccal cast film for CPX delivery was carried out by Kanango et al. [7]. In this case, the study reported a release of CPX for up to 6 h, with a mucoadhesion time of approximately 211 min. A similar study based on the oral mucosa release of metronidazole reported a release time of up to 7 h, with an average mucoadhesion of approximately 2 h [10]. Mucoadhesive electrospun patches for the release of clobetasol have also been reported in the literature, where authors reported a clobetasol release close to 100% after 360 min, along with a patch residence time of approximately 120 min [28]. According to these studies, it appears that the release kinetics of the API are often designed for mucoadhesive platforms to match the relatively short average mucoadhesion time of the patch.

This work presents a multilayer CPX drug delivery system developed to simultaneously adhere to the mucosa, support drug unidirectionality and treat antimicrobial infections in the oral cavity. We previously reported a multilayer approach based on carvedilol (CVD)-loaded fibers, in which a trilayer system modulated the adhesion and release of CVD [17]. For the work presented here, a reservoir layer containing CPX, a mucoadhesive layer (ADH) and a backing layer (BL) were assembled independently to obtain a sustained drug delivery system. Firstly, a blending strategy using two polymers, poly-ε-caprolactone (PCL) and poly(lactic acid) (PLA), was used to finely tune the release of CPX. The most optimum formulation in terms of release rate was chosen as the reservoir layer and was characterized by scanning electron microscope (SEM), attenuated total reflectance Fourier transformed infrared spectroscopy (ATR-FTIR), wide angle x-ray scattering (WAXS) and differential scanning calorimetry (DSC). The reservoir layer was then embedded into a sandwich-like structure within the adhesive and the backing layer. Lastly, the release kinetics of the multilayer, as well as its antimicrobial and adhesive characteristics, were analyzed to assess the effectiveness of the antibiotic multilayer system.

2. Materials and Methods

2.1. Materials

Ciprofloxacin hydrochloride monohydrate (CPX) was obtained from Uquifa (Castellbisbal, Spain). Poly-ε-caprolactone (PCL, Mw 80000 Da) was supplied by Perstorp Caprolactones Ltd (Warrington, United Kingdom), and poly(lactic acid) (PLA viscosity midpoint 2.0 dL/g) was supplied by Natureworks®(Naarden, Netherlands). For the mucoadhesive layer, polyethylene oxide (PEO, Mw 200000 Da) was purchased from the Dow Chemical Company (Montomeryville, PA, USA), and Eudragit RS100 (PAC, copolymer of ethylacrylate, methyl methacrylate and trimethylammonioethyl meth-acrylate chloride) was purchased from Evonik Industries (Essen, Germany). Chloroform (ACS reagent, ≥99.8%) was supplied by Sigma-Aldrich (Madrid, Spain), whilst methanol (≥99%) was supplied by Panreac Química S.L.U. (Castellar del Vallès, Barcelona). The solvent 1,1,1,3,3,3-hexafluoro-2-propanol (HFIP) was supplied by Fluorochem (Hadfield, United Kingdom) and N,N,-dimethylformamide (DMF, ≥99.8%) was purchased from VWR Chemicals (Leuven, Belgium). All the polymers and reagents were used as received without further purification.

2.2. Solution Preparation

Solutions were prepared by dissolving each polymer in its corresponding solvent, as indicated in Table 1. A concentration of 8 wt.% was used for the different reservoir layers and the backing layer (BL), however the concentration was 13 wt.% for the mucoadhesive layer (ADH). In some cases, the surface tension was measured using a DynoTester tensiometer from Krüss GmbH (Hamburg, Germany). In all cases, an amount of 2 wt.% in a solution of CPX was added, so the loading of CPX in the materials was 20%.

Table 1. Composition of PCL-PLA polymer blend solutions, backing layer (BL) and adhesive layer (ADH).

Sample ID	Polymer Matrix and Ratio of the Polymer Blend (*w/w*)	Ratio Polymer/CPX (*w/w*)	Solvents and Ratio (*w/w*)
PCL	PCL	80/20	HFIP
80PCL/20PLA	PCL/PLA (80/20)	80/20	HFIP
70PCL/30PLA	PCL/PLA (70/30)	80/20	HFIP
60PCL/40PLA	PCL/PLA (60/40)	80/20	HFIP
50PCL/50PLA	PCL/PLA (50/50)	80/20	HFIP
20PCL/80PLA	PCL/PLA (20/80)	80/20	HFIP
PLA	PLA	80/20	HFIP
BL	PCL	-	Chloroform/Methanol (90/10)
ADH	PEO/PCL/PAC (70/17.5/12.5)	-	Chloroform/DMF (80/20)

2.3. Electrospinning

The electrospinning process was carried out in a high throughput Fluidnatek^{TM} LE-100 equipped with a multi-emitter injector from Bioinicia S.L. (Valencia, Spain) and coupled with an air-conditioned unit system. Table 2 shows the electrospinning parameters used for each solution. The environmental conditions were kept at 25 °C and 30% relative humidity (RH) for all the electrospinning processes.

Table 2. Electrospinning parameters of the PCL-PLA polymer blends solutions with and without CPX, backing layer (BL) and adhesive layer (ADH).

Sample ID	Flow-Rate (mL/h)	Voltage V+/V− (kV)	Needle-to Collector Distance (cm)
PCL	5	30/−25	15
80PCL/20PLA	10	15/−5	15
70PCL/30PLA	10	35/−25	15
60PCL/40PLA	10	35/−25	15
50PCL/50PLA	20	30/−15	15
20PCL/80PLA	10	25/−5	15
PLA	10	27/−20	15
BL	20	15/−2	15
ADH	15	25/−10	30

To prepare the multilayer patch, a three-layer structure was prepared. For this, the mucoadhesive layer and reservoir layer were electrospun in a "layer-by-layer" approach, where one layer was electrospun on top of the other one (see Figure 1a,b). Then, a hydrophobic backing layer (BL) made of electrospun PCL fibers was electrospun separately (Figure 1c) and laminated to the previously prepared bilayer patch. The lamination was carried out using a hot press (Carver 4122, Wabash, IN, USA), programmed at 50 °C for 10 s without pressure at the top plate facing the backing layer, meaning that no temperature on the bottom plate was applied in the adhesive layer zone to assemble the whole multilayer patch (Figure 1d,e). The backing layer of the patch is designed to act as an impermeable layer due to the coalescence of the fibers to promote drug unidirectionality towards the mucosa, and so it is pivotal to the structure of the patch. The surface density was optimized at 20 g/m^2 for the backing layer, 60 g/m^2 for the reservoir layer and 100 g/m^2 for the adhesive layer.

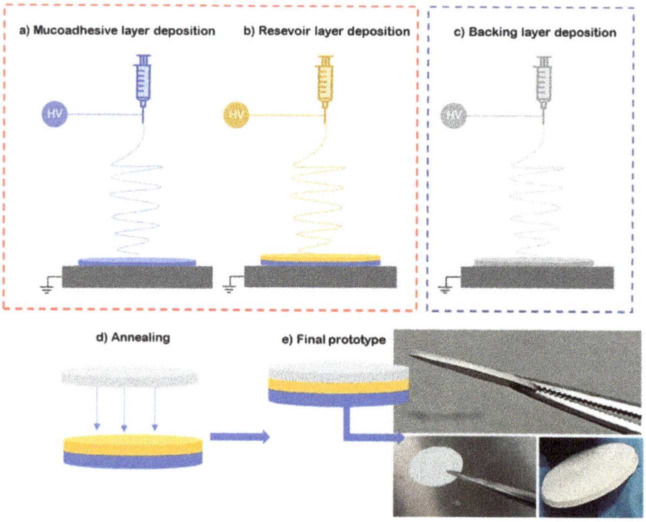

Figure 1. Diagram of the multilayer assembling. (**a**) Electrospinning of adhesive layer (blue, ADH); (**b**) electrospinning of reservoir layer over the adhesive layer (yellow); (**c**) backing layer electrospun separately from the previous layers (grey, BL); (**d**) lamination by low-temperature annealing of the backing layer against the bilayer patch; (**e**) resultant prototype of the multilayer approach.

2.4. Fiber Morphology (SEM)

Fiber morphology was analyzed by scanning electron microscopy (SEM) using a Phenom XL G2 Desktop microscope (Thermo Fisher Scientific, Waltham, MA, USA) with an electron beam acceleration of 5 kV. Microanalysis was performed by energy-dispersive X-ray spectroscopy with a Hitachi S-4800 FE-SEM (EDS, Hitachi High Technologies Corp., Hitachi, Japan). Average fiber diameter based on at least 100 fibers was determined using Phenom ProSuite Software on SEM images.

2.5. Fourier Transform Infrared (FTIR)

The placebo and CPX electrospun blends were evaluated with Fourier transformed infrared spectroscopy and measured with a Bruker Tensor 37 FT-IR Spectrometer (Bruker, Ettlingen, Germany) coupled with the attenuated total reflectance (ATR) sampling accessory Golden Gate (Specac Ltd., Orpington, UK). Spectra were collected from an average of 64 scans in the range of 600–4000 cm^{-1}, with a resolution of 4 cm^{-1}.

2.6. Differential Scanning Calorimetry (DSC)

The electrospun fibers were studied by differential scanning calorimetry (DSC) on a DSC-8000 analyzer from PerkinElmer, Inc. (Waltham, MA, USA), equipped with a cooling accessory Intracooler 2 also from PerkinElmer, Inc. Approximately 3 mg of each sample were placed in standard aluminum pans and heated from 0 to 300 °C and at a rate of 10 °C/min using a nitrogen flow of 20 mL/min as the sweeping gas.

2.7. Wide-Angle X-ray Scattering (WAXS)

Samples were scanned by wide-angle X-ray scattering at room temperature in reflection mode using a Bruker AXS D4 Endeavor diffractometer (Bruker, Ettlingen, Germany). The samples were analyzed using incident Cu K-alpha radiation (Cu $K\alpha$ = 1.54 Å) while the generator was set up at 40 kV and 40 mA. The data were collected over a range of scattering angles (2Θ) in the 5–40° range.

2.8. In Vitro Drug Release

Drug release was evaluated using a UV-spectrophotometer DINKO UV4000 (Barcelona, Spain). The release of the CPX-loaded monolayer and multilayer patches (2.19 cm^2) into an aqueous phosphate-buffered solution (pH 6.8) medium was monitored by measuring the absorbance at 270 nm at predetermined times whilst stirring at 100 rpm at 37 °C. The reading was compared against a calibration curve produced using standard samples of 1–8 μg/mL of CPX in buffer solution (pH 6.8). The placebo patches were also measured to ensure that the polymeric matrix did not interfere with the CPX reading. A total of 1 mL aliquot of the solution was withdrawn at each time point for UV–vis analysis, and an equal volume of fresh buffer solution was added to maintain the sink conditions. The patches were attached to supports and lowered into the solution media. In the case of the multilayer approach, the patch was placed with the adhesive layer facing toward the buffer solution to somehow mimic the initial contact with the mucosa. Since the purpose of the study was to generate a patch for oral mucosa delivery, a relatively low release time (8 h) was intended, taking into consideration that the mucoadhesion of the patch may, in principle, last for a few hours for patient comfortability. The release experiments and the standard curves were carried out in triplicate, and the cumulative release rate was reported as mean ± S.D.

2.9. Determination of Experimental Loading Capacity

To determine the experimental loading of CPX within the fibers, the CPX-loaded monolayers (2.19 cm^2), weighing approximately 2 mg, were dissolved in 60 mL of HFIP to fully dissolve both CPX and the polymeric matrix. The resulting solution was stirred at 100 rpm for an hour and then analyzed by UV-spectrophotometer DINKO UV4000 (Barcelona, Spain). The reading was compared against a calibration curve produced using standard samples of 1–8 μg/mL of CPX in HFIP. The absorbances at 270 nm were recorded, and the experimental CPX loading (%) in the fibers was calculated using Equation (1):

$$\text{CPX Loading }(\%) = \frac{m_d}{m_p} \times 100, \tag{1}$$

where m_d is the mass of the drug obtained experimentally as described above, and m_p is the total mass of the sample analyzed. Similarly, the process yield was calculated as follows:

$$\text{Process yield}(\%) = \frac{\text{experimental L}}{\text{theoretical L}} \times 100 \tag{2}$$

where process yield is calculated as the ratio between the theoretical and experimental loading of the drug in the solution and the patch, respectively.

2.10. Kinetic Model of In Vitro Drug Release

To analyze the kinetics of the in vitro drug release behavior of the fibers, the semi-empirical mathematical model of Korsmeyer–Peppas was applied as follows:

$$Q = kt^n \tag{3}$$

where Q is the amount of drug released in time t, K is the Korsmeyer–Peppas release rate constant and n is the release exponent, which depends on the type of drug polydispersity, geometry and transport. Depending on the release exponent, diffusional release mechanisms were classified as; $n< 0.5$ pseudo-Fickian diffusional behavior, $n = 0.5$ Fickian diffusion, $0.5 < n < 1$ non-Fickian diffusion, $n = 1$ case II transport (zero-order release) and $n > 1$ super case II transport [29].

2.11. In Vitro Patch Residence Time Study

For the in vitro adhesion studies, a qualitative study was carried out in which 1 mL of aqueous phosphate-buffered solution (pH 6.8) was initially deposited on 60 × 15 mm size Petri dishes. Thereafter, the electrospun multilayer of 2.19 cm^2 size (with the adhesive layer facing the Petri dish) was applied on the wet plastic surface of the Petri dishes by pressing firmly on top of the patch (backing layer side) for 5 s. The test was carried out at 37 °C. A visual inspection of the adhesion of the patch to the surface of the Petri dish was carried out at 30 min and 90 min.

2.12. Mucosa In Vivo Patch Residence Time

In order to determine the overall in vivo adhesion time and patch acceptability, multilayer patches were tested by six healthy human volunteers (three males and three females) ages between 25–50 years old. Similarly to other studies [30–32], the volunteers were asked to apply the multilayer patches in the gingiva region for 5 s with applied pressure. The residence time of the patch was defined as the time interval between the application of the patch and the time point where it moved, detached or could not be felt any more at the site of application. During the test period, volunteers were allowed to drink, eat and speak.

2.13. Antimicrobial Activity

Staphylococcus aureus (*S. aureus*) CECT240 (ATCC 6538p) and Escherichia coli (*E. coli*) CECT434 (ATCC 25922) strains were obtained from the Spanish Type Culture Collection (CECT, Valencia, Spain). The bacteria were thawed at 37 °C under agitation at 180 rpm for 24 h and were then diluted in a 1:1000 proportion in a Mueller–Hinton broth until obtaining a concentration of 3–5$\times 10^5$ colony-forming unit (CFU)/mL [33].

The antimicrobial activity of the multilayer patch was studied by the disc diffusion method, following the protocols of the Clinical and Laboratory Standards Institute (CLSI) with some modifications [33,34]. Patches of 2.19 cm^2 with (CPX multilayer patch, approximately 2.6 mg of CPX) and without CPX (placebo multilayer patch, control) were deposited onto the Mueller–Hinton solid agar surface previously inoculated with 100 µL of *S. aureus* and *E. coli* (3–5 × 10^5 CFU/mL). The samples were analyzed in triplicate and incubated at 37 °C for 24 h. Inhibition diameters were measured after incubation, and the results are presented as the mean ± S.D.

The antimicrobial performance of the patches was also determined based on the guidelines of the macro-dilution protocol, as described in the Methods for Dilution Antimicrobial Susceptibility Tests for Bacteria that Grow Aerobically [35]. For this, patches with and without CPX (placebo) with sizes of 2.19 cm^2 were placed in a tube previously inoculated with *S. aureus* and *E. coli* (3–5 × 10^5 CFU/mL). The tubes were incubated at 37 °C, and aliquots were taken at 1, 3, 6 and 8 h. Thereafter, the aliquots were 10-fold serially diluted and incubated at 37 °C for 24 h to quantify the number of viable bacteria by a conventional plate count. Each test was conducted in triplicate. The results are presented as bacterial density expressed as Log CFU/mL.

3. Results and Discussion

3.1. Reservoir Layer

3.1.1. Effect of Polymer Blends on Release Kinetics of CPX

Blends of PCL and PLA containing CPX were electrospun to generate different reservoir layers in an attempt to modulate the release kinetics of CPX. Although the electrospinning parameters were modified slightly for each blend, all of them had a similar smooth fiber morphology and a fiber diameter between 0.5 to 1.5 µm (see Figure 2).

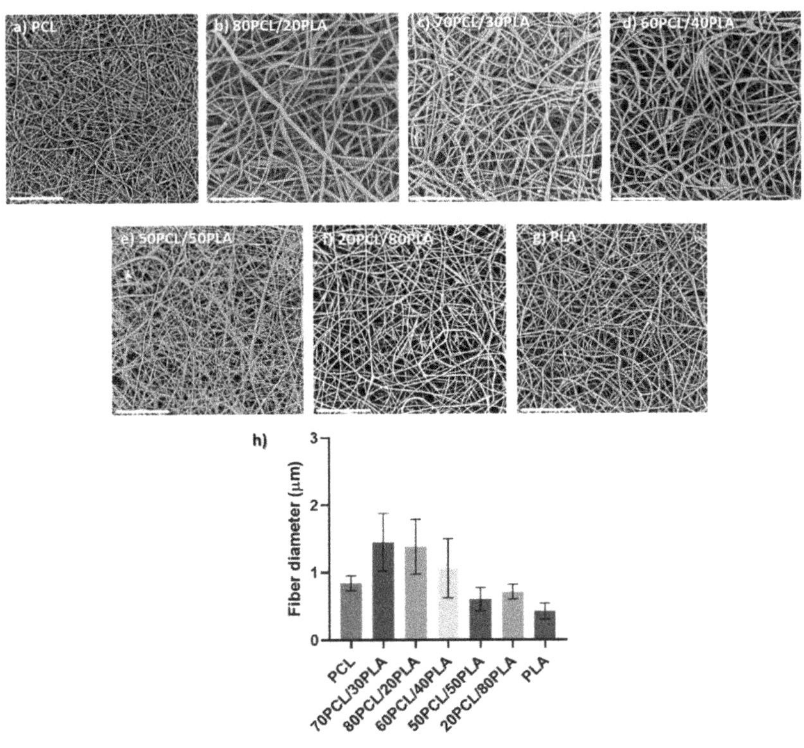

Figure 2. (**a–g**) Scanning electron microscopy (SEM) micrographs of the different blends prepared by electrospinning containing CPX (20%) and (**h**) their average fiber diameter (µm). Scale bar= 30 µm, Magnification (×2500) for all the samples.

Thereafter, the loading of CPX was then measured to ensure the presence of CPX in the matrices. Table 3 gathers the results obtained on the experimental CPX loadings for the different electrospun fibers. All the monolayers presented experimental loadings close to the theoretical ones (20%), which led to close to 100% process yield, indicating the suitability of electrospinning for the processing of APIs to generate efficient solid pharmaceutical forms.

Table 3. Values of experimental CPX loadings in the different electrospun fibers as well as the yield of the process (%).

Sample ID	CPX Loading (%)	Yield (%)
PCL	19.9 ± 1.4	99.4 ± 1.4
80PCL/20PLA	19.6± 1.1	97.8 ± 0.5
70PCL/30PLA	19.5 ± 0.6	97.4 ± 2.8
60PCL/40PLA	19.4 ± 0.9	97.1 ± 1.4
50PCL/50PLA	19.8 ± 1.2	98.0 ± 1.5
20PCL/80PLA	19.7 ± 1.1	98.2 ± 1.1
PLA	19.3 ± 0.2	96.2 ± 0.9

Figure 3 shows the release behavior of CPX-loaded electrospun fibers prepared with PCL, 80PCL/20PLA, 70PCL/30PLA, 60PCL/40PLA, 50PCL/50PLA, 20PCL/80PLA and PLA. As can be observed in Figure 3a, the pure PLA and PCL encapsulating materials presented antagonist behavior. The release of CPX in the electrospun PLA fibers showed very slow release over time, whilst PCL presented a burst release with complete release after 2 h. In the case of PCL, the well-known high drug permeability of the PCL polymer was in good agreement with previous studies [21,36,37]. On the other hand, the slow release of PLA, also reported previously, was attributed to its higher intermolecular cohesion and rigidity [36]. Such differing release rates could be used to obtain a tailor-made delivery by blending the two materials. When blending both biopolymers, it was observed that the blend 20PCL/80PLA, which contained the highest amount of PLA, exhibited similar behavior to neat PLA fibers. On the other hand, blends with a higher PCL content (80PCL/20PLA) showed a similar behavior to PCL but with somewhat arrested release compared to pure PCL (Figure 3a). Surprisingly, when the 50PCL/50PLA was analyzed, a limited burst with slower drug release than expected was observed, which was more similar to the behavior of the neat PLA, hence resulting in a negative deviation from the simple rule of mixtures.

Other intermediate blends, i.e., 70PCL/30PLA and 60PCL/40PLA, were also prepared to further modulate drug release (Figure 3a,b). Interestingly, when the blend of 60PCL/40PLA was analyzed, a burst followed by suspended drug released behavior was observed (Figure 3b), similar to what was observed for the 50PCL/50PLA blend. In this case, the CPX was not released entirely during the time of the study. The 70PCL/30PLA blend showed more sustained release than the blend of 80PCL/20PLA, reaching approximately 100% of drug release after 8 h. For the delivery of antibiotics at the local site of action, an initial burst can be ideal for inhibiting bacterial growth before proliferation. Thereafter, more arrested release is convenient to prevent bacteria proliferation of the organisms that resisted the initial burst [37]. The blend 70PCL/30PLA was selected as the reservoir layer to be employed for the design of the multilayer patch.

Polymer blending was previously used as an important strategy to tailor drug release [37–40]. Basar et al. (2017) reported the release modulation of ketoprofen by preparing blends of PCL and gelatin [21]. Malagón et al. (2015) used blends of PCL and PLA to analyze the different release kinetics of amoxicillin. In agreement with this study, rapid release occurred for the electrospun pure PCL-loaded amoxicillin, whereas slow release was reflected for the pure PLA-loaded fibers. Interestingly, the release in the blends was not seen to follow the rule of mixtures either, and the effect was attributed to better compatibility of the antibiotic with the PLA [37]. Similarly, a study by Chou et al. [41] reported an increase in Young's modulus of blended polymer fibers made of PLGA and PCL when PLGA composition increased from 0% to 100%. However, this trend varied significantly and did not follow the rule of mixtures either when the polymer blend fibers were loaded with a 15 wt.% of tenofovir (TFV).

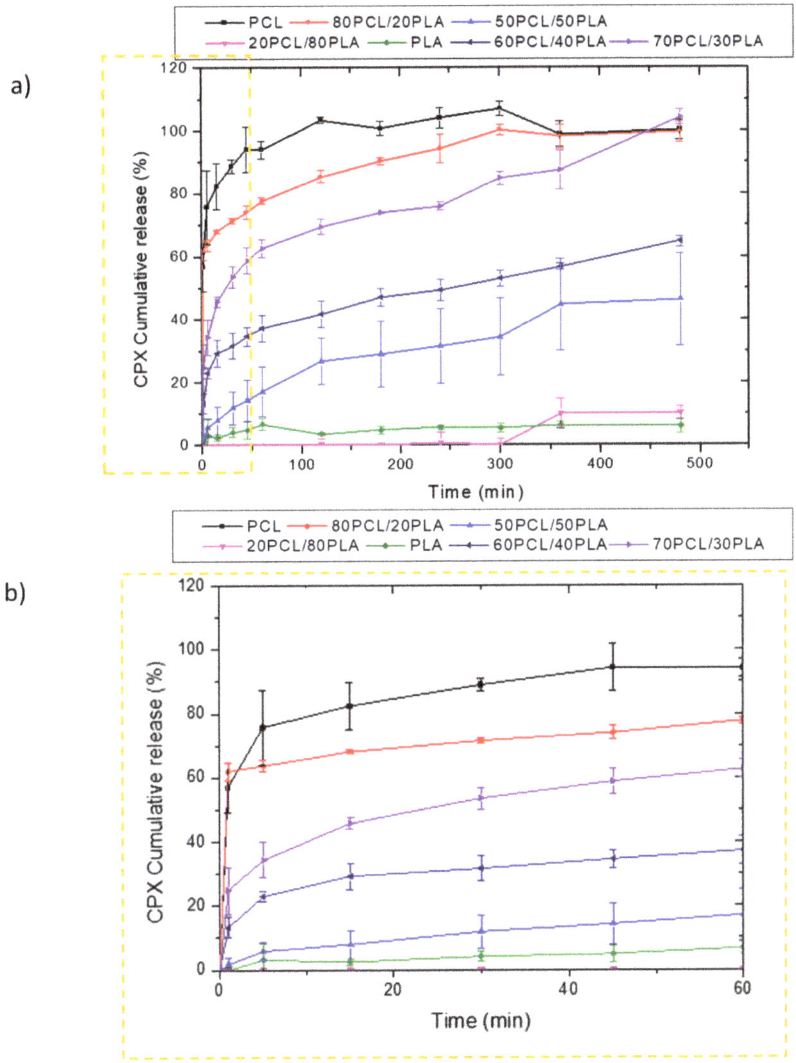

Figure 3. Release profiles of CPX from electrospun PCL/PLA blends. (**a**) Blends PCL, 80PCL/20PLA, 70PCL/30PLA, 60PCL/40PLA, 50PCL/50PLA, 20PCL/80PLA and PLA; (**b**) zoomed zone of the first hour to analyze the initial burst effect. The graphs show the mean ± S.D. ($n = 3$).

In our study, a clear difference can be seen in the release of CPX when PCL becomes the predominant phase in the blend. However, intermediate blends such as 50PCL/50PLA and 60PCL/40PLA deviate very strongly from the rule of mixtures. Thus, it is visible that the blends containing a major ratio of PLA undergo a release arrest of CPX, hence suggesting better compatibility of CPX with PLA. There are, in fact, many potential parameters involved in the release of drugs, such as the morphology of the nanofibers, the crystalline morphology at the mesoscale of the blend components, the physical state of the drug and also the different drug–polymer affinities that may ultimately impact its release [37,41].

3.1.2. Characterization of the Selected Reservoir Layer

The selected 70PCL/30PLA electrospun material was characterized further to obtain information regarding the physical state of CPX and the polymeric blend. Figure 4a shows the DSC thermograms of the selected reservoir layer (70PCL/30PLA), as well as its placebo counterpart (without CPX) and pure CPX. The thermogram of the CPX showed a broad endothermic peak around 150 °C when it ran up to 300 °C, ascribed to dehydration and the loss of moisture corresponding to water molecules that bound directly to the cationic ciprofloxacin, which dehydrates between 140–160 °C [42–47]. Studies in the literature reported that ciprofloxacin hydrochloride monohydrate sequentially melts and degrades in the range of 310–340 °C [45,47], whereas others reported that anhydrous ciprofloxacin melted around 270–280 °C [24]. In this thermogram, a small endothermic peak was present at around 285 °C, suggesting that there may be a part of anhydrous CPX present in the sample, perhaps resultant of the initial water loss. The peaks beyond 300 °C were not analyzed because the blend components would have degraded.

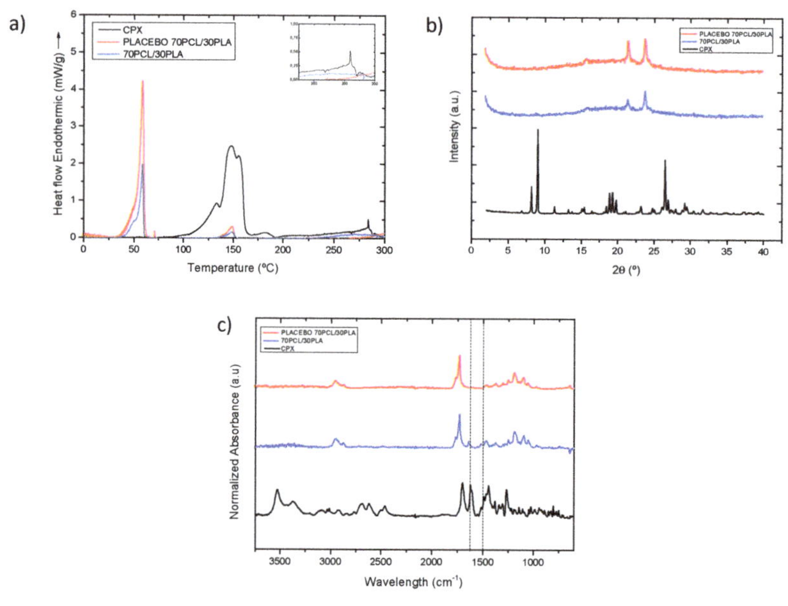

Figure 4. (**a**) Normalized to the polymeric content DSC thermograms and inset with the zoomed out area in the temperature range 250–300 °C, (**b**) WAXS diffractogram and (**c**) normalized intensity ATR-FTIR spectra of samples of CPX powder (black line), placebo electrospun blend (red line) and electrospun CPX containing blend (blue line). The dashed vertical lines indicate the CPX characteristic peaks at 1622 and 1492 cm^{-1}.

For the thermogram of the placebo electrospun blend (70PCL/30PLA), a clear thermal endothermic peak at 59.78 °C, corresponding to the melting point of PCL crystals, was found. Additionally, a small endothermic feature could be seen at 150.2 °C, which was attributed to the melting point of PLA. As per the CPX-containing blend, the signal of PCL and PLA can also be discerned at 59.50 °C and 149.73 °C, respectively. In this case, both peaks, after normalization of the endotherm for the number of polymers present, were smaller in area when compared to the placebo blend. This suggests that API impedes the development of crystallinity in both polymeric phases.

As per the physical state of the drug in the polymeric matrix, this could not be analyzed via DSC since, on the one hand, the degradation of the polymers could influence the endotherm signal beyond 300 °C, and the PCL (T_m ca. 60 °C) and PLA (T_m ca. 150 °C) melting before the CPX (T_m ca. 300–340 °C) could dissolve the CPX crystals [48]. Thus, to assess the physical state of the drug, WAXS analysis was carried out instead (Figure 4b).

The diffractograms in Figure 4b clearly show the X-ray diffraction patterns of the neat CPX powder, exhibiting a clear crystalline nature presented by various smaller peaks and three main sharp ones at around 2-Theta = 8.2°, 9.1° and 26.5°, in agreement with previous studies [49]. For the blend containing CPX and its placebo, the only crystalline peaks that were unambiguously discerned were those associated with the crystals of the PCL in the polyester electrospun blend (70PCL/30PLA), also in agreement with other studies [50]. Interestingly, the placebo spectra show sharper peaks than the blend containing CPX, again suggesting a higher degree of crystallinity for the blend without API. Nevertheless, the lack of CPX representative peaks in the CPX-containing blend confirmed that the CPX was most likely present in an amorphous solid form of the API within the fibers, hindering the arrangement of macromolecular chains in the fibers.

Figure 4c shows a comparison of the ATR-FTIR spectra of the CPX powder, the placebo blend and the CPX-loaded blend. The placebo and CPX-loaded blend showed the main characteristic bands of PCL at 2946, 2870, and 2821 cm^{-1} assigned to CH_2 vibrations, as well as C=O and C-O-C stretching, which were seen at 1720 cm^{-1}, 1238 cm^{-1} and 1161 cm^{-1}, respectively. In addition, the main characteristic peak of PLA at 1080 cm^{-1} associated with the C-O-C stretching was also observed [51]. The CPX powder presented characteristic peaks at 1622 and 1492 cm^{-1} (dashed lines in Figure 4c), associated with C=O and C-H stretching, respectively [52,53]. Regarding the blend 70PCL/30PLA, the more intense characteristic peaks of CPX can be clearly seen in the blend, as suggested in the dashed lines. Therefore, the ATR-FTIR results confirm the presence of CPX within the polymer blend.

3.2. CPX Multilayer Patch

3.2.1. Patch Morphology Characterization

As described in Figure 1, the developed patch consisted of a backing layer based on annealed occlusive electrospun PCL fibers to direct the drug delivery towards the mucosa and a mucoadhesive layer to promote patch adhesion to the oral cavity. The different layers of the CPX multilayer patch made with the 70PCL/30PLA reservoir layer were analyzed under SEM (see Figure 5). The electrospun reservoir layer with and without CPX had a fibrous morphology randomly distributed; however, subtle changes in fiber size were observed when adding CPX (see Figure 5a,b,e). The placebo 70PCL/30PLA fiber size was 2.24 ± 0.7 µm, and for 70PCL/30PLA it was 1.45 ± 0.43 µm. The addition of active ingredients into a polymer solution often results in changes in the solution properties, leading to a change in processability and final fiber morphology. The addition of CPX resulted in a slight increase in the surface tension of the solution (placebo 70PCL/30PLA= 35.7 mN/m; 70PCL/30PLA = 38.4 mN/m), which could be responsible for the decrease in fiber diameter. In terms of processability, both formulas were electrospun under the same conditions, concluding that the addition of CPX did affect fiber diameter but did not affect the productivity or processability of the materials.

Figure 5c,d show the morphology of the adhesive layer (ADH) and the backing layer, respectively. The backing layer exhibited fused PCL fibers due to the annealing step (Figure 5d), whilst the adhesive layer showed a fine random fibrous morphology (Figure 5c). Lastly, Figure 5f shows the EDS mapping of Nitrogen and Fluor elements and the EDS spectrum of the electrospun CPX-containing fiber layer. The spectrum showed the presence of Carbon (C) and Oxygen (O), characteristic elements of the PCL, PLA and CPX, but also Nitrogen and Fluor were detected, elements characteristic of the CPX. The EDS mapping analysis of the F and N elements confirmed the presence and good dispersion of the CPX in the fibers.

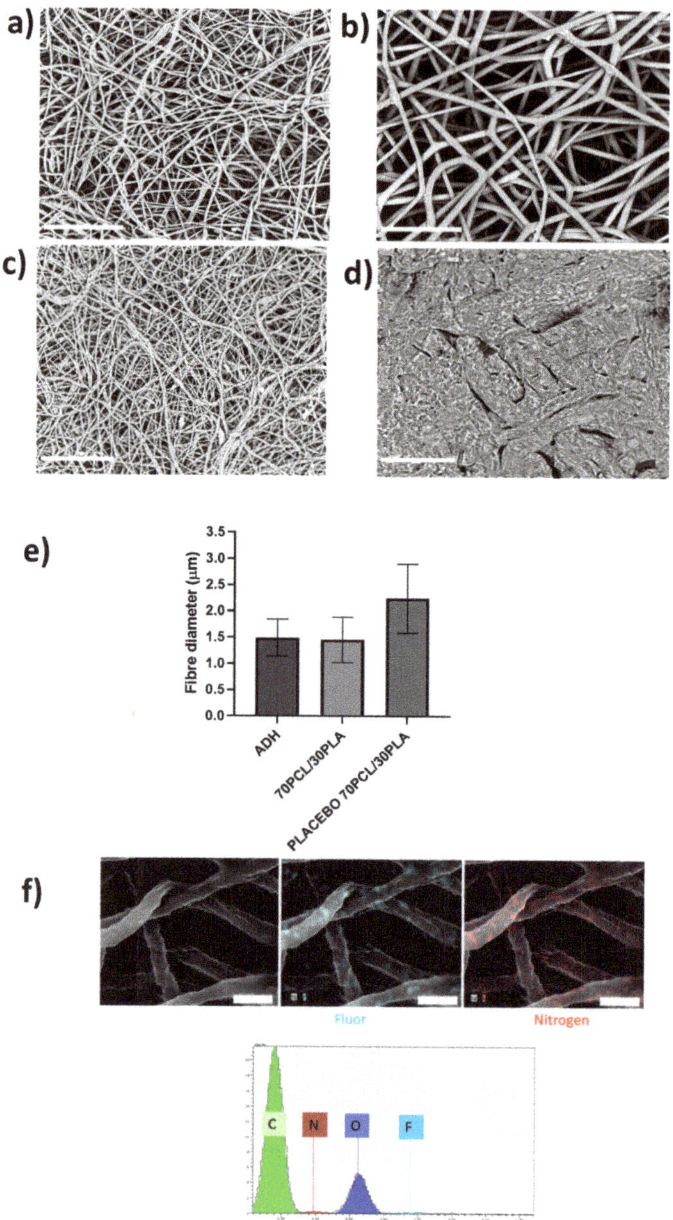

Figure 5. Scanning electron microscopy (SEM) micrographs. (**a**) Blend 70PCL/30PLA containing CPX, (**b**) placebo blend 70PCL/30PLA, (**c**) adhesive layer ADH and (**d**) backing layer after the annealing process. Scale bar = 30 µm, magnification (×2500). (**e**) Fiber diameter of the adhesive layer (ADH), the reservoir layer 70PCL/30PLA and the placebo layer (placebo 70PCL/30PLA). (**f**) Energy-dispersive elemental mapping micrographs of the characteristic elements of CPX. EDS microanalysis spectrum with the main components found is also included (Scale bar = 4 µm).

3.2.2. Effect of the Multilayer Structure in Drug Release

Figure 6 illustrates the cumulative release of the reservoir layer as a monolayer and within the multilayer patch. The release curves were fitted to the Korsmeyer–Peppas fitting model parameters (Table 4). Changes in the release rate among both systems were mainly attributed to the attenuated diffusion of the CPX through the adhesive layer in the multilayer patch. For both mono and multilayer, the values of the regression coefficient (r^2) were high for the model used (Korsmeyer–Peppas), suggesting both a good fit and that more than one type of phenomenon of drug release was involved in the kinetics. In fact, the corresponding n values of the evaluated samples were below 0.5, which indeed indicated that the drug release appeared to follow pseudo-Fickian diffusional behavior.

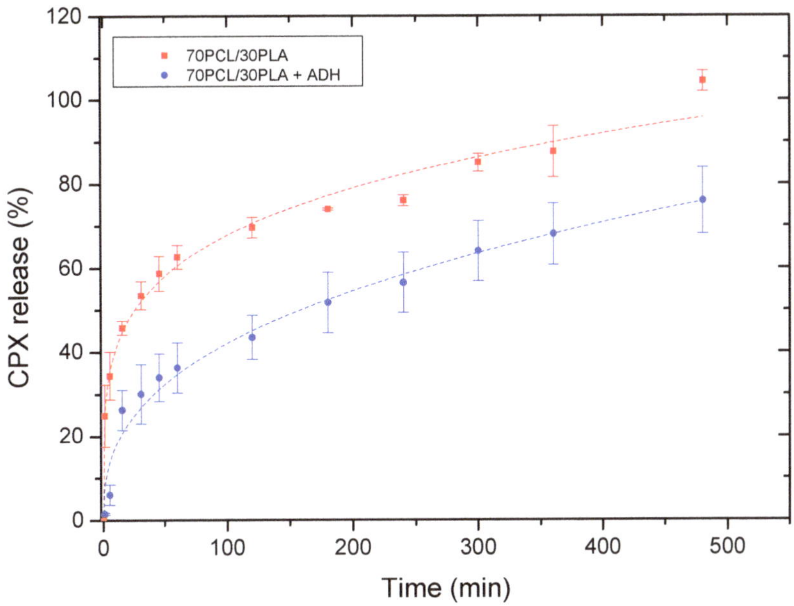

Figure 6. Drug release data comparing the monolayer reservoir layer (70PCL/30PLA) and the multilayer patch containing ADH (PEO/PCL/PAC). Dashed lines correspond to the Korsmeyer–Peppas fitting. Values are presented as the mean ± SD (n = 3).

Table 4. Model parameters of the CPX release profiles for the monolayer 70PCL/30PLA and multilayer patch obtained from the Korsmeyer–Peppas model.

Sample ID	K	n	r^2
Monolayer	24.61	0.22	0.98
Multilayer	7.46	0.38	0.98

As stated above, the multilayer patch led to a slower drug release rate compared to the reservoir monolayer. This observation could be mainly ascribed to the presence of a hydrophobic polymer (PCL) in the adhesive layer, which may hinder the CPX mobility across the adhesive layer, thus resulting in a slower drug release rate. This phenomenon is quantitatively characterized by the modeled parameter K (Korsmeyer–Peppas release rate), which is higher in the monolayer than in the multilayer approach.

3.2.3. Adhesion Test

Mucoadhesion refers to the state in which material and the mucosa are attached together by means of interfacial forces [30]. This parameter is crucial to acknowledge the feasibility of a system to adequately adhere to the mucosa for a desired amount of time [54]. The adhesive formula presented in this work is a combination of hydrophilic (PEO) and hydrophobic (PCL and PAC) polymers since it is well reported in the bibliography that blends of polymers with opposite solubility can maintain layer consistency whilst improving the adhesive properties in the buccal environment [55,56]. The placebo multilayer structure was placed over the surface of a Petri dish containing a buffer solution, and its adhesion was checked after 30 and 90 min to assess the adhesive capabilities of the patch, as previously described in another study [11]. Figure 7a,b present the in vitro adhesion of the patch after 30 and 90 min, respectively. The patch remained strongly attached to the surface of the Petri dish after 30 and 90 min, to the point where it was possible to lift the Petri dish by pulling up the patch (see Figure 7b) due to the adhesion. In the adhesive layer (ADH), the presence of PEO, known to become an adhesive hydrogel in contact with water, and PAC with its ammonium-charged quaternary groups promoting ionic interactions with the negatively charged substrate [57–59], are thought to be the responsible materials to promote the observed strong adhesion. In light of these results, in vivo mucoadhesive study with healthy human volunteers was carried out (Figure 7c).

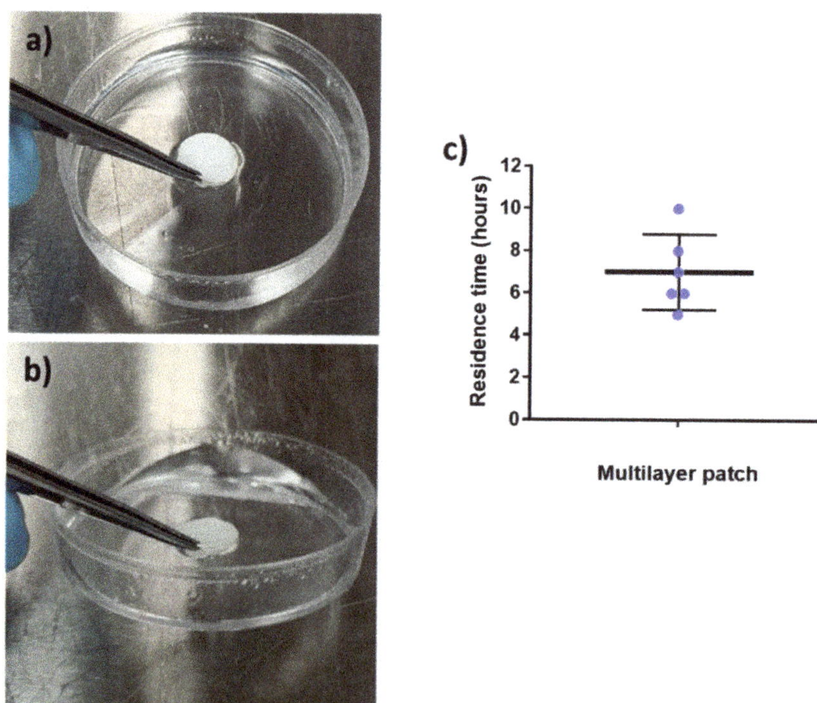

Figure 7. In vitro adhesion tests over time. (**a**) Multilayer placebo patch at time 30 min and (**b**) multilayer placebo patch at time 90 min, showing the lifting of the Petri dish. (**c**) In vivo mucoadhesive performance of the placebo multilayer patch, placed on the gingiva zone. Blue points indicate the individual results of all volunteers involved. The graph presents the mean ± SD (n = 6).

Placebo multilayer patches were placed in the gingiva zone of the mouth since previous studies had shown a better residence time in this area compared to the cheek or the tongue [28]. The patch residence time was ca. 7 h on average, with a variable distribution across the volunteers, probably due to the fact that no restrictions were given to the volunteers in terms of eating and drinking during the study (see Figure 7c). As shown in the in vitro adhesion study, the combination of the hydrophilic PEO and hydrophobic polymers PAC and PCL allowed the synergic prolonged adhesive behavior observed. The different solubility of the polymers that comprise the adhesive layer may have favored the consistency of the layer and, consequently, mucoadhesion. Additionally, as mentioned above, the cationic characteristics of PAC and the possible Van der Waals forces formed between the adhesive layer and the mucus area probably contributed to the adhesiveness [55,56,60–62]. In terms of the data on the controlled release mentioned above, it can be concluded that on average, the adhesive layer ADH adhered during the time required for a significant release of the CPX present in the patch.

3.2.4. Antibacterial Activity

The multilayer patch was also characterized in terms of its antibacterial activity against the Gram-positive and negative bacteria *E. coli* and *S. aureus* after 24 h. Figure 8a represents the inhibition zones presented by both the multilayer patches with CPX (CPX patch) and without CPX (placebo patch). The multilayer patches containing CPX showed a clear inhibition zone for both the Gram-positive and Gram-negative bacteria, with an inhibition halo of 5.92 $\pm$ 0.01 and 5.20 $\pm$ 0.01 cm, respectively, indicating the strong inhibition for both strains. These inhibition zones were not observed in the placebo multilayer patch, indicating the strength of CPX as an antimicrobial. The antibacterial activity was also measured at 1, 3, 6 and 8 h to simulate different patch residence times. Figure 8b shows the antimicrobial results of the multilayer patches with and without CPX. For the patches containing CPX, a high Log reduction was obtained after 1 h and also throughout the timeframe of the experiment for *E. coli*, whilst a lower inhibition was obtained against *S. aureus*, which growth was completely inhibited after 6 h. These results indicate that not only the CPX retains its properties after the electrospinning process but also that a strong antibacterial effect is observed even at low exposure times (less than 8 h). The effectiveness of the loaded electrospun CPX was also observed in other studies, with similar halo sizes to the ones reported here [34,49]. For instance, Li, H. et al. (2019) [34] carried out a study with CPX-loaded poly(vinylpyrrolidone) (PVP) and CPX-loaded ethyl cellulose (EC) fibers containing either 5 or 15% (*w*/*w*) of CPX with respect to the polymer concentration. The inhibition zones of the CPX-loaded PVP fibers at 5 and 15% CPX for *E. coli* and *S. aureus* after 24 h were 5.30 $\pm$ 0.61 and 5.71 $\pm$ 0.60 cm, whereas CPX-loaded EC fibers showed a smaller inhibition zone (4.29 $\pm$ 0.77–4.72 $\pm$ 0.23 cm), most likely due to the faster drug release rates of the PVP nanofibers compared to the EC material [34]. In another study reported by the same group, fibrous blends of poly (di(ethylene glycol) methyl ethermethacrylate) (PDEGMA) and poly(L-lactic acid-co-ε-caprolactone) (P(LLA-CL)) containing CPX showed inhibition zones for *E. coli* and *S. aureus* of 5.35 $\pm$ 0.51 cm and 5.21 $\pm$ 0.44 cm after 24 h, respectively. Similar values were obtained after 72 h, with halo sizes of approximately 5 cm [63]. These studies confirmed that CPX-loaded fibers could efficiently act as antimicrobial monolayer systems. Here, we have additionally shown that, even if enclosed in the middle layer of a multilayer patch, the CPX released from the fibers can gradually diffuse through the external layer, thus exerting an effective antimicrobial effect.

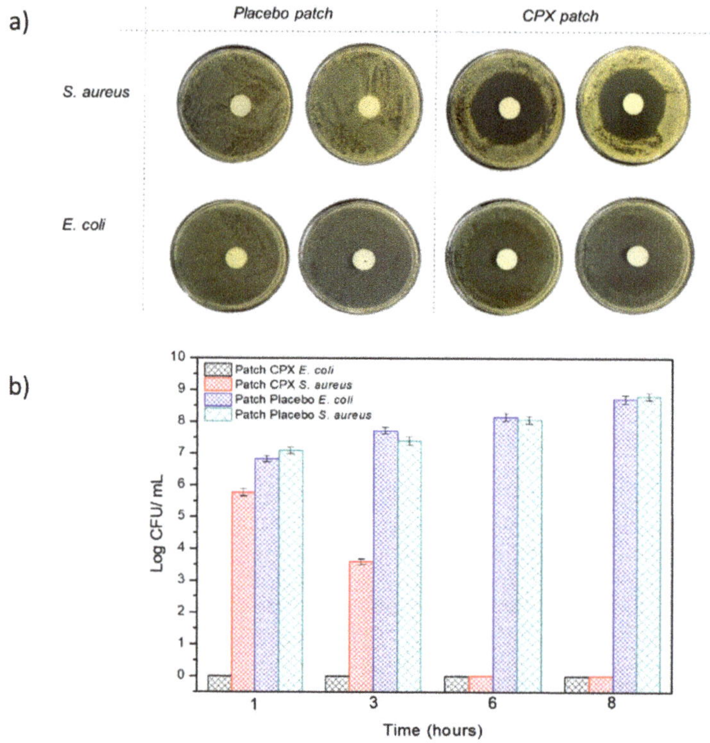

Figure 8. (**a**) Representative photographs of the growth inhibition against Escherichia coli (*E. coli*), and the Staphylococcus aureus (*S. aureus*) multilayer patch with and without CPX (n = 3) after 24 h. (**b**) Antibacterial reduction for Staphylococcus aureus (*S. aureus*) and Escherichia coli (*E. coli*) of the electrospun multilayer patches with CPX and without CPX (placebo) over a period of 1, 3, 6 and 8 h. Values are presented as the mean ± SD (n = 3).

4. Conclusions

This work further demonstrates the feasibility of using electrospinning to generate fully functional drug delivery platforms, as is the case of a CPX-loaded multilayer patch. In this work, it was confirmed that using polymeric blends (in this case, PCL and PLA) and tuning the polymer ratio, it was possible to modulate the drug release rate. For demonstration purposes, the mixture 70PCL/3PLA was selected to generate the multilayer structure and was embedded between a backing and an adhesive layer to promote mucoadhesion and drug directionality. The release of the multilayer structure showed that the presence of an adhesive layer could also be used to further modulate the release rate of the API, acting as a rate-controlling membrane.

The multilayer patch containing the electrospun blend 70PCL/30PLA interlayer was assessed in terms of adhesion and in vitro antimicrobial activity. The patch showed good adhesion in vitro as well as in vivo, with an average adhesion time in the gingiva zone of 7 h. The excellent antimicrobial properties of CPX were also corroborated in the multilayer structure across different time intervals. The results presented here illustrate the development of a model multilayer platform that can be potentially used as a buccal drug delivery system. Such drug delivery platforms could be further tuned with these or other polymers for the delivery of different BCS class II and IV APIs with use in multiple types of delivery strategies. Furthermore, electrospinning technology, now available at an industrial scale, could be quickly transferred to the pharmaceutical industry, opening new avenues for application in the pharmaceutical field.

5. Patents

The patch design developed in this research paper is based on a patent application PCT/ES2021/070294, in which some of the authors are inventors.

Author Contributions: Conceptualization, J.M.L., M.P.-F. and J.T. methodology, J.T. and M.P.-F.; analysis and characterization, M.P.-F., C.P., J.T. and K.J.F.-L.; investigation, J.T. and M.P.-F.; data curation, J.T. and M.P.-F.; writing—original draft preparation, J.T. and M.P.-F.; writing—review and editing, M.P.-F., C.P. and J.T.; funding acquisition, J.M.L. All authors have read and agreed to the published version of the manuscript.

Funding: This research was funded by the Spanish Ministry of Science and Universities (project RTI-2018-097249-B-C21), the Valencian Innovation Agency BIOENCAP project (reference number INNCAD00-18-31), the H2020 EU projects FODIAC (reference number 778388), CAPSULTEK (reference number 873827), the CYTED thematic network (code 319RT0576) and BIOINICIA's internal project ASOPHARM.

Institutional Review Board Statement: Not applicable.

Informed Consent Statement: Informed consent was obtained from all subjects involved in the study.

Conflicts of Interest: Authors declare no conflict of interest.

References

1. Wu, Z.L.; Zhao, J.; Xu, R. Recent advances in oral nano-antibiotics for bacterial infection therapy. *Int. J. Nanomed.* **2020**, *15*, 9587–9610. [CrossRef] [PubMed]
2. Baskakova, A.; Awwad, S.; Jiménez, J.Q.; Gill, H.; Novikov, O.; Khaw, P.T.; Brocchini, S.; Zhilyakova, E.; Williams, G.R. Electrospun formulations of acyclovir, ciprofloxacin and cyanocobalamin for ocular drug delivery. *Int. J. Pharm.* **2016**, *502*, 208–218. [CrossRef] [PubMed]
3. Garhwal, R.; Shady, S.F.; Ellis, E.J.; Ellis, J.Y.; Leahy, C.D.; Mccarthy, S.P.; Crawford, K.S.; Gaines, P. Sustained ocular delivery of ciprofloxacin using nanospheres and conventional contact lens materials. *Investig. Ophthalmol. Vis. Sci.* **2012**, *53*, 1341–1352. [CrossRef]
4. Arias, M.A.; De Bagües, M.P.J.; Aguiló, N.; Menao, S.; Hervás-Stubbs, S.; De Martino, A.; Alcaraz, A.; Simon, M.M.; Froelich, C.J.; Pardo, J. Elucidating Sources and Roles of Granzymes A and B during Bacterial Infection and Sepsis. *Cell Rep.* **2014**, *8*, 420–429. [CrossRef]
5. Mehra, S.; Nisar, S.; Chauhan, S.; Singh, V.; Rattan, S. Soy Protein-Based Hydrogel under Microwave-Induced Grafting of Acrylic Acid and 4-(4-Hydroxyphenyl)butanoic Acid: A Potential Vehicle for Controlled Drug Delivery in Oral Cavity Bacterial Infections. *ACS Omega* **2020**, *5*, 21610–21622. [CrossRef] [PubMed]
6. Wu, W.; Chen, W.; Jin, Q. Oral mucoadhesive buccal film of ciprofloxacin for periodontitis: Preparation and characterization. *Trop. J. Pharm. Res.* **2016**, *15*, 447–451. [CrossRef]
7. Choudhury, A.; Das, S.; Dhangar, S.; Kapasiya, S.; Kanango, A. Development and characterization buccoadhesive film of ciprofloxacin hydrochloride. *Int. J. PharmTech Res.* **2010**, *2*, 1050–1057.
8. Ramineni, S.K. *Mucoadhesive Films for Treatment of Local Oral Disorders: Development, Characterization and in vivo Testing*; University of Kentucky: Lexington, KY, USA, 2014.
9. Jones, D.; Lawlor, M.; Woolfson, A. Formulation and Characterisation of Tetracycline-Containing Bioadhesive Polymer Networks Designed for the Treatment of Periodontal Disease. *Curr. Drug Deliv.* **2004**, *1*, 17–25. [CrossRef]
10. El-Kamel, A.H.; Ashri, L.Y.; Alsarra, I.A. Micromatricial metronidazole benzoate film as a local mucoadhesive delivery system for treatment of periodontal diseases. *AAPS PharmSciTech* **2007**, *8*, E1–E11. [CrossRef]
11. Santocildes-Romero, M.E.; Hadley, L.; Clitherow, K.H.; Hansen, J.; Murdoch, C.; Colley, H.E.; Thornhill, M.H.; Hatton, P.V. Fabrication of Electrospun Mucoadhesive Membranes for Therapeutic Applications in Oral Medicine. *ACS Appl. Mater. Interfaces* **2017**, *9*, 11557–11567. [CrossRef]
12. Bahri-Najafi, R.; Tavakoli, N.; Senemar, M.; Peikanpour, M. Preparation and pharmaceutical evaluation of glibenclamide slow release mucoadhesive Buccal film. *Res. Pharm. Sci.* **2014**, *9*, 213–223. [PubMed]
13. Kim, T.H.; Ahn, J.S.; Choi, H.K.; Choi, Y.J.; Cho, C.S. A novel mucoadhesive polymer film composed of carbopol, poloxamer and hydroxypropylmethylcellulose. *Arch. Pharm. Res.* **2007**, *3*, 381–386. [CrossRef] [PubMed]
14. McMullan, B.J.; Andresen, D.; Blyth, C.C.; Avent, M.L.; Bowen, A.C.; Britton, P.N.; Clark, J.E.; Cooper, C.M.; Curtis, N.; Goeman, E.; et al. Antibiotic duration and timing of the switch from intravenous to oral route for bacterial infections in children: Systematic review and guidelines. *Lancet Infect. Dis.* **2016**, *8*, 139–152. [CrossRef]

15. Olivera, M.E.; Manzo, R.H.; Junginger, H.E.; Midha, K.K.; Shah, V.P.; Stavchansky, S.; Dressman, J.B.; Barends, D.M. Biowaiver monographs for immediate release solid oral dosage forms: Ciprofloxacin hydrochloride. *J. Pharm. Sci.* **2011**, *100*, 22–23. [CrossRef]
16. Fülöp, G.; Balogh, A.; Farkas, B.; Farkas, A.; Szabó, B.; Démuth, B.; Borbás, E.; Nagy, Z.K.; Marosi, G. Homogenization of amorphous solid dispersions prepared by electrospinning in low-dose tablet formulation. *Pharmaceutics* **2018**, *10*, 114. [CrossRef]
17. Pardo-Figuerez, M.; Teno, J.; Lafraya, A.; Prieto, C.; Lagaron, J.M. Development of an Electrospun Patch Platform Technology for the Delivery of Carvedilol in the Oral Mucosa. *Nanomaterials* **2022**, *12*, 438. [CrossRef]
18. Kajdič, S.; Vrečer, F.; Kocbek, P. Preparation of poloxamer-based nanofibers for enhanced dissolution of carvedilol. *Eur. J. Pharm. Sci.* **2018**, *117*, 331–340. [CrossRef]
19. Zupančič, Š.; Sinha-Ray, S.; Sinha-Ray, S.; Kristl, J.; Yarin, A.L. Long-Term Sustained Ciprofloxacin Release from PMMA and Hydrophilic Polymer Blended Nanofibers. *Mol. Pharm.* **2016**, *13*, 295–305. [CrossRef]
20. Pant, B.; Park, M.; Park, S.J. Drug delivery applications of core-sheath nanofibers prepared by coaxial electrospinning: A review. *Pharmaceutics* **2019**, *11*, 305. [CrossRef]
21. Basar, A.O.; Castro, S.; Torres-Giner, S.; Lagaron, J.M.; Turkoglu Sasmazel, H. Novel poly(ε-caprolactone)/gelatin wound dressings prepared by emulsion electrospinning with controlled release capacity of Ketoprofen anti-inflammatory drug. *Mater. Sci. Eng. C* **2017**, *81*, 459–468. [CrossRef]
22. Günday, C.; Anand, S.; Gencer, H.B.; Munafò, S.; Moroni, L.; Fusco, A.; Donnarumma, G.; Ricci, C.; Hatir, P.C.; Türeli, N.G.; et al. Ciprofloxacin-loaded polymeric nanoparticles incorporated electrospun fibers for drug delivery in tissue engineering applications. *Drug Deliv. Transl. Res.* **2020**, *10*, 706–720. [CrossRef] [PubMed]
23. Davis, R.; Markham, A.; Balfour, J.A. Ciprofloxacin: An Updated Review of its Pharmacology, Therapeutic Efficacy and Tolerability. *Drugs* **1996**, *51*, 1019–1074. [CrossRef] [PubMed]
24. Uhljar, L.É.; Kan, S.Y.; Radacsi, N.; Koutsos, V.; Szabó-Révész, P.; Ambrus, R. In Vitro Drug Release, Permeability, and Structural Test of Ciprofloxacin-Loaded Nanofibers. *Pharmaceutics* **2021**, *13*, 556. [CrossRef] [PubMed]
25. Blakney, A.K.; Ball, C.; Krogstad, E.A.; Woodrow, K.A. Electrospun fibers for vaginal anti-HIV drug delivery. *Antiviral Res.* **2013**, *100*, S9–S16. [CrossRef]
26. Moydeen, A.M.; Ali Padusha, M.S.; Aboelfetoh, E.F.; Al-Deyab, S.S.; El-Newehy, M.H. Fabrication of electrospun poly(vinyl alcohol)/dextran nanofibers via emulsion process as drug delivery system: Kinetics and in vitro release study. *Int. J. Biol. Macromol.* **2018**, *116*, 1250–1259. [CrossRef]
27. Wu, J.; Zhang, Z.; Gu, J.; Zhou, W.; Liang, X.; Zhou, G.; Han, C.C.; Xu, S.; Liu, Y. Mechanism of a long-term controlled drug release system based on simple blended electrospun fibers. *J. Control. Release* **2020**, *320*, 337–346. [CrossRef]
28. Colley, H.E.; Said, Z.; Santocildes-Romero, M.E.; Baker, S.R.; D'Apice, K.; Hansen, J.; Madsen, L.S.; Thornhill, M.H.; Hatton, P.V.; Murdoch, C. Pre-clinical evaluation of novel mucoadhesive bilayer patches for local delivery of clobetasol-17-propionate to the oral mucosa. *Biomaterials* **2018**, *178*, 134–146. [CrossRef]
29. Mathematical models of drug release. In *Strategies to Modify the Drug Release from Pharmaceutical Systems*; Elsevier: Amsterdam, The Netherlands, 2015; pp. 63–86. ISBN 9780081000922.
30. Baus, R.A.; Haug, M.F.; Leichner, C.; Jelkmann, M.; Bernkop-Schnürch, A. In Vitro-in Vivo Correlation of Mucoadhesion Studies on Buccal Mucosa. *Mol. Pharm.* **2019**, *16*, 2719–2727. [CrossRef]
31. Nafee, N.A.; Ismail, F.A.; Boraie, N.A.; Mortada, L.M. Mucoadhesive buccal patches of miconazole nitrate: In vitro/in vivo performance and effect of ageing. *Int. J. Pharm.* **2003**, *264*, 1–14. [CrossRef]
32. Voronova, A.; Prieto, C.; Pardo-Figuerez, M.; Lagaron, J.M.; Sanyal, A.; Demir, B.; Hubert, T.; Plaisance, V.; Pawlowski, V.; Vignoud-Despond, S.; et al. Photothermal Activatable Mucoadhesive Fiber Mats for On-Demand Delivery of Insulin via Buccal and Corneal Mucosa. *ACS Appl. Bio Mater.* **2022**, *5*, 771–778. [CrossRef]
33. Figueroa-Lopez, K.J.; Andrade-Mahecha, M.M.; Torres-Vargas, O.L. Spice oleoresins containing antimicrobial agents improve the potential use of bio-composite films based on gelatin. *Food Packag. Shelf Life* **2018**, *17*, 50–56. [CrossRef]
34. Li, H.; Zhang, Z.; Godakanda, V.U.; Chiu, Y.J.; Angkawinitwong, U.; Patel, K.; Stapleton, P.G.; De Silva, R.M.; De Silva, K.M.N.; Zhu, L.M.; et al. The effect of collection substrate on electrospun ciprofloxacin-loaded poly(vinylpyrrolidone) and ethyl cellulose nanofibers as potential wound dressing materials. *Mater. Sci. Eng. C* **2019**, *104*, 109917. [CrossRef] [PubMed]
35. Clinical Laboratory Standards Institute. Methods for Dilution Antimicrobial Susceptibility Tests for Bacteria That Grow Aerobically; Approved Standard—Ninth Edition. CLSI document M07-A9. *Clin. Lab. Standars Inst.* **2018**, *32*, 18.
36. Cai, Q.; Bei, J.; Wang, S. In vitro study on the drug release behavior from polylactide-based blend matrices. *Polym. Adv. Technol.* **2002**, *13*, 534–540. [CrossRef]
37. Valarezo, E.; Tammaro, L.; Malagón, O.; González, S.; Armijos, C.; Vittoria, V. Fabrication and characterization of poly(lactic acid)/poly(ε-caprolactone) blend electrospun fibers loaded with amoxicillin for tunable delivering. *J. Nanosci. Nanotechnol.* **2015**, *15*, 4706–4712. [CrossRef] [PubMed]
38. Shen, Y.; Sun, W.; Zhu, K.J.; Shen, Z. Regulation of biodegradability and drug release behavior of aliphatic polyesters by blending. *J. Biomed. Mater. Res.* **2000**, *50*, 528–535. [CrossRef]
39. Li, F.; Li, X.; He, R.; Cheng, J.; Ni, Z.; Zhao, G. Preparation and evaluation of poly(D, L-lactic acid)/poly(L-lactide-co-ε-caprolactone) blends for tunable sirolimus release. *Colloids Surfaces A Physicochem. Eng. Asp.* **2020**, *590*, 124518. [CrossRef]

40. Wang, L.; Zhang, Z.; Chen, H.; Zhang, S.; Xiong, C. Preparation and characterization of biodegradable thermoplastic Elastomers (PLCA/PLGA blends). *J. Polym. Res.* **2010**, *17*, 77–82. [CrossRef]
41. Chou, S.-F.; Woodrow, K.A. Relationships between mechanical properties and drug release from electrospun fibers of PCL and PLGA blends. *J. Mech. Behav. Biomed. Mater.* **2017**, *65*, 724–733. [CrossRef]
42. Putra, O.D.; Pettersen, A.; Yonemochi, E.; Uekusa, H. Structural origin of physicochemical properties differences upon dehydration and polymorphic transformation of ciprofloxacin hydrochloride revealed by structure determination from powder X-ray diffraction data. *CrystEngComm* **2020**, *22*, 7272–7279. [CrossRef]
43. Hanafy, A.F. In-vitro bioequivalence, physicochemical and economic benefits study for marketed innovator and generic ciprofloxacin hydrochloride tablets in Saudi Arabia. *J. Appl. Pharm. Sci.* **2016**, *6*, 063–068. [CrossRef]
44. Turel, I.; Bukovec, P. Comparison of the thermal stability of ciprofloxacin and its compounds. *Thermochim. Acta* **1996**, *287*, 311–318. [CrossRef]
45. Okoye, E.I.; Okolie, T.A. Development and in vitro characterization of ciprofloxacin loaded polymeric films for wound dressing. *Int. J. Health Allied Sci.* **2015**, *4*, 234–242. [CrossRef]
46. Sobhani, Z.; Samani, S.M.; Montaseri, H.; Khezri, E. Nanoparticles of chitosan loaded ciprofloxacin: Fabrication and antimicrobial activity. *Adv. Pharm. Bull.* **2017**, *7*, 427–432. [CrossRef] [PubMed]
47. Karimi, K.; Pallagi, E.; Szabó-Révész, P.; Csóka, I.; Ambrus, R. Development of a microparticle-based dry powder inhalation formulation of ciprofloxacin hydrochloride applying the quality by design approach. *Drug Des. Devel. Ther.* **2016**, *10*, 3331–3343. [CrossRef]
48. Pisal, S.; Zainnuddin, R.; Nalawade, P.; Mahadik, K.; Kadam, S. Molecular properties of ciprofloxacin-Indion 234 complexes. *AAPS PharmSciTech* **2004**, *5*, 84–92. [CrossRef]
49. Xia, L.; Lu, L.; Liang, Y.; Cheng, B. Fabrication of centrifugally spun prepared poly(lactic acid)/gelatin/ciprofloxacin nanofibers for antimicrobial wound dressing. *RSC Adv.* **2019**, *9*, 35328. [CrossRef]
50. Cabedo, L.; Feijoo, J.L.; Villanueva, M.P.; Lagarón, J.M.; Giménez, E. Optimization of biodegradable nanocomposites based on aPLA/PCL blends for food packaging applications. *Macromol. Symp.* **2006**, *233*, 191–197. [CrossRef]
51. Mbarki, K.; Boumbimba, R.M.; Sayari, A.; Elleuch, B. Influence of microfibers length on PDLA/cellulose microfibers biocomposites crystallinity and properties. *Polym. Bull.* **2019**, *76*, 1061–1079. [CrossRef]
52. Wu, Q.; Li, Z.; Hong, H.; Yin, K.; Tie, L. Adsorption and intercalation of ciprofloxacin on montmorillonite. *Appl. Clay Sci.* **2010**, *50*, 204–211. [CrossRef]
53. Li, H.; Williams, G.R.; Wu, J.; Wang, H.; Sun, X.; Zhu, L.M. Poly(N-isopropylacrylamide)/poly(L-lactic acid-co-ϵ-caprolactone) fibers loaded with ciprofloxacin as wound dressing materials. *Mater. Sci. Eng. C* **2017**, *79*, 245–254. [CrossRef] [PubMed]
54. Preis, M.; Woertz, C.; Kleinebudde, P.; Breitkreutz, J. Oromucosal film preparations: Classification and characterization methods. *Expert Opin. Drug Deliv.* **2013**, *10*, 1303–1317. [CrossRef] [PubMed]
55. Perumal, V.A.; Lutchman, D.; Mackraj, I.; Govender, T. Formulation of monolayered films with drug and polymers of opposing solubilities. *Int. J. Pharm.* **2008**, *358*, 184–191. [CrossRef]
56. Morales, J.O.; McConville, J.T. Manufacture and characterization of mucoadhesive buccal films. *Eur. J. Pharm. Biopharm.* **2011**, *77*, 187–199. [CrossRef]
57. Di Prima, G.; Conigliaro, A.; De Caro, V. Mucoadhesive Polymeric Films to Enhance Barbaloin Penetration Into Buccal Mucosa: A Novel Approach to Chemoprevention. *AAPS PharmSciTech* **2019**, *20*, 18. [CrossRef] [PubMed]
58. Bravo-Osuna, I.; Vauthier, C.; Farabollini, A.; Palmieri, G.F.; Ponchel, G. Mucoadhesion mechanism of chitosan and thiolated chitosan-poly(isobutyl cyanoacrylate) core-shell nanoparticles. *Biomaterials* **2007**, *28*, 2233–2243. [CrossRef]
59. Reda, R.I.; Wen, M.M.; El-Kamel, A.H. Ketoprofen-loaded Eudragit electrospun nanofibers for the treatment of oral mucositis. *Int. J. Nanomed.* **2017**, *12*, 2335–2351. [CrossRef] [PubMed]
60. Chaves, P.D.S.; Frank, L.A.; Frank, A.G.; Pohlmann, A.R.; Guterres, S.S.; Beck, R.C.R. Mucoadhesive Properties of Eudragit®RS100, Eudragit®S100, and Poly(ϵ-caprolactone) Nanocapsules: Influence of the Vehicle and the Mucosal Surface. *AAPS PharmSciTech* **2018**, *19*, 1637–1646. [CrossRef]
61. Yehia, S.; El-Gazayerly, O.; Basalious, E. Fluconazole Mucoadhesive Buccal Films: In Vitro/In Vivo Performance. *Curr. Drug Deliv.* **2009**, *6*, 17–27. [CrossRef]
62. Pérez-González, G.L.; Villarreal-Gómez, L.J.; Serrano-Medina, A.; Torres-Martínez, E.J.; Cornejo-Bravo, J.M. Mucoadhesive electrospun nanofibers for drug delivery systems: Applications of polymers and the parameters' roles. *Int. J. Nanomed.* **2019**, *14*, 5271–5285. [CrossRef]
63. Li, H.; Williams, G.R.; Wu, J.; Lv, Y.; Sun, X.; Wu, H.; Zhu, L.M. Thermosensitive nanofibers loaded with ciprofloxacin as antibacterial wound dressing materials. *Int. J. Pharm.* **2017**, *517*, 135–147. [CrossRef] [PubMed]

Journal of
Functional
Biomaterials

MDPI

Article

A Novel Hydrophilic, Antibacterial Chitosan-Based Coating Prepared by Ultrasonic Atomization Assisted LbL Assembly Technique

Xiaoyu Wang [1,†], Yuyang Zhou [2,3,†], Melissa Johnson [1], Cameron Milne [1], Sigen A [1], Yening Li [2], Wenxin Wang [1], Nan Zhang [2,*] and Qian Xu [1,*]

1 Charles Institute of Dermatology, School of Medicine, University College Dublin, D04 V1W8 Dublin, Ireland
2 Centre of Micro/Nano Manufacturing Technology (MNMT-Dublin), School of Mechanical and Materials Engineering, University College Dublin, D04 KW52 Dublin, Ireland
3 National Engineering Laboratory for Modern Silk, College of Textile and Clothing Engineering, Soochow University, Suzhou 215123, China
* Correspondence: nan.zhang@ucd.ie (N.Z.); qian.xu@ucd.ie (Q.X.)
† These authors contributed equally to this work.

Abstract: To explore the potential applicability of chitosan (CTS), we prepared aldehyde chitosan (CTS-CHO) with chitosan and sodium periodate via oxidation reaction and then a chitosan-based hydrophilic and antibacterial coating on the surface of poly (lactic acid) (PLA) film was developed and characterized. The oxidation degree was determined by Elemental analyser to be 12.53%, and a Fourier transform infrared spectroscopy was used to characterize the structure of CTS-CHO. It was evident that CTS-CHO is a biocompatible coating biomaterial with more than 80% cell viability obtained through the Live/Dead staining assay and the alamarBlue assay. The hydrophilic and antibacterial CTS-CHO coating on the PLA surface was prepared by ultrasonic atomization assisted LbL assembly technique due to Schiff's base reaction within and between layers. The CTS-CHO coating had better hydrophilicity and transparency, a more definite industrialization potential, and higher antibacterial activity at experimental concentrations than the CTS coating. All of the results demonstrated that the ultrasonic atomization-assisted LbL assembly CTS-CHO coating is a promising alternative for improving hydrophilicity and antibacterial activity on the PLA surface. The functional groups of CTS-CHO could react with active components with amino groups via dynamic Schiff's base reaction and provide the opportunity to create a drug releasing surface for biomedical applications.

Keywords: chitosan; PLA; hydrophilic; antibacterial; coating

1. Introduction

PLA is an aliphatic polyester and an environmentally friendly polymer. PLA is constructed from lactic acid (2-hydroxy propionic acid) building blocks [1,2]. Given its renewability, absorbability [1], biodegradability [3], and biocompatibility [4], it is widely applied in the biomedical field, such as absorbable surgical sutures [5], scaffolds [6–8], drug delivery systems [9,10], personal protective equipment [11,12], food packaging [13,14], and clothing fabrics and textiles [15]. PLA has been studied widely in the biomedical field during the global COVID-19 pandemic. However, the poor hydrophilicity limits its application in some fields, such as clothing, and medical devices [16], because the hydrophobic property leads to the absorption of non-specific protein and promotes bacterial adhesion [17,18]. Modification of the PLA surface can significantly improve the surface properties such as wettability, biocompatibility, and functionality of PLA [19–21].

Numerous surface modification strategies have been explored to improve the hydrophilicity of PLA, including physical, chemical, plasma, and radiation treatments. Among these methods, plasma-treatment is an effective tool for surface activation before grafting of bioactive components onto material surfaces [22–28]. For example, in Park et al.'s study [29], plasma treatment and hydrophilic acrylic acid grafting made hydrophilic functional groups successfully adapt on the surface of scaffolds [30]. Gutierrez-Villarreal et al. grafted N-vinylpyrrolidone onto PLA using benzophenone as the initiator and improved the hydrophilicity of PLA [31].

The LbL assembly technique allows coatings to be built based on the interactions of selected materials. Interactions exploited in the LbL method include covalent interactions, hydrogen bonds, and electrostatic attraction [32]. Ultrasonic atomization technology, which can convert the liquid into aerosols, has also been explored for developing multi-layered coatings [33]. The LbL assembly technique has been considered one of the most appropriate methods for preparing multilayer films incorporated with therapeutic molecules.

PLA's antibacterial activity is one of the most important considerations, particularly in the fields of medical devices and food packaging. Among the various antibacterial materials which are commonly used on the PLA surface, natural polymers show great potential due to their excellent biocompatibility and degradability. Over the past decade, increasing research has gained insight into the antimicrobial activity of CTS, which is composed of N-acetyl-D-glucosamine and D-glucosamine units. In Munteanu et al.'s study, PLA films were coated with chitosan oil by coaxial electrospinning, combining the mechanical properties and biodegradability of PLA substrates with the antioxidant and antimicrobial properties of the chitosan–oil nano coatings [16]. However, the affinity of CTS to the surface of PLA is limited due to its poor solubility, high viscosity, and easy aggregation. Additionally, acidic solvents used to dissolve CTS are not suitable for industrial production. CTS-derived polymers fabricated through chemical functionalization have achieved the desired properties of polymer and coating, as well as industrial production. In particular, those CTS-derived polymers with antimicrobial activity have been extensively studied for the use on PLA surfaces for medical devices or food packaging [34,35]. However, the antibacterial coating on PLA surface prepared with aldehyde-chitosan (CTS-CHO) using ultrasonic atomization assisted LbL assembly technique has not been reported.

In a recent study, the CTS-CHO was fabricated through chemical functionalization. CTS-CHO demonstrated the potential for industrial production of antibacterial coating due to its excellent properties, such as antibacterial activity, and solubility. Then an LbL assembly coating was prepared by ultrasonic atomization-assisted technique. The study process, including the preparation and characterization in this work is outlined in Scheme 1. The characterization of CTS-CHO was performed using Fourier transform infrared spectroscopy (FT-IR) and an Exeter elemental analyser. The solubility, zeta-potential, stability, viscosity, and aggregation profiles of CTS and CTS-CHO were evaluated. Furthermore, the biocompatibility of CTS-CHO and CTS was assessed using Live/Dead staining assay and alamarBlue assay. After plasma treatment, active groups, such as hydroxyl and carboxyl groups, were generated on the PLA film surface. Then the bioactive inks prepared with CTS-CHO and CTS were sprayed on the surface of the PLA layer-by-layer through ultrasonic atomization, respectively. Due to the presence of aldehyde groups and amino groups in the structure of CTS-CHO, Schiff's reaction occurred within and between layers. The transparency, antibacterial activity, and hydrophilicity of ultrasonic atomization-assisted LbL CTS-CHO coating and CTS coating on the PLA surface were then compared.

2. Materials and Methods

2.1. Materials

Chitosan with medium molecular weight, LB agar, and LB broth were purchased from Sigma-Aldrich (Dublin, Ireland). PLA film (0.5 mm) was purchased from Esun (Shenzhen, China). Sodium periodate and ethylene glycol were purchased from Thermo Fisher Scientific (Dublin, Ireland). Glacial acetic acid was supplied by Aladdin (Dublin, Ireland). Dialysis tubing (cut-off molecular weight: 8 kDa) were supplied by Spectrum Lab (Dublin, Ireland). *E. coli* and HEK 293 cells were supplied by ATCC. Cell culture medium was purchased from Invitrogen (Dublin, Ireland). Live/Dead staining kit was supplied by Biosciences (Dublin, Ireland) and an alamarBlue cell viability assay kit was purchased from Sigma-Aldrich (Dublin, Ireland), respectively.

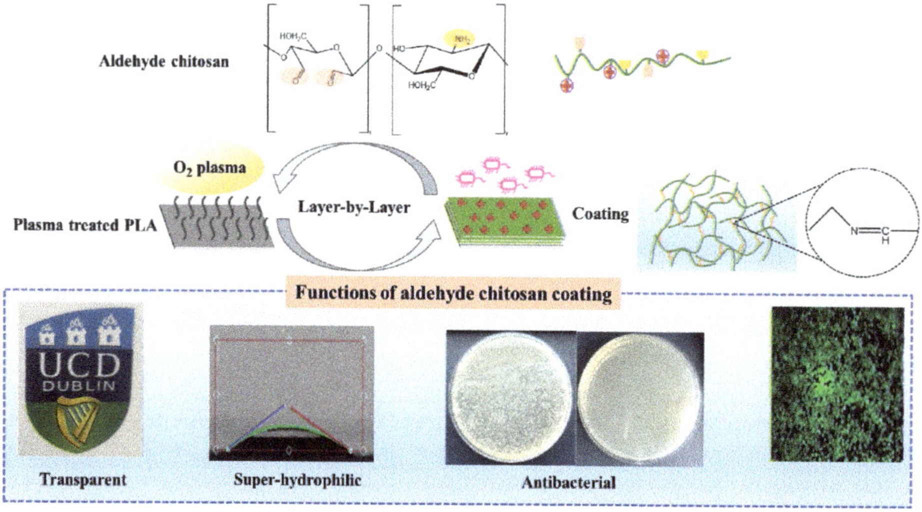

Scheme 1. The molecular structure of aldehyde chitosan and the functions of aldehyde chitosan coating.

2.2. Fabrication of Antibacterial PLA Film

2.2.1. Preparation of CTS-CHO

CTS-CHO was fabricated using chitosan (CTS) and sodium periodate via oxidation reaction, as reported previously [36].

2.2.2. Bioactive Ink Formulation

The CTS-CHO freeze-dried sponge was dissolved in deionized water to the desired concentrations and vortexed for 30 min. 0.1 mol/L acetic acid solution was used to dissolve the CTS. Then the CTS solution was stirred for 24 h to ensure complete dissolution.

2.2.3. Preparation of Coatings

The coating was prepared with a coating workstation (UAC120 Ultrasonic Atomizer System, Hangzhou, China). Prior to coating, PLA films were treated by plasma for 30~60 s under 30~80 W power. The plasma treatment was carried out in the oxygen atmosphere holding in a cylindrical chamber. The infusion rate was 0.5 mL/min, and the guide gas pressure was 0.01 MPa. After 20 times repeated coating, the films were placed in the open air to dry.

2.3. Characterizations

2.3.1. CTS-CHO

Aldehyde chitosan was characterized by Fourier transform infrared spectrometry and an Exeter elemental analyser.

The infrared spectrograms of CTS and CTS-CHO were obtained by an ALPHA FT-IR spectrometer with an ATR accessory (Bruker, Dublin, Ireland). The samples were placed in the sampling area. The resolution was set to 4 cm^{-1}. The spectrogram (32 scans) was recorded from 4000 cm^{-1} to 400 cm^{-1}. The sample spectra were then subtracted from the background.

In this study, quantitative flash combustion was used for element analysis. After freeze-drying, CTS-CHO was kept in a desiccator before elemental analysis. An Exeter elemental analyser (CE440, Coventry, UK) was used to conduct this measurement. The oxidation degree (F_{ox}) was calculated as below:

$$\frac{N}{C} = \frac{F_A + (1 - F_A)\cdot(1 - F_{ox})}{2F_{ox} + 6} \quad (1)$$

where F_{ox} is the oxidation degree, F_A is acetylated unit content, C is the carbon percentage, N is the nitrogen percentage.

2.3.2. Bioactive Ink

The properties of bioactive inks were characterized by a zetasizer, viscometer, and microscope.

The viscosity of the ink was measured at 25 °C and 100 rpm with a rotational viscometer (AMETEK, Brookfield, MA, USA). The particle size of the inks was measured using a zetasizer before and after filtering with a 0.45 μm filter (Zetasizer Pro, Malvern, Ireland). Aggregation profiles of the ink were observed under a microscope (Olympus, Ireland). The zeta potential of the inks was tested using a zetasizer (Zetasizer Pro, Malvern, Ireland). The particle size of the ink was tested at predetermined time points using a zetasizer (Zetasizer Pro, Malvern, Ireland).

2.3.3. Coating

The properties of the coatings were characterized by a digital camera, and contact angle goniometer, etc.

A digital camera was used to record the transparency of films, including the PLA film before and after plasma treatment, CTS and CTS-CHO coating on the PLA film surface. The measurement of the water contact angle was conducted using a Contact Angle Goniometer (Ossila, London, UK).

The antibacterial activity of plasma-treated PLA film, PLA films with CTS and CTS-CHO coating were tested according to a modified method based on ISO 22196. Briefly, a colony of *E. coli* was cultivated in LB broth overnight at 37 °C. The bacterial suspension was diluted with LB broth to a 0.5 McFarland concentration (~1.5×10^8 CFU/mL). The bacterial solution was diluted to 1.5×10^5 CFU/mL with LB broth to conduct the further experiment. 10 mL of bacterial solution was added into an ultrasonic atomizing sprayer. The PLA films with CTS and CTS-CHO coating were then cut into 5 cm × 5 cm squares and placed in the sterilized dishes. As a control, plasma treated PLA film without any coating was used and operated in the same way as described above. The bacterial solution was sprayed onto the Z-shaped films 3 times. Then 10 mL of LB broth was added to the dish with plasma-treated PLA film after inoculation. Then, 10-fold serial dilutions of the bacterial solution were performed with LB broth. 1 mL of each diluent was placed into two dishes, and 20 mL of LB agar was poured in. After gently swirling, the dishes were incubated for 2 days at 35 °C. After the bacterial solution was sprayed onto the films, 4 cm × 4 cm sterilized PE films were cut and placed onto the PLA films with coating and the plasma treated PLA films. 2 mL of sterilized water was dropped around the PLA films with coating and plasma treated PLA film to avoid bacterial solution drying. Then the dishes were incubated for 24 h at 37 °C. A pipette was used to remove the water from around the films. To recover the bacteria, 10 mL of LB broth was added to the dishes. 10-fold serial dilutions of the bacterial solution were performed with LB broth. 1 mL of each diluent was placed into two dishes and followed by 20 mL of LB agar. After gently swirling the dishes, they were incubated at 35 °C for 2 days. Then the antibacterial activity was calculated according to the equations in ISO 22196.

AlamarBlue assay and Live/Dead staining assay were used to evaluate the cytotoxicity of materials (CTS, CTS-CHO) against HEK293 cells. CTS and CTS-CHO were dissolved in sodium acetate buffer (25 mM, pH 5.2) and the stock solution was obtained after extraction for 24 h at 37 °C. Then 0.22 μm filters were used to filter the stock solutions for sterilization and the sterilized stock solutions were diluted with complete cell culture medium to various concentrations. 1×10^5 cells/well of HEK 293 cells were inoculated in a 96-well microplate with complete medium at 37 °C (5% CO_2). After overnight incubation, CTS or CTS-CHO solutions were used to replace the culture medium. After 24 h of incubation, 20 µL of alamarBlue reagent was added to each well. The fluorescence excitation wavelength was read at 570 nm by a microplate reader after 3 h of incubation. The negative control group consisted of cells grown in medium containing alamarBlue reagent. Live/Dead cell staining assay was performed according to the manufacturer's protocol after 24 h incubation. 100 µL of staining solution was used to replace the culture medium at predetermined time points. Then DPBS was used to wash staining reagent away after 30 min incubation (25 °C). A fluorescence microscope was used to record the images.

3. Results and Discussion

3.1. Characterization of CTS-CHO

To confirm that the functionalization was successful, FT-IR was used to characterize the CTS and the CTS-CHO. The characteristic bands were shown in Figure 1. The stretching vibrations at 3283, 2924, 1647, and 1558 cm^{-1} are attributed to the O-H, C-H, C=O, N-H, and C-O-C linkages, which is consistent with previous literature reports. The band at 1725 cm^{-1} in CTS-CHO was the characteristic peak of aldehyde groups. Other bands, such as those at 3283, 2924, 1647, and 1558 cm^{-1}, were not significantly altered in the oxidation reaction. These results were consistent with those reported in the literature [37–40]. Therefore, the C_2-C_3 linkage was cleaved in the GlcN unit, and the dialdehyde was formed in the structure of chitosan, as shown in Figure 1.

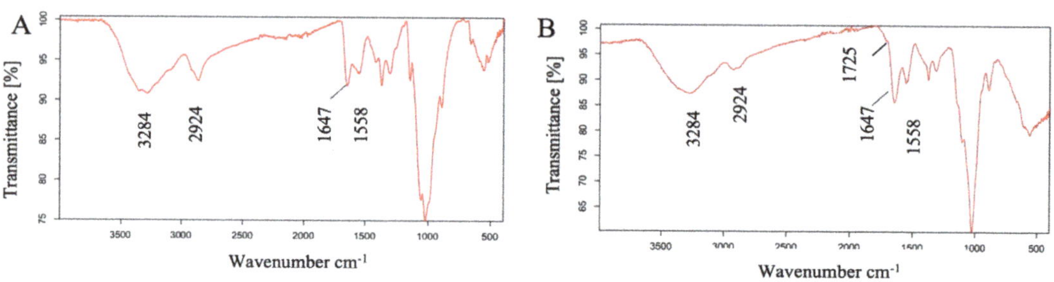

Figure 1. FT-IR spectra. (**A**) CTS. (**B**) CTS-CHO.

An elemental analyser was used to test the percentages of C, H, and N in the structure of CTS and CTS-CHO. The oxidation degree is defined as the dialdehyde percentage per 100 GlcN units. According to the literature, the oxidation degree was calculated with Equation (1). The oxidation degree was 12.53% (Table S1).

3.2. Characterization of Bioactive Inks

To select the appropriate concentrations of CTS and CTS-CHO to conduct further study, the viscosity was measured by a rotational viscometer. A promising property of CTS-CHO is that its water solubility improved significantly compared to CTS. Presumably the hydration of aldehyde groups improved the solubility dramatically. Therefore, the CTS solution and CTS-CHO solution were prepared by dissolving materials in acetic acid solution and deionized water respectively. As shown in Table 1, the viscosity of the CTS solution increased with concentrations (from 1 mg/mL to 10 mg/mL). However, there was no obvious difference in the viscosity of the CTS-CHO solution (from 1 mg/mL to 10 mg/mL). The viscosity of the CTS-CHO solution was significantly lower than that of CTS solution at the same concentration. The appropriate ink viscosity is critical for ultrasonic atomization spray coating. High viscosity ink may cause ultrasonic atomizer pipe clogging, and uneven coating. Therefore, 10 mg/mL CTS-CHO solution and 1 mg/mL CTS solution were used in this study.

Table 1. Viscosity of bioactive inks, including CTS solution and CTS-CHO solution.

Sample	Concentration (mg/mL)	Viscosity (cp)
CTS	1	47.64
	5	269.6
	10	399.1
CTS-CHO	1	7.64
	5	7.73
	10	7.82

Chitosan can only be dissolved in acidic solutions at a pH below 6.0. However, according to the literature, a certain degree of aggregation exists even in a dissolved chitosan solution [41]. The CTS solutions consist of numerous intermolecular aggregates and molecularly dispersed polymer chains. Therefore, the uniformity of the deposited the CTS coating may be affected. Moreover, polysaccharide solutions usually exhibit a strong tendency to aggregate, including the CTS molecules in aqueous solvents. Ultracentrifugation, extensive filtering of solutions, and changes in solvent conditions such as temperature of exposure to acidic proteases, ionic strength, and pH are normally used to remove large aggregates. However, strong aggregation still cannot be prevented [29,42–46].

To observe the aggregation profiles of the CTS and CTS-CHO solution at a concentration of 1 mg/mL and 10 mg/mL, the particle size was measured using a zetasizer and microscope. As shown in Figure 2A–D, the obvious aggregation phenomenon of CTS was observed in the original solution and even the filtered solution. There are some particles over 20 μm in size after filtering with a 0.45 μm filter. The same results were observed for the particle size obtained from the zetasizer in Figure 2E,F. As the relative amount of amide groups decreased, the aggregation of CTS-CHO was significantly reduced, as shown in Figure 2G–L. After filtering, the majority of CTS-CHO particles were around 141 nm in size, but quite a few CTS particles were around 2 μm. Compared with CTS, the slight aggregation of CTS-CHO reduced the risk of pipe blockage and uneven coating.

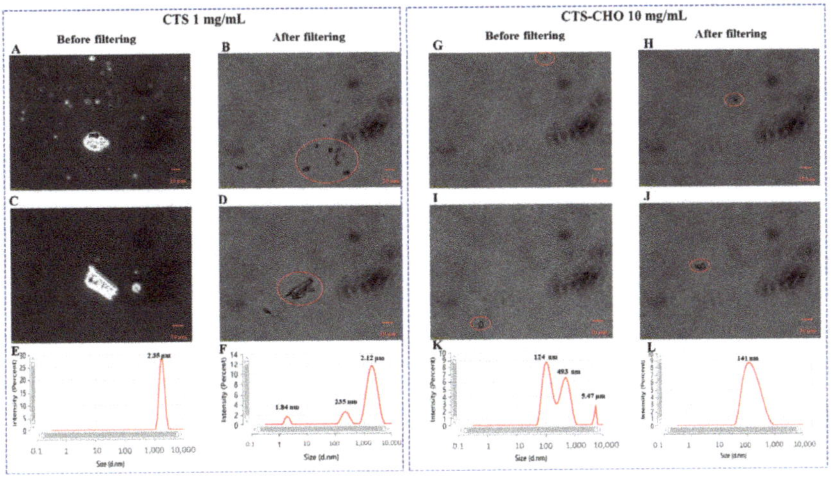

Figure 2. Aggregation profiles of CTS and CTS-CHO solution before and after filtering with a 0.45 μm filter. (**A–D**) Aggregation profiles of CTS solution (1 mg/mL) under a microscope. (**G–J**) Aggregation profiles of CTS-CHO (10 mg/mL) under a microscope. (**E,F**) Particle size of CTS solution (1 mg/mL) measured by zetasizer. (**K,L**) Particle size of CTS-CHO solution (1 mg/mL) measured by a zetasizer. Scale bar: 20 μm. Particles in red circles indicated the aggregation.

The antibacterial activity of CTS depends on its positive charge. Positive charges bind to the negatively charged bacterial cell wall, causing damage to the cell wall and the alteration of the permeability of the cell membrane [47]. Chitosan then attaches to the DNA of bacterial cells and inhibits DNA replication, leading to bacteria death. Therefore, the zeta potential of the CTS solution and CTS-CHO solution was evaluated using a zetasizer. The results are shown in Table S2. The potential of the 1 mg/mL CTS solution was 10.9 mv while the 10 mg/mL CTS-CHO solution has a potential of 28.8 mv. The results demonstrated that both CTS and CTS-CHO have positive charges, and thus possess potential antibacterial activity. These results were consistent with our previous report [36].

The stability of the inks also affects the ultrasonic atomization coating. As this study is the first report on the application of the CTS-CHO as an antibacterial coating material, the particle size of the solutions at predetermined time points was measured by zetasizer to observe the stability of CTS-CHO solution. The particle size was around 140 nm, and the PDI was around 0.25 (as shown in Figure 3). Both particle size and PDI showed no significant changes at 8 h, and only a slight increase at 24 h.

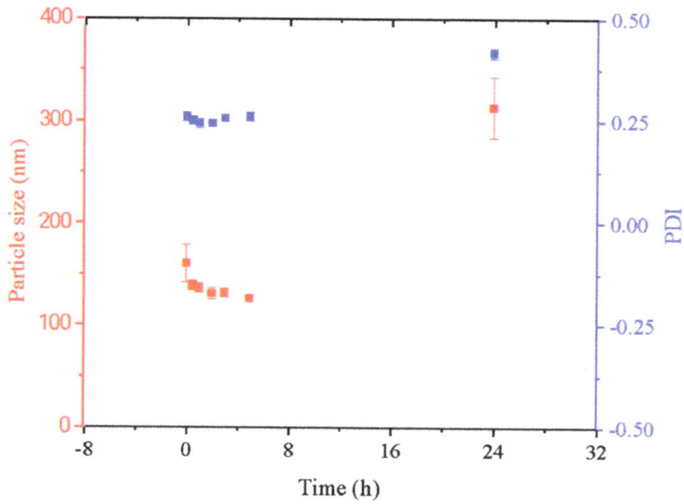

Figure 3. Stability of the CTS-CHO solution.

All of the results demonstrated that the bioactive inks prepared with CTS-CHO are a promising candidate for antibacterial coating material in the biomedical, food packaging and personal protection fields.

3.3. Characterization of Coatings

The photos of pristine PLA film, plasma treated PLA film, CTS coating and CTS-CHO coated PLA film were taken with a digital camera. The pristine PLA film and plasma treated PLA film showed high visible light transparency (see Figure 4A,B). Interestingly, with the 20 bilayers of the CTS-CHO coating, it is still possible to see the background beneath the film without any visible shelter or obscured area (see Figure 4D). However, the CTS coated PLA film showed poor transparency (see Figure 4C). The reduction of molecular weight and the improvement of solubility after the oxidation reaction enable the CTS-CHO coating to possess high transparency.

To evaluate the surface hydrophilicity, the water contact angle was measured with a contact angle goniometer. The results were shown in Figure 4E, where the contact angle of pristine was 77.9°, and that of plasma treated PLA film was reduced significantly to 14°. 83°. Water contact angles of CTS coating and CTS-CHO coating were 83.0 and 28.1°, respectively, which means that the hydrophilicity of the CTS-CHO coating was higher than that of the CTS coating.

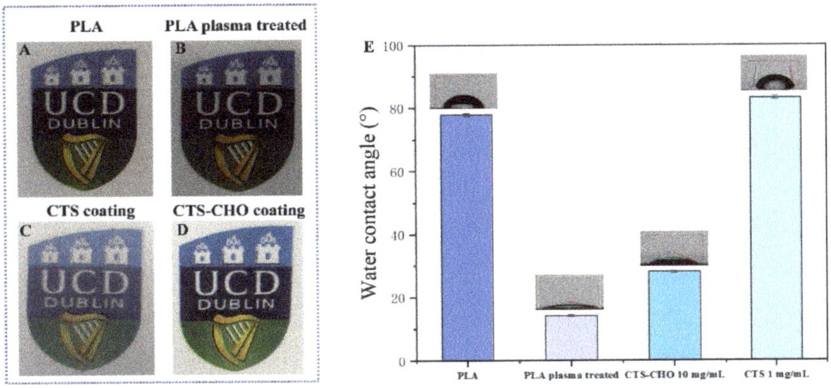

Figure 4. Transparency and water contact angles. (**A**) Pristine PLA film. (**B**) PLA film after plasma treatment. (**C**) CTS coated PLA film. (**D**) CTS-CHO coated PLA film. (**E**) Water contact angles.

A modified method based on ISO 22196 was used to evaluate the antibacterial activity in this study. As shown in Figure 5A–C, there were no bacterial colonies on the dishes after 48 h incubation for both the CTS-CHO coatings sprayed 10 times and 20 times. The antibacterial activity (R) of the CTS-CHO coating was around 4 in the experimental condition in this study. Therefore, when the CTS-CHO coating thickness reaches a certain level, the antibacterial activity will not increase with the spraying times and coating thickness. Figure 5D–F showed that the antibacterial activity of the CTS-CHO coating was significantly higher than that of the CTS coating. A large number of positively charged amino groups enable chitosan to have excellent antibacterial activity. After the oxidation reaction, the CTS−CHO still contains many amino groups which contribute to the antibacterial activity.

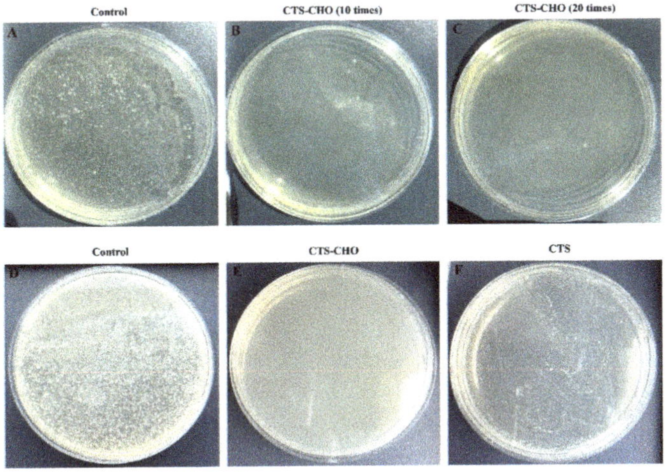

Figure 5. Antibacterial activity of CTS coating PLA film and CTS−CHO coating PLA film against E. coli. (**A**,**D**) Plasma treated PLA films. (**B**) CTS-CHO coating PLA film (10 times). (**C**) CTS-CHO coating PLA film (20 times). (**E**) CTS-CHO coating PLA film (20 times). (**F**) CTS coating on the surface of PLA film (20 times).

AlamarBlue measurement and Live/Dead staining assay were used to assess the cytotoxicity of the materials. The sodium acetate buffer (25 mM, pH = 5.2) was used to dissolve CTS and CTS-CHO to make sure that the experimental conditions were consistent. The cell viability results (>90%) indicated that the cytotoxicity of CTS-CHO didn't increase after oxidation (Figure 6A,B).

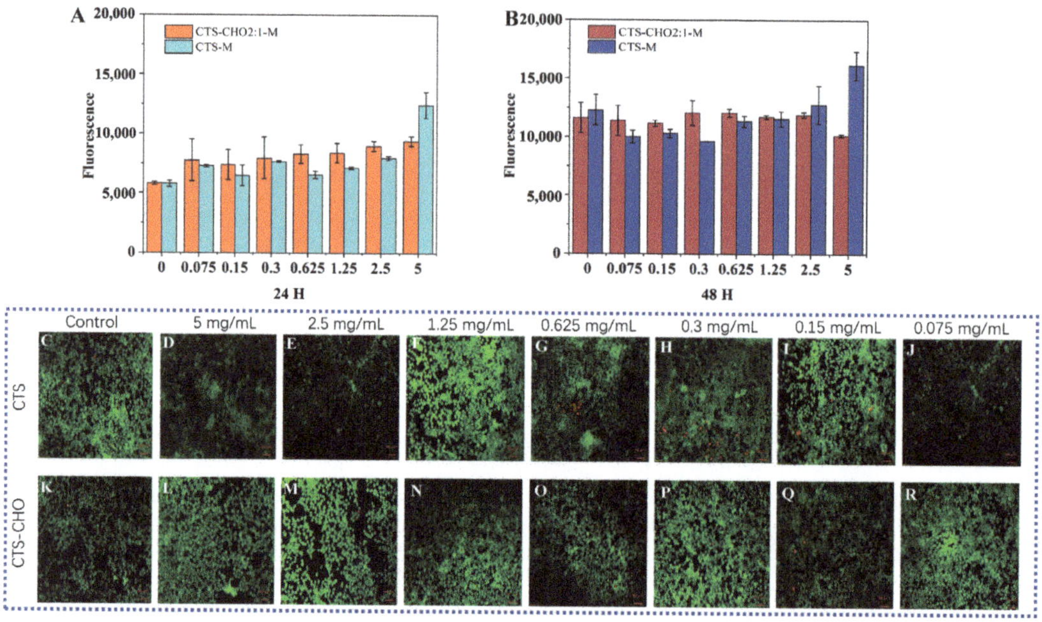

Figure 6. Cytocompatibility. (**A,B**) AlamarBlue measurement (n = 3). (**C–J**) Live/Dead staining assay of CTS (24 h). (**K–R**) Live/Dead staining assay of CTS–CHO (24 h). Scale bar: 50 μm. Red fluorescence indicated dead cells. Green fluorescence indicated living cells.

Live/Dead assay was conducted after co-culturing CTS and CTS-CHO solution for 24 h. A fluorescence microscope was used to observe the outcomes. After 24 h following treatment with CTS solution and CTS−CHO solution, most HEK 293 cells were viable (Figure 6C–R). According to ISO 10993, the materials were non-cytotoxic.

4. Conclusions

A hydrophilic, antibacterial coating based on aldehyde chitosan was developed using nebulization assisted LbL assembly technology via Schiff's base reaction. Aldehyde chitosan was fabricated via an oxidation reaction with chitosan and sodium periodate. According to the FT-IR spectra, aldehyde groups were introduced into chitosan successfully after the oxidation reaction. The oxidation degree of aldehyde chitosan in this study was 12.53%. The results of viscosity, zeta potential, particle size, and stability showed that aldehyde chitosan was a promising candidate for bioactive inks used in antibacterial coating fields. An ideal coating on the surface of the PLA film with hydrophilic, transparent properties and antibacterial activity was designed and characterized. The better transparency, lower water contact angle, higher antibacterial activity, and biocompatibility demonstrated that CTS-CHO coating will be an alternative to CTS as a material for antibacterial coating in the biomedical field, food packaging field, and personal protective field. Drug embedded layers can be assembled to realize drug loadings on the surface for sustained release. This study also represents one of the steps before further investigation for clinical use.

Supplementary Materials: The following supporting information can be downloaded at: https://www.mdpi.com/article/10.3390/jfb14010043/s1, Table S1: Element analysis results of CTS-CHO; Table S2: Zeta potential results of CTS solution and CTS-CHO solution.

Author Contributions: All authors have contributed to this manuscript and approved its final version. Conceptualization, X.W. and Y.Z.; methodology, X.W. and Y.Z.; software, C.M.; validation, C.M.; formal analysis, X.W. and Y.Z.; investigation, Y.L.; resources, W.W. and N.Z.; data curation, X.W. and Y.Z.; writing—original draft preparation, X.W. and Y.Z.; writing—review and editing, M.J.; visualization, X.W. and Y.Z.; supervision, S.A., N.Z. and Q.X.; project administration, S.A.; funding acquisition, Q.X. All authors have read and agreed to the published version of the manuscript.

Funding: This research was funded by the Science Foundation Ireland (SFI) (Funding Agency Ref No: 19/FFP/6522), and the China Scholarship Council (CSC202009110089).

Data Availability Statement: The data presented in this study are available on request from the corresponding author.

Conflicts of Interest: The authors declare no conflict of interest.

References

1. Lim, L.T.; Auras, R.; Rubino, M. Processing technologies for poly(lactic acid). *Prog. Polym. Sci.* **2008**, *33*, 820–852. [CrossRef]
2. Qi, Y.; Ma, H.L.; Du, Z.H.; Yang, B.; Wu, J.; Wang, R.; Zhang, X.Q. Hydrophilic and Antibacterial Modification of Poly(lactic acid) Films by gamma-ray Irradiation. *ACS Omega* **2019**, *4*, 21439–21445. [CrossRef] [PubMed]
3. Zaaba, N.F.; Jaafar, M. A review on degradation mechanisms of polylactic acid: Hydrolytic, photodegradative, microbial, and enzymatic degradation. *Polym. Eng. Sci.* **2020**, *60*, 2061–2075. [CrossRef]
4. Ramot, Y.; Haim-Zada, M.; Domb, A.J.; Nyska, A. Biocompatibility and safety of PLA and its copolymers. *Adv. Drug Deliv. Rev.* **2016**, *107*, 153–162. [CrossRef]
5. Chu, C.C. Materials for absorbable and nonabsorbable surgical sutures. In *Biotextiles as Medical Implants*; Elsevier: Amsterdam, The Netherlands, 2013; pp. 275–334.
6. Gregor, A.; Filova, E.; Novak, M.; Kronek, J.; Chlup, H.; Buzgo, M.; Blahnova, V.; Lukasova, V.; Bartos, M.; Necas, A.; et al. Designing of PLA scaffolds for bone tissue replacement fabricated by ordinary commercial 3D printer. *J. Biol. Eng.* **2017**, *11*, 31. [CrossRef]
7. Liao, S.S.; Cui, F.Z.; Zhang, W.; Feng, Q.L. Hierarchically biomimetic bone scaffold materials: Nano-HA/collagen/PLA composite. *J. Biomed. Mater. Res. B Appl. Biomater.* **2004**, *69*, 158–165. [CrossRef]
8. Singh, D.; Babbar, A.; Jain, V.; Gupta, D.; Saxena, S.; Dwibedi, V. Synthesis, characterization, and bioactivity investigation of biomimetic biodegradable PLA scaffold fabricated by fused filament fabrication process. *J. Braz. Soc. Mech. Sci. Eng.* **2019**, *41*, 121. [CrossRef]
9. Lassalle, V.; Ferreira, M.L. PLA nano- and microparticles for drug delivery: An overview of the methods of preparation. *Macromol. Biosci.* **2007**, *7*, 767–783. [CrossRef]
10. Rancan, F.; Papakostas, D.; Hadam, S.; Hackbarth, S.; Delair, T.; Primard, C.; Verrier, B.; Sterry, W.; Blume-Peytavi, U.; Vogt, A. Investigation of polylactic acid (PLA) nanoparticles as drug delivery systems for local dermatotherapy. *Pharm. Res.* **2009**, *26*, 2027–2036. [CrossRef]
11. Rendeki, S.; Nagy, B.; Bene, M.; Pentek, A.; Toth, L.; Szanto, Z.; Told, R.; Maroti, P. An Overview on Personal Protective Equipment (PPE) Fabricated with Additive Manufacturing Technologies in the Era of COVID-19 Pandemic. *Polymers* **2020**, *12*, 2703. [CrossRef]
12. Viera-Artiles, J.; Valdiande, J.J. 3D-printable headlight face shield adapter. Personal protective equipment in the COVID-19 era. *Am. J. Otolaryngol.* **2020**, *41*, 102576. [CrossRef] [PubMed]
13. Diez-Pascual, A.M. Antimicrobial Polymer-Based Materials for Food Packaging Applications. *Polymers* **2020**, *12*, 731. [CrossRef] [PubMed]
14. Frine, V.C.; Hector, A.P.; Manuel, N.S.; Estrella, N.D.; Antonio, G.J. Development and Characterization of a Biodegradable PLA Food Packaging Hold Monoterpene-Cyclodextrin Complexes against Alternaria alternata. *Polymers* **2019**, *11*, 1720. [CrossRef]
15. Yang, B.; Wang, R.; Ma, H.L.; Li, X.; Brunig, H.; Dong, Z.; Qi, Y.; Zhang, X. Structure Mediation and Properties of Poly(l-lactide)/Poly(d-lactide) Blend Fibers. *Polymers* **2018**, *10*, 1353. [CrossRef]
16. Munteanu, B.S.; Sacarescu, L.; Vasiliu, A.L.; Hitruc, G.E.; Pricope, G.M.; Sivertsvik, M.; Rosnes, J.T.; Vasile, C. Antioxidant/Antibacterial Electrospun Nanocoatings Applied onto PLA Films. *Materials* **2018**, *11*, 1973. [CrossRef] [PubMed]
17. Luque-Agudo, V.; Hierro-Oliva, M.; Gallardo-Moreno, A.M.; González-Martín, M.L. Effect of plasma treatment on the surface properties of polylactic acid films. *Polym. Test.* **2021**, *96*, 107097. [CrossRef]
18. Cai, K.; Yao, K.; Lin, S.; Yang, Z.; Li, X.; Xie, H.; Qing, T.; Gao, L. Poly(D,L-lactic acid) surfaces modified by silk fibroin: Effects on the culture of osteoblast in vitro. *Biomaterials* **2002**, *23*, 1153–1160. [CrossRef] [PubMed]

19. Hendrick, E.; Frey, M. Increasing Surface Hydrophilicity in Poly(Lactic Acid) Electrospun Fibers by Addition of Pla-b-Peg Co-Polymers. *J. Eng. Fibers Fabr.* **2014**, *9*, 153–164. [CrossRef]
20. Suganya, A.; Shanmugavelayutham, G.; Rodríguez, C.S. Study on plasma pre-functionalized PVC film grafted with TiO2/PVP to improve blood compatible and antibacterial properties. *J. Phys. D Appl. Phys.* **2017**, *50*, 145402. [CrossRef]
21. Minati, L.; Migliaresi, C.; Lunelli, L.; Viero, G.; Dalla Serra, M.; Speranza, G. Plasma assisted surface treatments of biomaterials. *Biophys. Chem.* **2017**, *229*, 151–164. [CrossRef]
22. Demina, T.S.; Piskarev, M.S.; Romanova, O.A.; Gatin, A.K.; Senatulin, B.R.; Skryleva, E.A.; Zharikova, T.M.; Gilman, A.B.; Kuznetsov, A.A.; Akopova, T.A.; et al. Plasma Treatment of Poly(ethylene terephthalate) Films and Chitosan Deposition: DC- vs. AC-Discharge. *Materials* **2020**, *13*, 508. [CrossRef] [PubMed]
23. Kolar, M.; Mozetic, M.; Stana-Kleinschek, K.; Frohlich, M.; Turk, B.; Vesel, A. Covalent Binding of Heparin to Functionalized PET Materials for Improved Haemocompatibility. *Materials* **2015**, *8*, 1526–1544. [CrossRef] [PubMed]
24. Aflori, M.; Drobota, M.; Dimitriu, D.G.; Stoica, I.; Simionescu, B.; Harabagiu, V. Collagen immobilization on polyethylene terephthalate surface after helium plasma treatment. *Mater. Sci. Eng. B* **2013**, *178*, 1303–1310. [CrossRef]
25. Recek, N.; Jaganjac, M.; Kolar, M.; Milkovic, L.; Mozetic, M.; Stana-Kleinschek, K.; Vesel, A. Protein adsorption on various plasma-treated polyethylene terephthalate substrates. *Molecules* **2013**, *18*, 12441–12463. [CrossRef]
26. Sophonvachiraporn, P.; Rujiravanit, R.; Sreethawong, T.; Tokura, S.; Chavadej, S. Surface Characterization and Antimicrobial Activity of Chitosan-Deposited DBD Plasma-Modified Woven PET Surface. *Plasma Chem. Plasma Process.* **2010**, *31*, 233–249. [CrossRef]
27. Novoa-Carballal, R.; Riguera, R.; Fernandez-Megia, E. Chitosan hydrophobic domains are favoured at low degree of acetylation and molecular weight. *Polymer* **2013**, *54*, 2081–2087. [CrossRef]
28. Vesel, A.; Mozetic, M.; Strnad, S. Improvement of adhesion of fucoidan on polyethylene terephthalate surface using gas plasma treatments. *Vacuum* **2011**, *85*, 1083–1086. [CrossRef]
29. Park, K.; Ju, Y.M.; Son, J.S.; Ahn, K.D.; Han, D.K. Surface modification of biodegradable electrospun nanofiber scaffolds and their interaction with fibroblasts. *J. Biomater. Sci. Polym. Ed.* **2007**, *18*, 369–382. [CrossRef]
30. Cheng, Y.; Deng, S.; Chen, P.; Ruan, R. Polylactic acid (PLA) synthesis and modifications: A review. *Front. Chem. China* **2009**, *4*, 259–264. [CrossRef]
31. Gutierrez-Villarreal, M.H.; Ulloa-Hinojosa, M.G.; Gaona-Lozano, J.G. Surface functionalization of poly(lactic acid) film by UV-photografting ofN-vinylpyrrolidone. *J. Appl. Polym. Sci.* **2008**, *110*, 163–169. [CrossRef]
32. Carosio, F.; Fontaine, G.; Alongi, J.; Bourbigot, S. Starch-Based Layer by Layer Assembly: Efficient and Sustainable Approach to Cotton Fire Protection. *ACS Appl. Mater. Interfaces* **2015**, *7*, 12158–12167. [CrossRef] [PubMed]
33. Stewart-Clark, S.S.; Lvov, Y.M.; Mills, D.K. Ultrasonic nebulization-assisted layer-by-layer assembly for spray coating of multilayered, multicomponent, bioactive nanostructures. *J. Coat. Technol. Res.* **2010**, *8*, 275–281. [CrossRef]
34. Doshi, B.; Repo, E.; Heiskanen, J.P.; Sirvio, J.A.; Sillanpaa, M. Effectiveness of N,O-carboxymethyl chitosan on destabilization of Marine Diesel, Diesel and Marine-2T oil for oil spill treatment. *Carbohydr. Polym.* **2017**, *167*, 326–336. [CrossRef] [PubMed]
35. Sangsuwan, J.; Rattanapanone, N.; Rachtanapun, P. Effect of chitosan/methyl cellulose films on microbial and quality characteristics of fresh-cut cantaloupe and pineapple. *Postharvest Biol. Technol.* **2008**, *49*, 403–410. [CrossRef]
36. Wang, X.; Song, R.; Johnson, M.; Asigen, S.; He, Z.; Milne, C.; Wang, X.; Lara-Saez, I.; Xu, Q.; Wang, W. An Injectable Chitosan-Based Self-Healable Hydrogel System as an Antibacterial Wound Dressing. *Materials* **2021**, *14*, 5956. [CrossRef]
37. Bam, P.; Bhatta, A.; Krishnamoorthy, G. Design of biostable scaffold based on collagen crosslinked by dialdehyde chitosan with presence of gallic acid. *Int. J. Biol. Macromol.* **2019**, *130*, 836–844. [CrossRef]
38. Vold, I.M.; Christensen, B.E. Periodate oxidation of chitosans with different chemical compositions. *Carbohydr. Res.* **2005**, *340*, 679–684. [CrossRef]
39. Yin, M.; Wang, Y.; Zhang, Y.; Ren, X.; Qiu, Y.; Huang, T.S. Novel quaternarized N-halamine chitosan and polyvinyl alcohol nanofibrous membranes as hemostatic materials with excellent antibacterial properties. *Carbohydr. Polym.* **2020**, *232*, 115823. [CrossRef]
40. Kong, M.; Chen, X.G.; Xing, K.; Park, H.J. Antimicrobial properties of chitosan and mode of action: A state of the art review. *Int. J. Food Microbiol.* **2010**, *144*, 51–63. [CrossRef]
41. Philippova, O.E.; Korchagina, E.V. Chitosan and its hydrophobic derivatives: Preparation and aggregation in dilute aqueous solutions. *Polym Sci Ser A* **2012**, *54*, 552–572. [CrossRef]
42. Pigaleva, M.A.; Portnov, I.V.; Rudov, A.A.; Blagodatskikh, I.V.; Grigoriev, T.E.; Gallyamov, M.O.; Potemkin, I.I. Stabilization of Chitosan Aggregates at the Nanoscale in Solutions in Carbonic Acid. *Macromolecules* **2014**, *47*, 5749–5758. [CrossRef]
43. Lee, K.Y.; Kwon, I.C.; Kim, Y.H.; Jo, W.H.; Jeong, S.Y. Preparation of chitosan self-aggregates as a gene delivery system. *J. Control. Release* **1998**, *51*, 213–220. [CrossRef] [PubMed]
44. Schatz, C.; Pichot, C.; Delair, T.; Viton, C.; Domard, A. Static Light Scattering Studies on Chitosan Solutions: From Macromolecular Chains to Colloidal Dispersions. *Langmuir* **2003**, *19*, 9896–9903. [CrossRef]
45. You, J.; Hu, F.Q.; Du, Y.Z.; Yuan, H. Polymeric Micelles with Glycolipid-like Structure and Multiple Hydrophobic Domains for Mediating Molecular Target Delivery of Paclitaxel. *Biomacromolecules* **2007**, *8*, 2450–2456. [CrossRef]

46. Yanagisawa, M.; Kato, Y.; Yoshida, Y.; Isogai, A. SEC-MALS study on aggregates of chitosan molecules in aqueous solvents: Influence of residual N-acetyl groups. *Carbohydr. Polym.* **2006**, *66*, 192–198. [CrossRef]
47. Yilmaz Atay, H. Antibacterial Activity of Chitosan-Based Systems. In *Functional Chitosan*; Springer: Singapore, 2019; pp. 457–489. [CrossRef]

Journal of
Functional Biomaterials

MDPI

Article

Ellagic Acid Inclusion Complex-Loaded Hydrogels as an Efficient Controlled Release System: Design, Fabrication and In Vitro Evaluation

Chengqun Yu [1,†], Abid Naeem [1,†], Yali Liu [2,3,*] and Yongmei Guan [1,*]

1 Key Laboratory of Modern Preparation of Traditional Chinese Medicines, Ministry of Education, Jiangxi University of Chinese Medicine, Nanchang 330004, China; yuchengqun@jxutcm.edu.cn (C.Y.); 20214003@jxutcm.edu.cn (A.N.)
2 Key Laboratory of Pharmacodynamics and Safety Evaluation, Health Commission of Jiangxi Province, 1688 Meiling Road, Nanchang 330006, China
3 Key Laboratory of Pharmacodynamics and Quality Evaluation on Anti-Inflammatory Chinese Herbs, Jiangxi Administration of Traditional Chinese Medicine, Nanchang Medical College, 1688 Meiling Road, Nanchang 330006, China
* Correspondence: liuyali@ncmc.edu.cn (Y.L.); 20081015@jxutcm.edu.cn (Y.G.)
† These authors contributed equally to this work.

Abstract: Oxidants play a crucial role in the development of oxidative stress, which is linked to disease progression. Ellagic acid is an effective antioxidant with applications in the treatment and prevention of several diseases, since it neutralizes free radicals and reduces oxidative stress. However, it has limited application due to its poor solubility and oral bioavailability. Since ellagic acid is hydrophobic, it is difficult to load it directly into hydrogels for controlled release applications. Therefore, the purpose of this study was to first prepare inclusion complexes of ellagic acid (EA) with hydroxypropyl-β-cyclodextrin and then load them into carbopol-934-grafted-2-acrylamido-2-methyl-1-propane sulfonic acid (CP-*g*-AMPS) hydrogels for orally controlled drug delivery. Fourier transform infrared spectroscopy (FTIR), X-ray diffraction (XRD), scanning electron microscopy (SEM), thermogravimetric analysis (TGA), and differential scanning calorimetry (DSC) were used to validate ellagic acid inclusion complexes and hydrogels. There was slightly higher swelling and drug release at pH 1.2 (42.20% and 92.13%) than at pH 7.4 (31.61% and 77.28%), respectively. Hydrogels had high porosity (88.90%) and biodegradation (9.2% per week in phosphate-buffered saline). Hydrogels were tested for their antioxidant properties in vitro against 2,2-diphenyl-1-picrylhydrazyl (DPPH) and 2,2′-azino-bis (3-ethylbenzothiazoline-6-sulfonic acid) (ABTS). Additionally, the antibacterial activity of hydrogels was demonstrated against Gram-positive bacterial strains (*Staphylococcus aureus* and *Escherichia coli*) and Gram-negative bacterial strains (*Pseudomonas aeruginosa*).

Keywords: hydrogels; polyphenol; phytoconstituents; inclusion complexation; anti-oxidants; bioavailability

1. Introduction

Ellagic acid (EA), a polyphenol with the molecular formula $C_{14}H_6O_8$, is found in a wide variety of fruits and nuts, such as pomegranates, strawberries, blueberries, and walnuts. It possesses strong anti-oxidant, anti-inflammatory, anti-viral, anti-microbial, anti-teratogenic, hepatoprotective, and anti-tumor properties, particularly in regard to colon cancer, esophageal cancer, breast cancer, and hepatocellular carcinoma [1]. Its low oral bioavailability and consequently low therapeutic potential is due to a combination of factors, including its low aqueous solubility, its permeability in the gastrointestinal tract (GIT), its permanent binding to DNA and proteins, and its first-pass metabolism. Furthermore, EA is rapidly absorbed in the GIT and eliminated within 2 to 6 h, depending on the composition of the food [2].

Previous studies investigated the in vivo and in vitro bioavailability of EA in humans, which revealed substantial interindividual variation (due to the low solubility of free EA in gastric conditions, the nature of the precursor, and insufficient intestinal absorption). Moreover, despite high intakes of free EA, plasma levels of EA were consistently low [3]. Research has demonstrated that EA undergoes extensive metabolism in the large intestine by the gut microbiota, resulting in urolithins that are 25–80 times more bioavailable and much more readily absorbed than EA [4,5]. Presently, research on ellagic acid focuses primarily on the distribution, extraction and purification, analysis of its content, and pharmacological properties of the compound. However, relatively few studies have been conducted on its formulations, including ellagic acid microspheres, phospholipid complexes, and nanoparticles [6–9]. These data have prompted an increase in interest in developing delivery systems, which are capable of increasing the solubility and bioavailability of EA in water, maintaining its structural integrity, and ensuring its controlled release at a physiological target [10].

Cyclodextrins (CDs) are cyclic oligosaccharides, consisting of (α-1,4) linked α-d-glucopyranose monomers. They have a lipophilic cavity, a 'molecular cage,' which may combine with the lipophilic part of the molecule via non-covalent interactions, while their hydrophilic surface aids in water solubilization [11]. In addition, this molecular inclusion enhances shelf life by protecting it against oxidation, light-induced decomposition, and heat-induced transformation. Unlike most other CDs, α-cyclodextrin lacks a sufficiently large cavity in which to encapsulate the majority of molecules, while γ-cyclodextrin does not offer economic viability because of its high price [12]. Therefore, β-cyclodextrin (β-CD) represents the most common form of the derivative. 2-Hydroxypropyl-β-cyclodextrin (HP-βCD) is an improved form of naturally occurring β-cyclodextrin, exhibiting enhanced safety characteristics. HP-βCD, which is generally recognized as safe by the FDA, is a water-soluble oligosaccharide that has shown promising results in increasing the solubility of various molecules [13].

Drug release can be controlled through the use of polymers that have known release profiles. As a result, drug release rate fluctuations may be minimized, and effective delivery can be achieved [14,15]. A controlled drug release system typically delivers the drug, over time, to the target area at a predetermined rate so as to maintain the concentration of the drug and to optimize therapeutic effectiveness [16]. Hydrogels are characterized by a cross-linked network of hydrophilic polymers that can absorb water without becoming soluble in it [17]. Hydrogels have found extensive applications in agriculture, biotechnology, food, and pharmacy. As a result of their swelling properties, hydrogels can absorb and release substantial amounts of drugs. There is a direct correlation between the swelling behavior of the hydrogel and its release rate [18]. Carbopol polymers are generally considered to be safe by the US Food and Drug Administration (FDA) [19]. In addition to being a hydrophilic polymer, carbopol-934 becomes highly ionized upon neutralization, causing electrostatic repulsion among polymer chains to produce a gel. The high stability, compatibility, and low toxicity of carbopol make it ideal for use in oral preparations, such as suspensions, tablets, and topically applied formulations [20]. 2-acrylamido-2 methylpropane sulfonic acid (AMPS) possesses high hydrophilicity and is commonly utilized in hydrogel formulations. AMPS shows pH-independent swelling characteristics due to the presence of sulfonic groups, which are easily ionized and dissociated at different pH values [21]. Furthermore, the increase in AMPS monomer concentration increases the swelling ratio of the hydrogels, owing to the presence of more ionizable sulfonic groups [22]. Ethylene glycol dimethacrylate (EGDMA) is a chemical crosslinker widely utilized for crosslinking of different polymers and monomers [23].

The aim of this study was to successfully encapsulate a hydrophobic molecule (ellagic acid) in hydrogels for orally controlled drug delivery to improve its bioavailability. Because most of the hydrophobic drugs cannot be very easily loaded into hydrogels, the first inclusion complexes were formed and then loaded in the hydrogels. This type of formulation provides a basis for encapsulating other hydrophobic phytochemicals/drugs in hydrogels for controlled release purposes for improving their bioavailability. In this study, first, the inclusion complexes of the hydrophobic drug (ellagic acid) with 2-hydroxypropyl-β-cyclodextrin (EIC), were developed to improve the solubility and stability of the drug. Then, these inclusion complexes were loaded inside carbopol-934-grafted-AMPS hydrogels. Various characterization techniques were utilized for characterizing the inclusion complexes and hydrogels, such as Fourier transform infrared spectroscopy (FTIR), differential scanning calorimetry (DSC), X-ray diffraction (XRD), thermogravimetric analysis (TGA), hydrogel porosity and sol–gel fraction, and biodegradation. The swelling characteristics and drug release behavior of the formulated hydrogels were determined using phosphate buffer (pH 7.4 and 1.2). Furthermore, the antioxidant (ABTS and DPPH) and antimicrobial activities (*Pseudomonas aeruginosa*, *Staphylococcus aureus*, and *Escherichia coli*) of ellagic acid inclusion complexes-loaded hydrogels were also investigated. As a result of their excellent water absorption, biodegradability, and controlled release behavior, these hydrogels are capable of being used as controlled oral drug delivery systems for hydrophilic and hydrophobic drugs, respectively.

2. Materials and Methods

2.1. Materials

Ellagic acid (EA; MW: 302.19 g/moL; Lot#R016669), ethylene glycol dimethacrylate (EGDMA; MW: 198.22 g/moL; Lot#335681), ammonium persulfate (APS; Lot#MKCM6448), and 2-acrylamido-2-methyl-1-propanesulfonic acid (AMPS; MW: 207.25 g/moL; Lot#STBK4291) were obtained from Sigma-Aldrich, Saint Louis, MI, USA. Sodium bisulfite (SHS; Lot#G2223206) was from Shanghai Aladdin Biochemical Technology, Shanghai, China. HP-βCD (HPβCD; MW:1541.5 g/moL; Lot#O1027C), cefepime HCL (Lot#N1118A), ABTS (Lot#A0807A), and DPPH (Lot#UFQ2I-WL) were acquired from Meilune Biological Company (Dalian, China). Carbopol-934 (CP; MW: 72.06 g/moL; Lot#C12467657) was obtained from Macklin Biochemical Co., Ltd. (Shanghai, China).

Escherichia coli (*E. coli*: ATCC25922HBJZ087), *Staphylococcus aureus* (*S. aureus*: ATCC25923HBJZ005), and *Pseudomonas aeruginosa* (*P. aeruginosa*: ATCC27853HBJZ017) were acquired from Qingdao Hope Biotechnology, Co., Ltd., Qingdao, China.

2.2. Synthesis of HP-βCD and Ellagic Acid Inclusion Complexes (EIC)

The EIC was prepared by using the mass ratio of HP-βCD to ellagic acid of 2:1 [24]. Briefly, HP-βCD was weighed and dissolved in a specified amount of ultrapure water, and ellagic acid was dissolved in an appropriate amount of anhydrous ethanol. The ellagic acid solution was then gradually added to the HP-βCD solution, and it was mixed well at 350 rpm/min for 72 h. A thorough mixing procedure was followed by centrifugation and storage in a −20 °C refrigerator for approximately 12 h. In the final step, the obtained sample was freeze-dried for two days in order to obtain pure HP-βCD and ellagic acid inclusion complexes.

2.3. Fabrication of CP-g-AMPS Hydrogels

The free radical polymerization technique was used for the synthesis of hydrogels, possessing slight modifications [22]. Briefly, carbopol-934, AMPS, EGDMA, and APS/SHS (APS was used as an initiator, and SHS was used as a co-initiator of the reaction) were weighed and placed separately in their corresponding bottles, as shown in Table 1. The labeled vials were filled with sufficient water and stirred vigorously to obtain a clear solution. The carbopol-934 was continuously stirred at 40 °C until it was well blended. A homogeneous mixture of APS/SHS and AMPS was prepared by mixing it evenly, and then it was added to the carbopol-934 solution. After mixing, the mixture was ultrasonically processed, and nitrogen was applied for 30 min to remove air bubbles. Following this, EGDMA was poured dropwise into the mixture. The final mixture was transferred to a water bath (50 °C), and it was slowly heated until the temperature reached 65 °C. After

24 h, the hydrogels were cut into discs of 8 mm, and they were vacuum dried at 40 °C for a week. Figure 1 illustrates the proposed chemical structure for CP-*g*-AMPS.

Table 1. Feed composition (g/mL water) of CP-*g*-AMPS hydrogels.

Formulation Codes	Carbopol-934 (g)	APS/SHS (g)	AMPS (g)	EGDMA (g)
KAE-1	0.5/15	0.3/0.3/4	20/15	**0.5**
KAE-2	0.5/15	0.3/0.3/4	20/15	**1**
KAE-3	0.5/15	0.3/0.3/4	20/15	**1.5**
KAE-4	0.5/15	0.3/0.3/4	**12**/15	0.5
KAE-5	0.5/15	0.3/0.3/4	**20**/15	0.5
KAE-6	0.5/15	0.3/0.3/4	**28**/15	0.5
KAE-7	**0.3**/15	0.3/0.3/4	20/15	0.5
KAE-8	**0.5**/15	0.3/0.3/4	20/15	0.5
KAE-9	**0.7**/15	0.3/0.3/4	20/15	0.5

Note: Bold letters refer to increased feeding amounts.

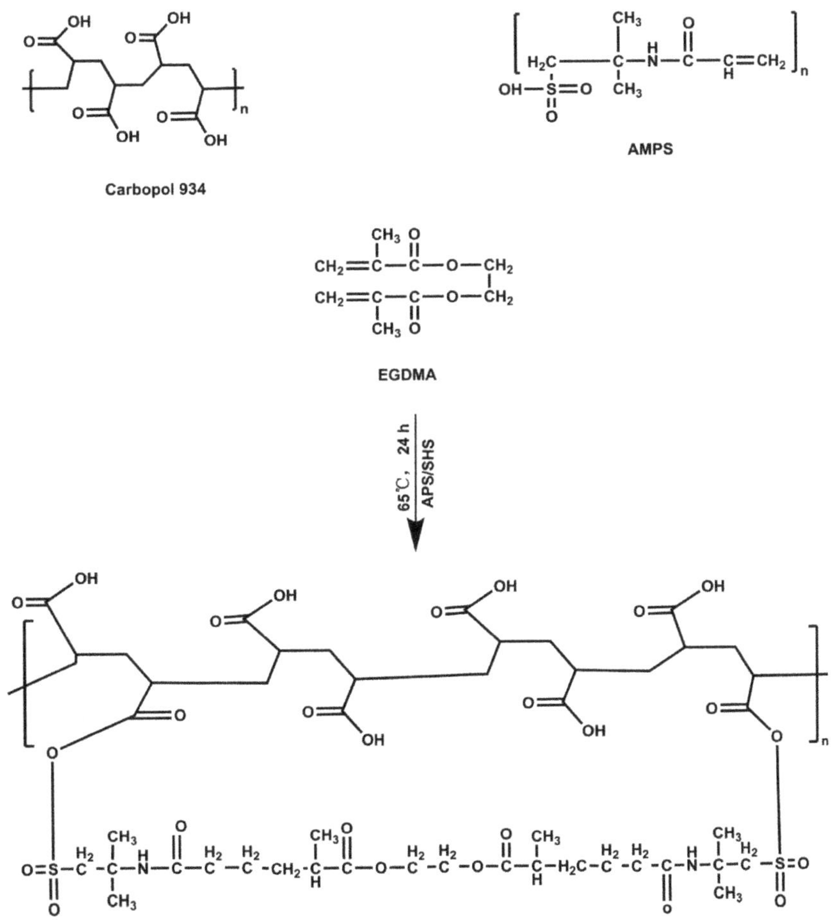

Figure 1. Proposed chemical structure of CP-*g*-AMPS hydrogels.

EIC Loading into Hydrogels

The EIC was loaded into the synthesized hydrogels by a swelling–diffusion procedure [25]. Briefly, 1% EIC solution was prepared in buffer pH 7.4, and, then, unloaded hydrogel discs (dried) were placed in it and stirred slowly for three days. Thereafter, the hydrogel discs were taken out, allowed to dry fully, weighed, and the amount of EIC-loaded in the hydrogel was determined by subtracting unloaded hydrogel weight from EIC-loaded hydrogel weight. In addition, UV-spectrometry was used to confirm the drug loading by extracting the drug from the hydrogel and analyzing it. Briefly, the drug-loaded hydrogel discs were immersed in freshly made 25 mL of pH 7.4 phosphate buffer for a period of 5 h. We changed the phosphate buffer solution after a predetermined time to a new 25 mL solution. Repeated testing was conducted until no drug was detected in the solution. A calibration curve for ellagic acid was used to measure the concentration of ellagic acid in the solution. A UV-visible spectrophotometer was used to determine the absorbance at a wavelength of 254 nm.

$$\text{EIC loading} = \text{EIC loaded hydrogels} - \text{Unloaded hydrogels} \quad (1)$$

2.4. In Vitro Characterization

2.4.1. FTIR Spectroscopy

Drug–formulation interactions were examined with the attenuated total reflectance method using a FTIR spectrometer (Spectrum Two FTIR Spectrometer, Perkin Elmer, Buckinghamshire, UK). The spectra of loaded and unloaded formulations and their components were acquired over a scanning range of 400 cm^{-1} to 4000 cm^{-1}.

2.4.2. Thermal Analysis

Thermal stability of the samples was assessed through the use of a thermogravimetric analyzer (TG/DTA6300, Seiko, Tokyo, Japan) and a differential scanning calorimeter (DSC 4000, Perkin Elmer, UK). An analysis of weight change with respect to temperature was conducted using a thermogravimetric instrument. A reference standard was used to calibrate the weight profile at the beginning. Carbopol-934, AMPS, EIC, and their respective formulations (0.4 to 6 mg) were individually tested in aluminum pans. A scanner operating at a temperature of 10 °C/min and a flow rate of 10 mL/min of inert nitrogen was used to measure the percentage weight loss. AMPS, EIC, carbopol-934, and synthesized formulations were analyzed using DSC to determine their melting points. A sapphire standard was employed for calibrating calorimeters for heat capacity. A standardization of cell constants and temperatures was achieved through the use of indium.

2.4.3. X-ray Diffraction

Crystallinity of the samples was determined by a diffractometer (TD-3500 X-ray diffractometer, Dandong, China), with CuKα irradiations at 30 kV and 20 mA. Scan speeds were set at 2 degrees per minute and 2θ between 10° and 60°. The crystallinity of an object can be determined by its peak. Normally, the presence of sharp and intensive peaks indicates the crystallinity of the sample. In contrast, diffuse peaks indicate an amorphous nature, as demonstrated by synthesized hydrogels. Measurements were conducted on carbopol-934, EIC, HP-βCD, ellagic acid, and unloaded and EIC-loaded hydrogels.

2.4.4. Scanning Electron Microscopy

The morphology, microstructural properties, and porosity of the hydrogel were investigated with the help of scanning electron microscopy (Quanta 250, Eindhoven, The Netherlands). The dried samples were first coated on aluminium stubs, and then they were sputtered with gold, and then they were evaluated in a cross-section, using an accelerated current of 15 kV.

2.4.5. Mechanical Characteristics

Tensile strength (TS) and elongation-at-break (EAB) of the hydrogels were measured for each formulation at 1 mm/s using a TA.XT plus texture analyzer (SMS TA.XT plus, Stable Micro Systems, Godalming, UK), which was equipped with a stainless steel cylindrical probe (P/5S) [26]. TS and EAB can be calculated using the following equations.

$$TS = \frac{Fm}{Th} \quad (2)$$

$$EAB = \frac{\sqrt{D^2 + R^2}}{R} - 1 \quad (3)$$

Fm represents the probe force, and Th represents the hydrogel thickness. D is the displacement of the probe after it first contacts the hydrogel, and R is the radius of the orifice plate.

2.4.6. Sol-Gel Fraction Determination

Sol-gel fraction analysis was conducted on the synthesized hydrogels with the aim of determining the levels of uncrosslinked and crosslinked constituents [27]. The hydrogels are composed of two different parts/portions: a gel fraction, which is an insoluble component, and a sol fraction, which is a soluble component. The Soxhlet extraction method was used to conduct the sol-gel fraction analysis. Unloaded hydrogels were added to a flask containing deionized water in a certain amount. The flask was equipped with a condenser. At 85 °C, the extraction was carried out for 14 h. Afterwards, the disc was extracted, dehydrated in a vacuum oven, and then weighed again. The given equations were used for determining the sol–gel fraction of hydrogel [28].

$$\text{Sol fraction } \% = \frac{S1 - S2}{S2} \times 100 \quad (4)$$

$$\text{Gel fraction} = 100 - \text{sol fraction} \quad (5)$$

The weight of a dried hydrogel (after extraction) is indicated by S1, whereas that of a fresh hydrogel is shown by S2.

2.4.7. Porosity Study

The porosity of each hydrogel formulation was assessed using a solvent replacement approach. Once the dried hydrogels (K1) had been accurately weighed, they were placed in ethanol (pure) for five days. After five days, the discs were lifted out of the ethanol, gently dried, and then weighed again (K2). Additionally, the diameter of the hydrogel disc, as well as its thickness, were measured. The equation given below was used to determine porosity [29].

$$\text{Porosity percentage } (\%) = \frac{K2 - K1}{\rho v} \times 100 \quad (6)$$

Here, ρ represents the absolute density of ethanol, and V indicates swollen hydrogel volume.

2.4.8. Polymer Network Parameters of CP-g-AMPS Hydrogels

The properties and structure of swollen hydrogels are determined by a number of important factors [30].

The diffusion coefficient (D) was calculated as follows:

$$D = \pi \left(\frac{h \cdot \theta}{4 \cdot qeq} \right)^2 \quad (7)$$

Whereas, qeq indicates equilibrium swelling, θ indicates slope of swelling curves, and h indicates disc thickness.

The polymeric volume fraction (V2, s) was determined as follows.

$$V2,\ s = \frac{1}{Veq} \quad (8)$$

Molecular weight across crosslinking connections (Mc) was determined as follows.

$$\mathrm{Mc} = \frac{\mathrm{dp\ Vs}\left(\mathrm{V}\,^{\frac{1}{3}}2,\mathrm{s} - \mathrm{V}2,\frac{\mathrm{s}}{2}\right)}{\ln(1 - \mathrm{V}2,\mathrm{s}) + \mathrm{V}2,\mathrm{s} + \chi\mathrm{V}^2 2,\mathrm{s}} \tag{9}$$

Whereas dp corresponds to polymer density, χ is the Flory-Huggins solvent polymer interaction parameter, and Vs refers to the volume of the solvent.

The polymer solvent interaction parameter (χ) can be determined with the following equation.

$$\chi = \frac{\ln(1 - \mathrm{V}2,\mathrm{s}) + \mathrm{V}2,\mathrm{s}}{\mathrm{V}^2 2,\mathrm{s}} \tag{10}$$

where; V2,s corresponds to the hydrogel volume after swelling.

The number of intercrosslink repeating units (N) were estimated by the following equation:

$$\mathrm{N} = \frac{2\mathrm{Mc}}{\mathrm{Mr}} \tag{11}$$

Mr denotes molar mass of the repeating units and is determined using the given equation:

$$\mathrm{Mr} = \frac{\mathrm{mCPMCP\ +\ mAMPSMAMPS\ +\ mEGDMAMEGDMA}}{\mathrm{mCP + mAMPS + mEGDMA}} \tag{12}$$

where "m" represents masses, and "M" shows the molar masses of carbopol-934, AMPS, and EGDMA, respectively.

2.4.9. Swelling Studies

Equilibrium-swelling ratios (ESR) were determined using phosphate buffers (pH 1.2 and 7.4) [31]. The weight of the hydrogels was measured after weighing and placing them in the buffers for a specified period of time. The weight of the hydrogel was measured and recorded at a number of different points until equilibrium was reached. The swelling percentage was calculated using the formula shown below.

$$\mathrm{ESR} = \frac{\mathrm{Yt\ -\ Yi}}{\mathrm{Yi}} \times 100 \tag{13}$$

The weight at time t is indicated by Yt, and the initial weight of the hydrogel is given by Yi.

2.4.10. In Vitro Release and Kinetics

Synthesized hydrogels were investigated for drug release in vitro at two pH levels, pH 1.2 and 7.4 [32]. Briefly, dried EIC-loaded hydrogel discs were immersed in pH 1.2 and 7.4 buffer solutions in a USP dissolution apparatus type II at 37 °C and 50 rpm. Each time, an aliquot of 5 mL was collected, and the same volume of fresh medium was infused into the sample at predetermined intervals. Samples were analyzed in triplicate using an ultraviolet-visible spectrophotometer (T6 New Century, Beijing, China) at a wavelength of 254 nanometers (the standard wavelength for ellagic acid).

$$\text{Percentage drug release} = \frac{(\text{drug released})}{(\text{drug loaded })} \times 100 \tag{14}$$

Among the most important parameters that can affect the rate of drug release in hydrogels are polymer chain stretching, matrix swelling, drug type, and the pH of the medium in which the drug is released. Swelling of hydrogels is fundamentally explained by solvent diffusion, as it is proportional to the penetration of solvents into the hydrogels, which causes them to swell. The following release kinetic models were used to identify the pattern of drug release.

$$\text{Zero} - \text{order kinetics Ft} = \text{K0t} \tag{15}$$

Ft represents the quantity of drug that has been released over time t, while K0 represents the apparent constant of the zero-order rate of drug release over time t.

$$\text{First order kinetics } \ln(1 - \mathrm{F}) = -\mathrm{K1t} \tag{16}$$

The amount of drug that is released at time t is denoted by the symbol F, and the first-order drug release rate constant is denoted by k1.

$$\text{Higuchi model } F = K2t^{\frac{1}{2}} \tag{17}$$

The Higuchi constant is denoted by the symbol K2 in this equation, while the release rate is denoted by the letter F.

$$\text{Korsmeyer} - \text{Peppas model } \frac{Mt}{M¥} = K3t^{n} \tag{18}$$

The quantity of water that is absorbed into a system when it is in a state of equilibrium is expressed by the symbol M∞, whereas the quantity that is absorbed at a particular time is represented by the symbol Mt. The geometrical and structural features of gels are the basis for the K3 constant, and the exponent of drug release is denoted by n.

2.4.11. Biodegradation Study

Biodegradation study of the fabricated hydrogel was carried out at 37 °C using a pH 7.4 phosphate buffer [33]. At different intervals, precisely weighed hydrogel discs were immersed in a buffer solution for one, three, five, and seven days, respectively. After taking out the hydrogel discs at the designated time, the hydrogel discs were dried under vacuum at 40 °C, reweighed, and then put into the buffer solution. Degradation of hydrogels was calculated using the following equation [34].

$$D = \frac{C1 - C2}{C1} \tag{19}$$

D shows degradation, and C1 shows dry weight, while C2 shows after-immersion weight.

2.5. Antioxidant Studies

2.5.1. DPPH Activity

The antioxidant activity of CP-*g*-AMPS hydrogel was measured using the DPPH free radical scavenging assay. After soaking a specified amount of sample in methanol, it was left at ambient temperature in the dark for 24 h. After that, all samples were added to the DPPH-methanol solution (0.1 M). Afterward, the mixture was thoroughly shaken and allowed to stand in the dark for 30 min. A UV-Vis spectrophotometer was used to measure the solution's absorbance at 517 nm, and the DPPH scavenging activity was calculated accordingly [35].

$$\text{DPPH}(\%) = \frac{A0 - A}{A0} \times 100 \tag{20}$$

Absorbance values A0 and A indicate the control and sample, respectively.

2.5.2. ABTS Activity

Hydrogels, containing EIC, were tested with the ABTS assay for their radical scavenging capability. The radicalization of ABTS was induced by adding 2.4 mm potassium persulfate ($K_2S_2O_8$) to a solution of 7.4 mM ABTS. After the hydrogels and the ABTS solution had been thoroughly combined, the mixture was allowed to sit in an incubator at 37 °C for half an hour. An absorbance measurement was performed at a wavelength of 730 nm. The scavenging effect of ABTS is calculated using the following formula [36].

$$\text{ABTS scavenging effect } (\%) = \frac{A0 - A1}{A0} \times 100 \tag{21}$$

The absorbance of ABTS is A0, whereas the absorbance of the samples is A1.

2.6. Antibacterial Activity

Nutrient agar was formulated with purified water, and it was subsequently autoclaved (121 °C/15 psi) for 30 min. Agar medium was applied to small Petri plates and allowed to solidify for a few hours at room temperature before use. Bacterial strains of *Pseudomonas aeruginosa*, *Escherichia coli*, and *Staphylococcus aureus* were cultured for 24 h, and then they were swabbed and grown on Petri dishes. Each of these plates was divided into four groups:

blank hydrogel, EIC-loaded hydrogel, cefipime (1 mg/mL, positive control), and negative control. Additionally, they were then incubated for 24 h at 37 °C before calculating the zone of inhibition (ZOI) [37]:

$$\text{Inhibition } (\%) = \frac{\text{ZOI of test sample (mm)}}{\text{ZOI of standard drug (mm)}} \times 100 \quad (22)$$

2.7. Statistical Analysis

Mean and standard deviations were used to quantitatively describe the data. Two-way analysis of variance and Tukey's post hoc test were used to find statistically significant differences between sets of neighbouring data. Statistical significance was determined by calculating the *p*-value, and the results were marked as follows: * $p < 0.05$, ** $p < 0.01$, and *** $p < 0.001$.

3. Results and Discussion

3.1. FTIR Analysis

The EA spectrum showed characteristic absorption bands similar to the ones previously described (Figure 2). A large sharp band at 3480 cm^{-1}, and a broad absorption band at 3360–2840 cm^{-1}, were assigned to the stretching vibrations of the -OH group. Absorption bands at 2933 cm^{-1} and 2851 cm^{-1} are due to asymmetric, as well as symmetric C-H, stretching vibrations for $-CH_3$. Stretching of the carbonyl group appeared at 1718 cm^{-1}. The bands observed at 1621 cm^{-1} and 1506 cm^{-1} are attributed to C=C–C vibrations, and bands at 1449 cm^{-1} are attributed to C–H bending vibrations. Whereas, 1328 cm^{-1} and 1198 cm^{-1} bands are due to C–O ester linkage stretching, and 1047 cm^{-1} bands are for aromatic C–H in-plane bending ester linkage. Bands at 925, 815, and 689 cm^{-1} are assigned to aromatic C–H out-plane bending [38]. In the case of CP, the FTIR spectrum showed bands in the range of 3000–1940 cm^{-1}, indicating stretching vibrations due to an –OH group of carboxylic acid and intramolecular H-bonding. A characteristic band at 1698 cm^{-1} was assigned to carbonyl group (C=O) stretching vibrations. Bands in the range of 1460–1400 cm^{-1} were assigned to –C–O and –OH bending vibrations. Bands at 1250–1200 cm^{-1} were due to the bending of –CH in methylene, and a prominent peak at 1155 cm^{-1} indicates stretching due to C–C bonding [39]. The HP-βCD exhibited –OH stretching vibration with a band of 3410 cm^{-1}, whereas C-H stretching vibration was symmetrical. The characteristic bands at 1160 cm^{-1} and 1030 cm^{-1} were attributed to the C–O stretching vibration arising from HP-βCD spectrum. AMPS exhibited stretching vibrations at 1461 cm^{-1}, 1360 cm^{-1}, 2981 cm^{-1}, and 1230 cm^{-1}, corresponding to CH_2, –C–O, –CH, and S=O stretching vibrations, respectively [40]. EGDMA showed bands at 1153, 1291, and 1633 cm^{-1}, corresponding to C–O and C=C stretching vibrations for both symmetrical and asymmetric ester chains, and it also showed a band at 1713 cm^{-1} for C=O stretching vibrations [41].

The EIC spectrum showed an -OH stretching vibration band at 3408 cm^{-1}, while the –OH characteristic band of EA disappeared. The band at 1635 cm^{-1} corresponds to the C=O stretching vibration band of EA. The characteristic absorption band of benzene ring disappeared or decreased, and the band at 1025 cm^{-1} belongs to the C-O stretching vibration band of HP-βCD. The band at 1051 cm^{-1} corresponds to the aromatic C-H plane curved ester bond in EA. In summary, this shows that ellagic acid is incorporated into the cavity of cyclodextrin to form EIC. For the physical mixture PM, the band at 3405 cm^{-1} corresponds to the tensile vibration of -OH, the band at 1447 cm^{-1} belongs to the C-H bending vibration of EA, the band at 577, 854 cm^{-1} corresponds to the aromatic C-H bending vibration of EA, and the band at 1027 cm^{-1} corresponds to the C-O stretching vibration of HP-βCD. Unloaded hydrogel displayed a different spectrum when compared with its parent components. The bands at 1442 cm^{-1} indicate the presence of bending vibration of –C–O and -OH in carbopol-934, respectively. The bands at 1359 and 1229 cm^{-1} correspond to the stretching vibration of –C–O in AMPS and a symmetric stretching vibration of a S=O functional group, respectively. The new bands and functional groups indicate that the polymer is successfully crosslinked. FTIR analysis of EIC-loaded hydrogel was also performed to confirm the presence of the drug. The bands at 1633 and 1158 cm^{-1} represent the tensile vibration band of C=O in EIC and the C–H bond in aromatic group, respectively. The appearance of these bands indicates that EIC has been successfully loaded into the hydrogel.

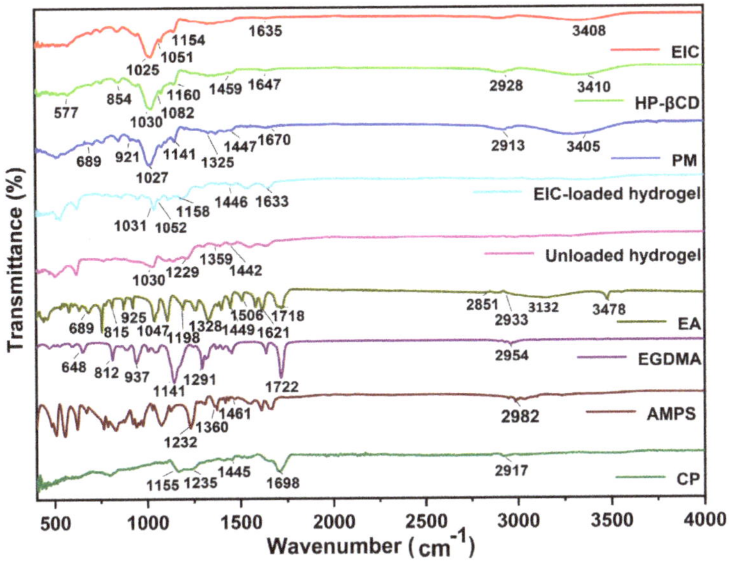

Figure 2. FTIR spectra of ellagic acid, EIC, HP-βCD, physical mixture (PM), CP, AMPS, EGDMA, unloaded, and EIC-loaded hydrogels.

3.2. Thermal Analysis

Hydrogels and polymers were thermally analyzed using TGA (Figure 3). The results showed that, as the CP temperature approaches 87 °C, it loses around 10% of its weight due to moisture evaporation. Similarly, the weight further drops by 21% when the temperature reaches 326 °C. The weight loss is a result of the decarboxylation of the polymer, resulting in unsaturated structures, as well as the depolymerization of the polymer, leading to degradation. CP began to degrade at 383 °C and eventually became completely decomposed [42]. TGA analysis of EA revealed a mass loss of 7.9% at 107 °C due to hydrogen bond separation from water. A subsequent weight loss of 36% was observed at 457 °C, in agreement with previous studies [43]. AMPS is shown to lose 6% of its weight at 208 °C based on thermogravimetric analysis. In the 210–250 °C temperature range, a further 20% weight loss was seen, indicative of the dehydration of AMPS. Additionally, the sulfonic acid group began to break down at 340 °C, with a weight loss of 20% recorded between 250 and 340 °C [44]. Consistent with prior findings, the current investigation indicated that HP-βCD samples lost weight below 80 °C due to water evaporation, whereas HP-βCD degradation occurred between 305 °C and 380 °C [45]. The inclusion complex exhibited a similar thermogram, and weight loss could be observed in three regions. The first and second regions, respectively, correspond to water loss and degradation of HP-βCD. There is also evidence for a slight modification in the degradation temperature of HP-βCD to inclusion complexes. These findings suggest that inclusion complexes have formed. It is evident that, when EA is complexed with HP-βCD, its thermal stability increases [46].

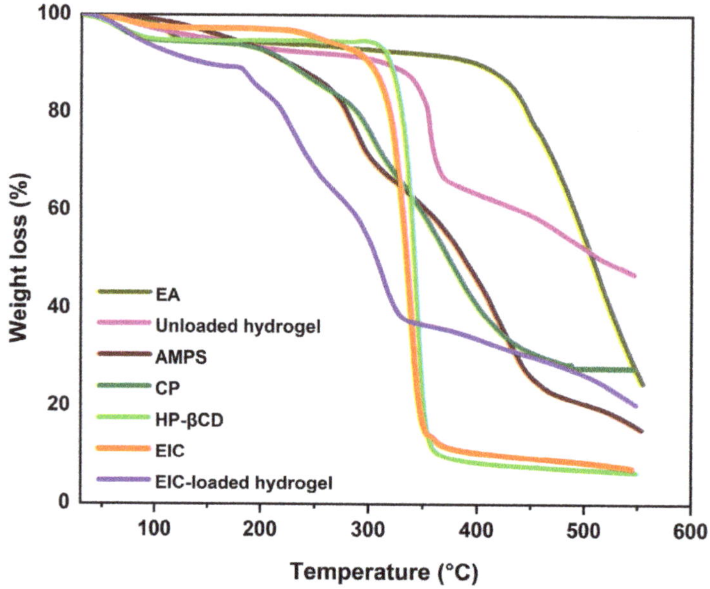

Figure 3. TGA of ellagic acid, HP-βCD, EIC, CP, AMPS, unloaded, and loaded hydrogels.

In the case of TGA analysis of EIC-loaded hydrogels, the initial weight loss was 15% due to dehydration at temperatures between 30 °C and 170 °C, followed by a 54% weight loss due to breakage of polymer bonds from 170 °C to 332 °C. Gradually, the polymer network began to degrade at 332 °C, continuing to degrade until all of the polymer skeletons had been completely destroyed. It was observed that the unloaded hydrogel lost 10% of its weight at 30–330 °C due to dehydration. In addition, it lost 26% at 330–362 °C due to a breakdown of the chemical bonds in the polymer. After 362 °C, the polymeric network gradually decomposes, and the polymer backbone degradation continues until complete degradation. Thermal profiles of hydrogels with a higher residual weight suggest that the polymeric matrix is more robust against thermal degradation over the entire temperature range investigated. Moreover, because of the increased strength and the contacts between the monomer and polymer, the degradation of the hydrogel occurs at higher temperatures and at a slower rate than with the individual reactants. Hydrogels' thermal stability is evidenced by the formation of rigid networks, which represent superior stability.

The DSC thermogram of EA displayed an endothermic peak at approximately 126.72 °C, which could be attributed to the incorporation of water during crystallization [47]. In the DSC thermogram curve of HP-βCD, the melting point is approximately 344.12 °C, whereas the endothermic peak located at 77.70 °C shows water evaporation. Hydrogen bonds may be responsible for this transition between the -H group of water and the -OH group of HP-βCD [48]. The first endothermic peak in the DSC thermogram curve of AMPS can be seen at 193 °C, which represents the melting point of the substance. Decomposition is indicated by the endothermic peak at approximately 202.64 °C. CP exhibited two endothermic peaks at 78.70 °C and 254.74 °C, according to DSC thermogram measurements. Endothermic peaks may be attributed to water evaporation from CP, while the latter peak may be the result of anhydride formation [49]. A DSC thermogram analysis of the synthesized hydrogels revealed a higher glass transition temperature for the formulation as a result of higher intermolecular hydrogen bonding, which indicates a greater degree of compatibility between the individual components and a more rigid network structure. As a result, the developed polymeric hydrogel network shows a higher level of thermal stability (Figure 4).

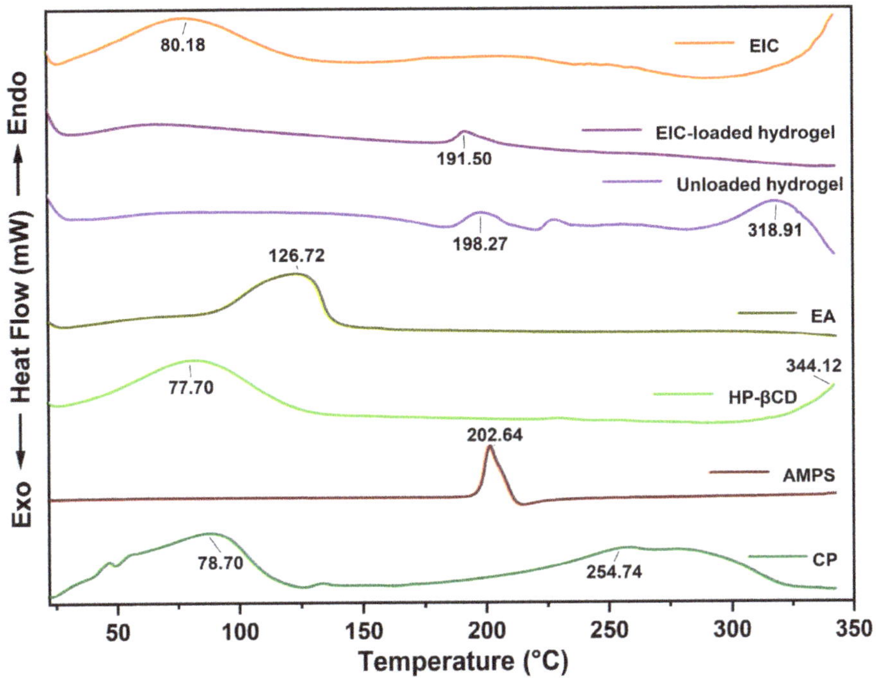

Figure 4. DSC thermogram of EIC, ellagic acid, AMPS, HP-βCD, CP, unloaded, and drug-loaded hydrogels.

3.3. XRD Study

Figure 5 illustrates XRD diffractograms of all components and hydrogel formulations. HP-βCD diffractogram showed a diffuse peak at 2θ of 21.1°, which suggested that HP-βCD is an amorphous form, which is similar to the results of others [50]. The XRD pattern of EA exhibited sharp peaks at diffraction angles (2θ) of 10.32°, 25.06°, and 28.10°, indicating the typical crystalline properties of EA [51]. Meanwhile, AMPS shows peaks at 2θ = 11.15°,15.02°, 23.42°, and 27.89°, which are suggestive of crystalline properties. It can be seen from the XRD pattern of physical mixture (PM) that the characteristic peak of ellagic acid can be found in the physical mixture, indicating that the characteristic peak of ellagic acid is simply superimposed, while the characteristic peak of ellagic acid does not appear in EIC, indicating that ellagic acid has been incorporated in the cavity of cyclodextrin to form the inclusion complex. The absence of new peaks indicated that no new crystals were formed between the EA and the carrier, maintaining the stability of the original components. The diffractogram of an unloaded hydrogel exhibits a broad diffuse peak at 2θ = 21.30°, whereas that of an EIC-loaded hydrogel exhibits only a broad diffuse peak at 2θ = 21.68°, with no other intense peaks of the drug seen in this region. This may have been caused by an interaction between the drug and the polymeric blend, resulting in a reduction in purity and crystal lattice properties.

3.4. SEM Analysis

According to SEM micrographs, the hydrogel system exhibits rough, irregular, and porous structures, containing macropores and micropores (Figure 6). Hydrogel networks have porous surfaces, which permit the passage of water directly through the interstitial spaces, which allows fluid to diffuse through the network and enhances swelling capacity, as well as providing a suitable environment for the encapsulation and transportation of drugs. Water is taken up by the hydrogel network through the pores on the surface, resulting in the network absorbing a large volume of aqueous fluid. Similarly, a polymeric network's stability is determined by solid mass and surface, as demonstrated by the hydrogel system [52].

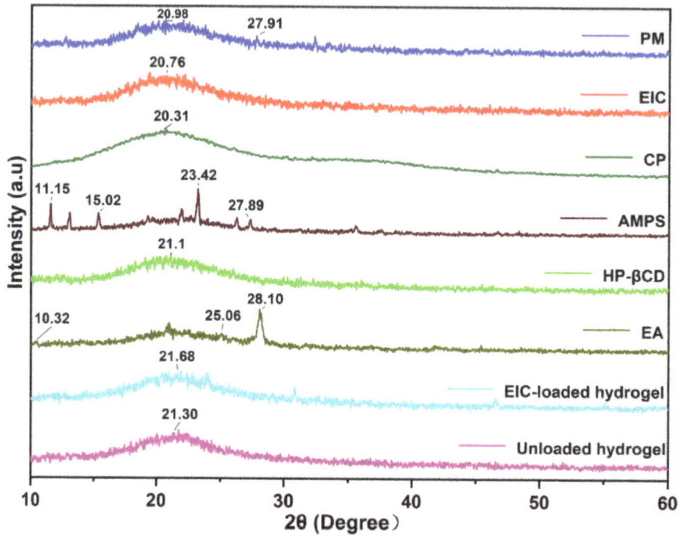

Figure 5. XRD of PM (physical mixture), EIC, CP, AMPS, HP-βCD, ellagic acid, EIC-loaded, and unloaded hydrogels.

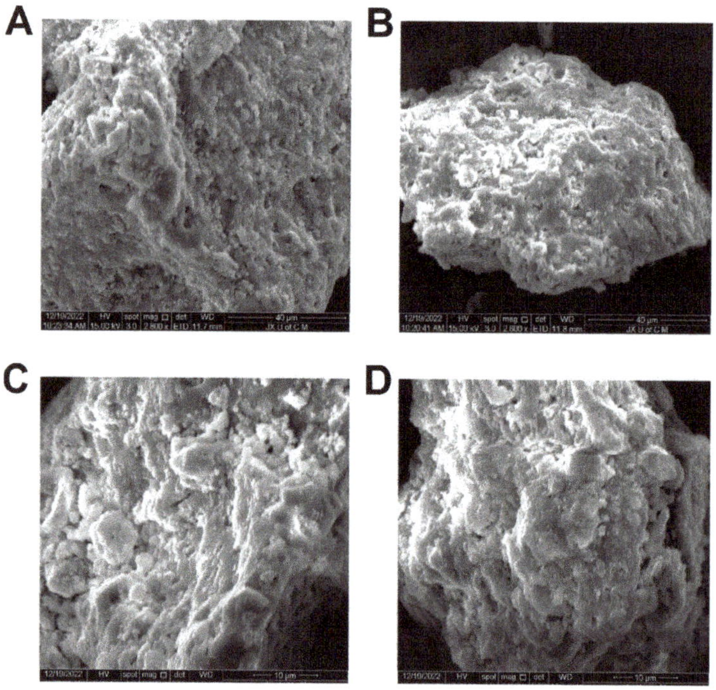

Figure 6. SEM micrographs of synthesized hydrogel at (**A**) 2800× from one angle, (**B**) 2800× from another angle, (**C**) 6000× from one side, and (**D**) 6000× from another side.

3.5. Mechanical Properties and Drug Loading

Table 2 shows hydrogel mechanical properties, such as their tensile strength (TS) and elongation-at-break (EAB), which are important parameters to consider when designing a drug delivery system. The increase in EGDMA increased the tensile strength [53]. As AMPS content increases, the gel's mechanical strength will decrease, possibly as a result of increasing electrostatic forces or osmotic pressure. Furthermore, synthetic polymer CP was incorporated into hydrogels for improved gelation and mechanical properties. The swelling of hydrogels affects its drug loading and release properties. So, hydrogels should have a sufficient mechanical strength so that, after higher swelling and drug loading, it is able to retain its structural integrity. If the crosslinking density is too high and hydrogels are mechanically too strong, then these factors will affect its swelling characteristics, and, therefore, lower drug loading will occur. Therefore, ideally, hydrogels used for drug delivery purposes should be evaluated for desired characteristics by varying the material ratios of the formulation and analyzing their effects on its swelling, drug loading, and release.

Table 2. Hydrogels' mechanical properties and EIC loading.

F. Codes	Thickness (mm)	TS (N/m^2)	EAB (%)	EIC-Loaded per 1 g Hydrogel (g)
KAE-1	1.15 ± 0.005	0.502 ± 0.103	46.3 ± 1.056	0.487 ± 0.013
KAE-2	1.25 ± 0.007	0.676 ± 0.086	59.9 ± 1.687	0.417 ± 0.006
KAE-3	1.37 ± 0.004	1.107 ± 0.076	72.6 ± 1.551	0.329 ± 0.010
KAE-4	1.05 ± 0.003	0.816 ± 0.059	63.2 ± 2.922	0.460 ± 0.008
KAE-5	1.15 ± 0.005	0.502 ± 0.103	46.3 ± 1.056	0.487 ± 0.013
KAE-6	1.08 ± 0.008	0.413 ± 0.237	38.6 ± 1.687	0.596 ± 0.098
KAE-7	1.09 ± 0.004	0.517 ± 0.211	50.8 ± 2.398	0.499 ± 0.069
KAE-8	1.15 ± 0.005	0.502 ± 0.103	46.3 ± 1.056	0.487 ± 0.013
KAE-9	1.47 ± 0.007	0.581 ± 0.051	60.7 ± 1.201	0.518 ± 0.029

3.6. Sol–Gel Analysis

Hydrogels are made when a polymerization reaction occurs, which results in a chain reaction, involving monomers, crosslinking agents, and polymers, and the part of the hydrogel that is not crosslinked is known as the "sol fraction", while that which is crosslinked is called the "gel fraction". The sol fraction occurs when high quantities of a component are used in hydrogels, and these parts remain uncrosslinked as a result of an insufficient number of reactive sites in the polymerization process. This requires the determination of the degree of crosslinking within the hydrogel as well as the degree of uncrosslinking within the hydrogel. Hydrogel formulations were all tested for sol–gel fractions (Figure 7A–C). As a result of the material ratio, the gel fraction percentage ranges from 83.70 to 96.80 percent. AMPS are hydrophilic monomers, and, as their concentration increases, more room is provided for chemical reactions, resulting in a higher gel fraction. A crosslinking agent, such as EGDMA, induces gel formation, and its content increases the gel fraction [54]. As the concentration of CP increases, the gel fraction increases as well, since free radicals are generated as a result of the rapid increase in polymer concentration. Thus, the gel fraction is also increased.

3.7. Porosity Evaluation

All of the hydrogels developed were tested for porosity. Porosity is a significant factor affecting hydrogel swelling properties, drug loading properties, and release characteristics. Therefore, it was essential to carefully monitor the porosity of the hydrogels in order to achieve the desired results. As pores become larger, swelling increases, which allows drugs to be loaded and released more effectively. Porosity is increased when a reaction mixture has a high viscosity, since this makes it more difficult for bubbles to escape. As a result, the porosity increases due to the establishment of interconnected channels. Porosity percentages ranged from 43.60% to 88.90% under different reagent ratios. The diameter of the pores decreases as the concentration of EGDMA increases due to the development of tight junctions and the increased cross-linking density, thereby reducing the network's flexibility [55]. A higher concentration of AMPS improves porosity because the sulfonate groups are able to generate stronger electrostatic forces. AMPS contains an alkyl group that is hydrophobic, which can lead to a reduction in hydrogen bond interactions through the formation of hydrophobic microregions. Thus, the pore and network sizes of the hydrogel are enhanced during the preparation process, which is in accordance with other research results [56]. Porosity percentage increases with increasing CP concentration. This may be a result of the viscosity of the reaction mixture, causing bubbles to become trapped. Thus, interconnected channels are formed, leading to an increase in porosity.

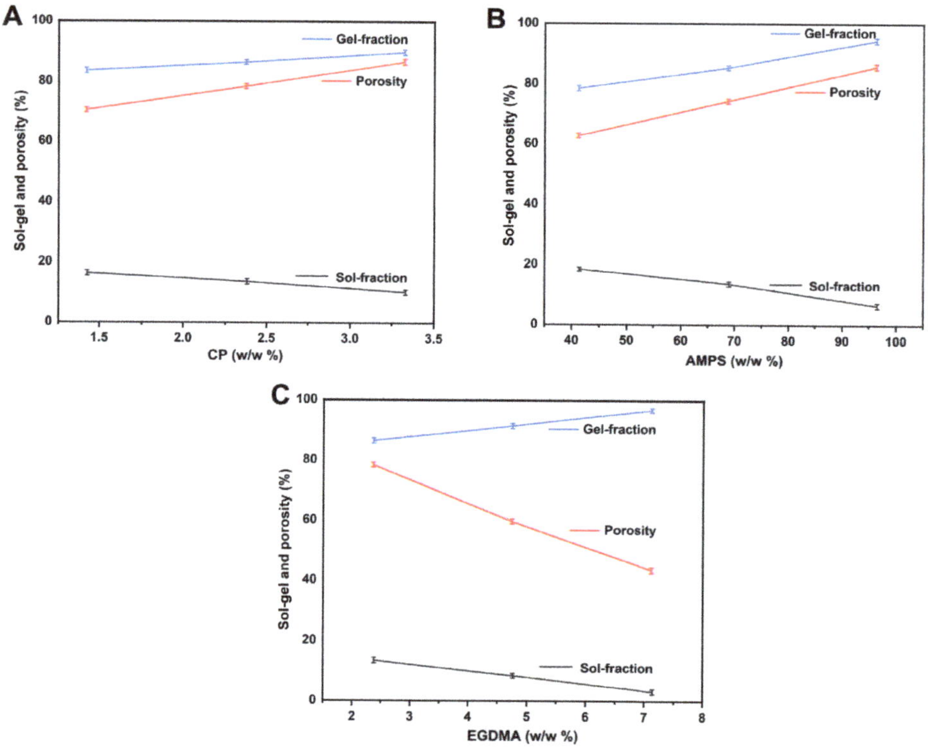

Figure 7. Influence of different concentrations of (**A**) CP, (**B**) AMPS, and (**C**) EGDMA on the sol–gel and porosity properties of CP-*g*-AMPS hydrogels.

3.8. Biodegradation Study

Figure 8 depicts the results of biodegradation tests performed to determine the hydrogel's degradation rate. Various weight ratios will influence the degradation of gel in a significant manner. Hydrogels with different proportions demonstrated physical degradability of 5.8% to 9.2%. EGDMA decreased hydrogel degradation speed, possibly as a result of the establishment of new functional groups and tight junctions, which improved water gel content. Our study showed that, when CP concentration increased, the produced hydrogel degraded at a slower rate. It is possible that free radicals have been produced, resulting in hypergelation and, subsequently, the formation of a highly cross-linked hydrogel network. Consequently, cross-linking between hydrogel components increases hydrogel volume density, which results in a slow degradation of hydrogels [57].

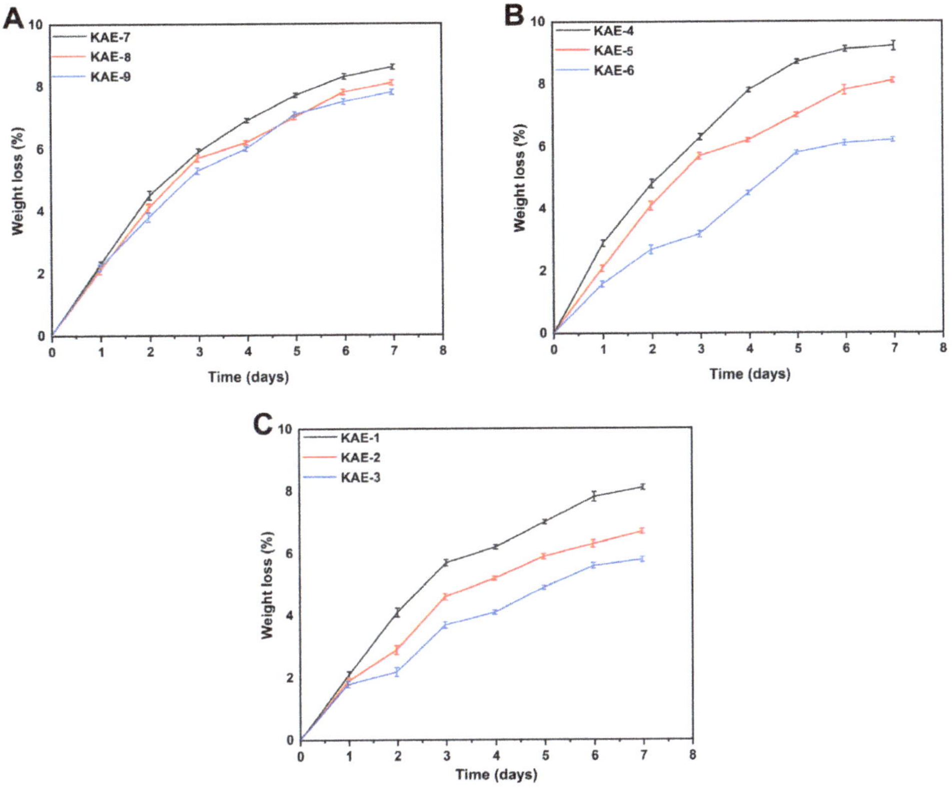

Figure 8. Influence of varying amounts of (**A**) CP (KAE-7,8,9), (**B**) AMPS (KAE-4,5,6), and (**C**) EGDMA (KAE-1,2,3) on the biodegradation of CP-*g*-AMPS hydrogels.

3.9. Structural Parameters of Hydrogels

The structural parameters of synthesized hydrogels were calculated. Table 3 provides information regarding various structural parameters. Hydrogel parameters are important to calculate, as they indicate compatibility of the polymers with the solvents and, consequently, higher water uptake and holding capacity of the hydrogel. V2, S, and χ values improved as the EGDMA concentration was enhanced, indicating that gel structures were becoming tighter and stiffer, which reduced the mesh size of the hydrogel [58]. Thus, the mesh size plays an important role in the mechanical strength, degradation properties, and diffusion properties of the material, and it can be modified by modifying the percentage of crosslinker in the reaction mixture [59]. A similar decrease in Mc and N was observed when EGDMA concentrations were increased because crosslinking density increased. Additionally, Wang and colleagues found that, when methylene bisacrylamide (MBA) was used as a crosslinker to synthesize hydrogels and when its concentration was increased, the Mc value decreased, and the water absorption decreased, as well [60].

3.10. Swelling Behavior

Hydrogels were synthesized using varying amounts of polymers/monomers and cross-linking agents to investigate the impact of their compositions upon swelling ratios across multiple pH media. Hydrogel composites swell when soaked in different media, since all polymers are hydrophilic and cross-linked. Figure 9 illustrates how swelling rates of hydrogels vary with pH over time. The synthesized hydrogels showed slightly higher swelling at a pH of 1.2 than at a pH of 7.4. The difference may be explained by the ionization of carboxylic acid groups to carboxylates at both pH. In the same manner, the $-SO_3H$ group also ionizes to the $-SO_3-$ group, regardless of the medium's pH. Electrostatic repulsion between carboxylate and SO_3- groups increases macromolecule expansion and reduces hydrogen bonding. Consequently, the formed hydrogel network swells more. Hydroxyl (–OH) functional groups of the hydrogels were ionized by water in the environment, resulting in increased swelling [61]. Swelling percentages for the hydrogel at a pH of 1.2 varied between 19.83% and 42.0%. Among these hydrogels, KAE-6 displayed the highest degree of swelling (42.20%), while KAE-3 displayed the lowest degree of swelling (19.83%) at a pH of 1.2. A swelling percentage of 12.95 to 31.6% was observed for the hydrogel at pH 7.4. KAE-6 had the highest swelling percentage (31.61%), while KAE-3 had the lowest swelling percentage (12.95%). Khalid et al. showed that CS-co-poly(AMPS) hydrogels show pH-independent swelling in different pH ranges, which is similar to our results [62]. Figure 9D, H shows the dried and swollen CP-g-AMPS hydrogels.

Table 3. Flory-Huggins network parameters of CP-g-AMPS hydrogels.

F. Codes	$V_{2,s}$	χ	M_c	M_r	N	$D \times 10^{-5}$ ($cm^2\ s^{-1}$)
KAE-1	0.030	0.510	3773.9	203.571	37.076	0.023
KAE-2	0.042	0.514	2356.7	224.307	21.013	0.031
KAE-3	0.050	0.517	1444.4	203.318	14.208	0.037
KAE-4	0.039	0.513	2358.4	201.461	23.412	0.028
KAE-5	0.030	0.510	3773.9	203.571	37.076	0.023
KAE-6	0.022	0.507	4363.8	204.517	42.674	0.015
KAE-7	0.031	0.510	2589.6	204.836	25.284	0.021
KAE-8	0.030	0.510	3773.9	203.571	37.076	0.023
KAE-9	0.024	0.508	3311.8	202.330	32.736	0.018

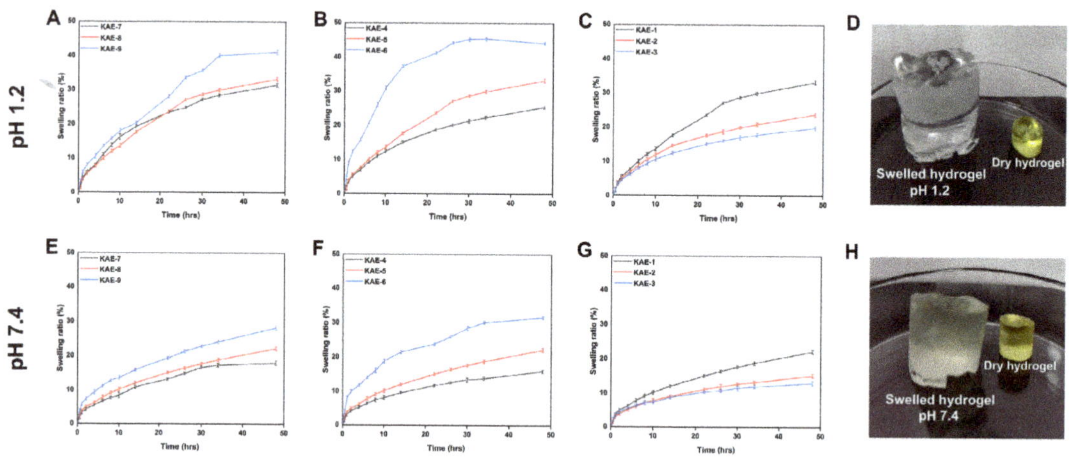

Figure 9. Effect of varying concentrations of components on hydrogels when swollen at pH 1.2 (**A**); CP, (**B**); AMPS, (**C**); EGDMA, (**D**); physical appearance and when hydrogels are swollen at pH 7.4 (**E**); CP, (**F**); AMPS, (**G**); EGDMA, and (**H**); physical appearance.

Figure 9A, E shows that water absorption (equilibrium swelling) increases with increasing CP content in KAE-7, KAE-8, and KAE-9 (1.428, 2.380, and 3.333 wt%, respectively), suggesting that there are more grafting sites available on the ends of the polymer chains. Low concentrations of CP assist monomer molecules in attaching to polymer reaction sites, and after monomer molecules have occupied the available reaction sites, they will be unable to attach further. This inhibition is due to the steric hindrance caused by the grafted chain and the redundant nature of the remaining monomer in the reaction system. In the case of excess monomers, they become homopolymers, which do not contribute to the absorption of water. As the polymer content increases, the homopolymer content decreases, providing a greater number of reaction sites for the monomer molecules and thus promoting water absorption. Additionally, increased CP content results in an increase in carboxylic acid groups, making the hydrogel more hydrophilic, thus increasing its swelling degree [39]. Since AMPS contains a large number of $-CONH_2$ and $-SO_3OH$ groups, increasing the amount of monomer AMPS will strengthen the equilibrium swelling degree of hydrogel provided that other chemical components remain the same. The ionization of these chains increases their ability to interact with water molecules, so the higher the concentration, the greater the water uptake by hydrogels. When the concentration of EGDMA is increased, the swelling of the hydrogel is reduced. A higher concentration of EGDMA results in a higher packing density in hydrogels, which reduces their porosity. Water penetration into the hydrogel network is reduced as EGDMA concentration increases, which results in a reduction in swelling [63].

3.11. Release and Kinetic Modelling Analysis

In vitro drug release studies provide insight into how much active constituent escapes from the dosage form and becomes soluble over time [64]. Figure 10 shows the percentage of drug released in the pH 1.2 buffer varied between 57.03 and 92.13%. Drug release rates were highest for KAE-6 (92.13%) at pH 1.2, while they were the lowest for KAE-3 (57.03%). The release rate of drugs in a buffer with a pH of 7.4 ranged from 46.00% to 77.28%. KAE-6 (77.28%) achieved the highest drug release rate, while KAE-3 (46.0%) achieved the lowest after 48 h of testing. The rate at which EA is released varies with buffer pH, with the maximum release rate after 48 h in a buffer, with a pH of 1.2 being 92.13%.

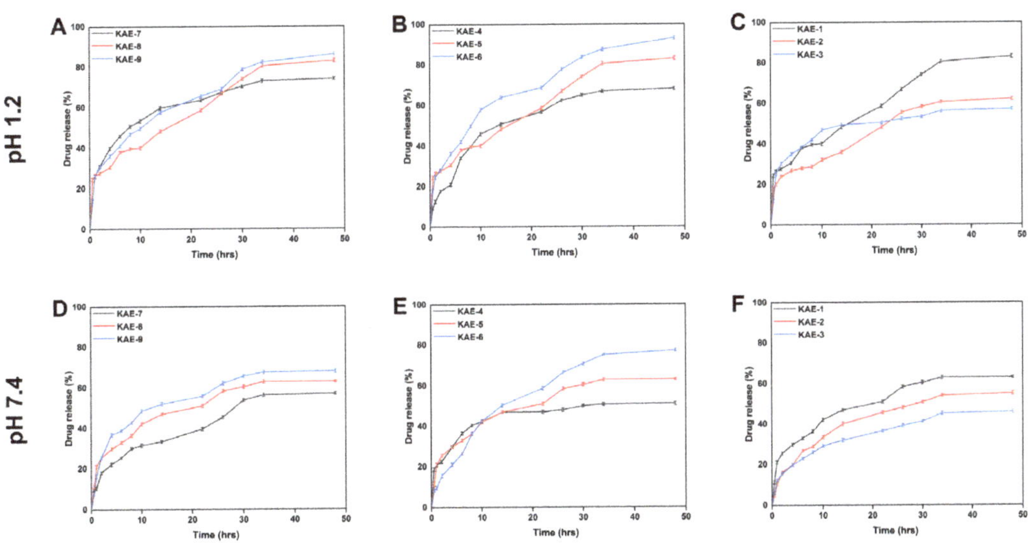

Figure 10. The drug release curve of CP-*g*-AMPS hydrogels and effect of components ((**A**); CP, (**B**); AMPS, and (**C**); EGDMA on release at pH 1.2 and at ((**D**); CP, (**E**); AMPS, and (**F**); EGDMA at pH 7.4.

The osmotic pressure difference between the polymeric hydrogel disc and the surrounding water causes water molecules to diffuse into hydrogel discs when submerged in water. In this way, hydrogel is able to contain water within its structure. As a result of water diffusion, the hydrogel discs swell, allowing the loaded drug to be released through the channels within the discs [65]. The value of the regression coefficient that was near to one was utilized to determine which model was the most appropriate and provided the best explanation for the drug release data. According to Table 4, samples (KAE-7, KAE-8, and KAE-9) with different concentrations of CP followed Higuchi release kinetics because their regression coefficients were greater than zero and greater than first-order models. Similarly, samples (KAE-1, -2, and -3), containing differing amounts of the crosslinker EGDMA, followed Higuchi release kinetics, as indicated by high regression coefficient values. All samples, including those with varying amounts of AMPS (KAE-4, -5, and -6), exhibit diffusion-controlled drug release, as demonstrated by the regression coefficient (r) in the Higuchi models [66]. Normally, the diffusion is of two types in controlled drug delivery devices, namely, Fickian diffusion ($0.45 < n < 0.5$) and non-Fickian or anomalous diffusion, if the "n" value is between 0.5 and 1. Similarly, the developed hydrogels were used in cylindrical form, so the Fickian diffusion mechanism is described by $0.45 < n < 0.50$. Overall, the hydrogels showed Fickian diffusion because the "n" values of all formulations ranged from 0.356 to 0.498 [67].

Table 4. Release kinetics of CP-*g*-AMPS hydrogels.

F. Codes	pH	Zero Order.		First Order		Higuchi Model		Korsmeyer-Peppas Model	
		K_o (h^{-1})	r^2	K_1 (h^{-1})	r^2	K_2 (h^{-1})	r^2	r^2	n
KAE-1	1.2 7.4	0.890 0.576	0.9640 0.9624	0.011 0.007	0.9801 0.9714	4.897 3.218	0.9942 0.9997	0.9949 * 0.9998 *	0.482 0.495
KAE-2	1.2 7.4	0.644 0.411	0.9467 0.9424	0.007 0.005	0.9599 0.9505	3.609 2.324	0.9972 0.9970	0.9976 * 0.9988 *	0.484 0.444
KAE-3	1.2 7.4	0.547 0.372	0.9372 0.9129	0.006 0.004	0.9492 0.9215	3.090 2.138	0.9956 0.9878	0.9974 * 0.9983 *	0.454 0.360
KAE-4	1.2 7.4	0.687 0.434	0.9513 0.9421	0.008 0.005	0.9650 0.9507	3.839 2.450	0.9978 * 0.9969	0.9977 0.9987 *	0.498 0.445
KAE-5	1.2 7.4	0.890 0.576	0.9640 0.9624	0.011 0.007	0.9801 0.9714	4.897 3.218	0.9942 0.9997	0.9949 * 0.9998 *	0.482 0.495
KAE-6	1.2 7.4	1.406 0.835	0.8748 0.8536	0.021 0.010	0.9294 0.8689	8.087 4.801	0.9669 * 0.9918	0.9963 0.9937 *	0.401 0.356
KAE-7	1.2 7.4	0.860 0.445	0.9462 0.9422	0.011 0.005	0.9469 0.9510	4.808 2.515	0.9954 0.9973	0.9952 * 0.9993 *	0.479 0.435
KAE-8	1.2 7.4	0.890 0.576	0.9640 0.9624	0.011 0.007	0.9801 0.9714	4.897 3.218	0.9942 0.9997	0.9949 * 0.9998 *	0.482 0.495
KAE-9	1.2 7.4	1.119 0.746	0.9638 0.9530	0.015 0.008	0.9825 0.9652	6.179 4.206	0.9919 0.9982	0.9927 * 0.9992 *	0.459 0.437

* Represent higher r^2 values.

3.12. Antioxidation Analysis

Figure 11 shows the scavenging efficiency of DPPH and ABTS in the presence of hydrogels as an indicator of their antioxidant activity. As a result of their higher swelling and higher release, four formulations (KAE-6, KAE-9, KAE-1, and KAE-7) demonstrated greater antioxidant activity than the others. Antioxidant rates for DPPH ranged from 40.43% to 83.56%, while those for ABTS ranged from 38.69% to 85.96%. The antioxidant phenolic compound ellagic acid is found naturally in a number of fruits and vegetables, particularly pomegranates, raspberries, persimmons, black raspberries, peaches, strawberries, feathers, nuts (almonds, walnuts), and wine. Many studies have examined the potential health benefits of ellagic acid due to its antioxidant properties [68]. EIC-loaded hydrogels showed strong antioxidant properties under different proportions of material in our experiments.

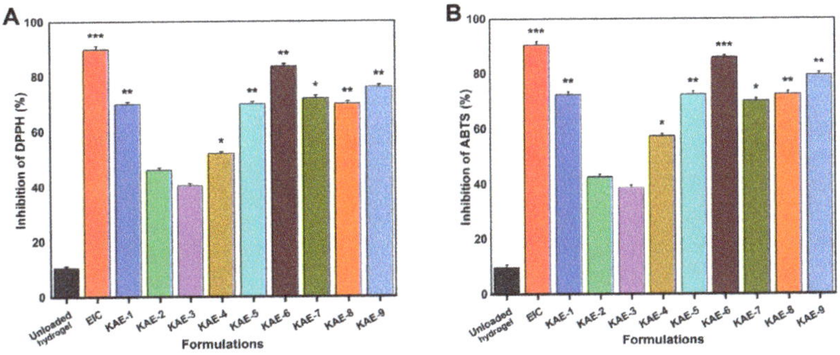

Figure 11. A comparison of the antioxidant properties of CP-*g*-AMPS hydrogels by using (**A**) DPPH and (**B**) ABTS (* $p < 0.05$, ** $p < 0.01$, *** $p < 0.001$).

3.13. Antibacterial Study

Figure 12 illustrates the antibacterial activity of hydrogel against Gram-positive (*E. coli* and *S. aureus*) and Gram-negative (*P. aeruginosa*) bacteria. Negative control and blank hydrogel groups showed no zone formation, whereas clear zones were observed for the positive control (34 mm, 32 mm, and 35 mm) and the EIC-loaded hydrogel (14, 29, and 31 mm) against *P. aeruginosa*, *S. aureus*, and *E. coli*, respectively. There have been several studies that indicate that the broad-spectrum antibiotic cefepime is effective against both Gram-positive and Gram-negative bacteria [69].

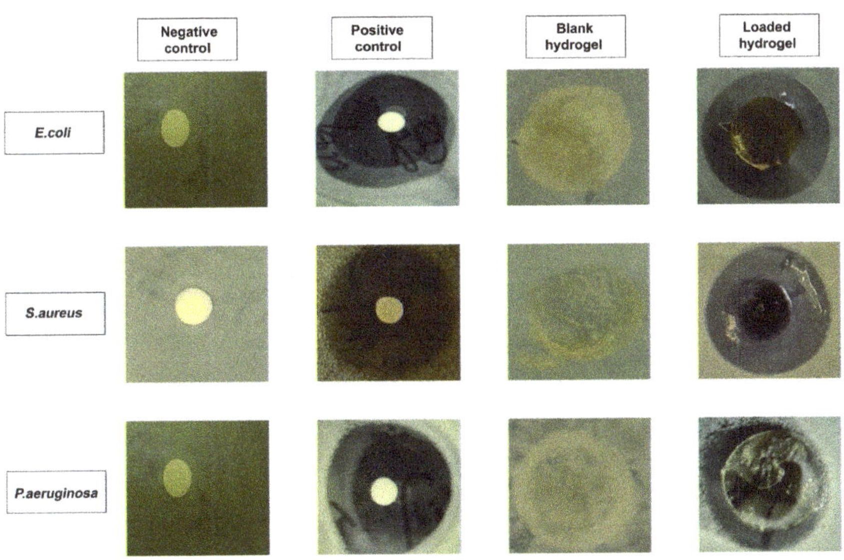

Figure 12. The zones of inhibition of samples against different bacterial strains.

Cefepime exhibited a smaller ZOI against Gram-negative bacteria compared to Gram-positive bacteria examined in the study. There could be a few different explanations for this behaviour, one of which being the composition of the cell wall of the bacteria. Gram-negative bacteria have a cell wall that is composed of three layers: the outer membrane, the peptidoglycan wall, and the cytoplasmic membrane. These layers are separated by an outer membrane [70]. The cell walls of Gram-positive bacteria are thick, but unlike Gram-negative bacteria, they do not have an outer membrane. Gram-negative bacteria are protected from the outside world by their outer membrane, which acts as a barrier against the effects of the external environment. Thus, the antibacterial effects of hydrogels and cefipime are much greater against Gram-positive bacteria than against Gram-negative bacteria.

The study has some limitations, such not being tested in vivo for the assessment of its toxicological and pharmacological effects, which are important for the evaluation of a new drug delivery system. A further investigation of the study will be conducted in the future.

4. Conclusions

In this study, HP-βCD and ellagic acid inclusion complexes (EIC) were developed, first, to increase the ellagic acid solubility. The results showed an entrapment efficiency of 83.96%, a drug loading of 27.31%, and a yield of 96.26% for ellagic acid in the EIC, which indicate a successful inclusion complexation process. The carbopol-934-g-AMPS controlled-release hydrogel was then synthesized through a free radical polymerization process. Different characterization techniques, such as FTIR, TGA, DSC, and XRD, provided confirmation of HP-βCD-ellagic acid inclusion complexes (EIC) formation, as well as successful incorporation of the drug into the hydrogel network. Additionally, morphological analysis by SEM revealed that the hydrogel has a rough and porous surface morphology. The hydrogels showed slightly higher swelling after 48 h at pH 1.2 (42.20%) compared with pH 7.4 (31.61%). Furthermore, the synthesized hydrogels released more drug at pH 1.2 (92.13%) than pH 7.4 (77.28%), suggesting that Fickian diffusion is the most likely mechanism for drug release. A substantial improvement in the mechanical properties and the release times of the drug was achieved by increasing the monomer concentration and polymer ratio. Additionally, the hydrogels exhibited high porosity (88.90%) and a high biodegradability (9.2% loss of weight in a week). A significant antioxidant effect was demonstrated by the developed hydrogels in the DPPH (inhibition rate 83.56%) and the ABTS testing (inhibition rate 85.96%). Moreover, hydrogels displayed excellent antibacterial properties against Gram-positive bacteria, such as *E. coli* (ZOI of 31 mm) and *S. aureus* (ZOI of 29 mm), as well as the Gram-negative bacteria *P. aeruginosa* (ZOI of 14 mm). In conclusion, the developed hydrogel system is capable of providing controlled delivery of both hydrophobic and hydrophilic drugs.

Author Contributions: Methodology, A.N. and C.Y.; conceptualization, A.N.; investigation, A.N. and C.Y.; data curation, C.Y. and A.N., writing—original draft preparation, C.Y. and A.N.; writing—review and editing, A.N.; supervision, A.N.; visualization, Y.G.; resources, Y.G.; funding acquisition, Y.L. and Y.G. All authors have read and agreed to the published version of the manuscript.

Funding: This study was supported by the Jiangxi Province high-level and high-skill leading personnel training project (No. 12623001), the Jiangxi university of traditional Chinese medicine 1050 youth talent project (No. 5142001007), the National Natural Science Foundation of China (No. 82260756), the Science and Technology Key Project of Jiangxi Provincial Department of Education (GJJ218915), and the Jiangxi University of Chinese Medicine Science and Technology Innovation Team Development Program (No. CXTD-22004).

Institutional Review Board Statement: Not applicable.

Informed Consent Statement: Not applicable.

Data Availability Statement: The data are contained within the article.

Conflicts of Interest: The authors declare no conflict of interest.

References

1. Ortenzi, M.A.; Antenucci, S.; Marzorati, S.; Panzella, L.; Molino, S.; Rufián-Henares, J.Á.; Napolitano, A.; Verotta, L. Pectin-based formulations for controlled release of an ellagic acid salt with high solubility profile in physiological media. *Molecules* **2021**, *26*, 433. [CrossRef] [PubMed]
2. Seeram, N.P.; Zhang, Y.; McKeever, R.; Henning, S.M.; Lee, R.-P.; Suchard, M.A.; Li, Z.; Chen, S.; Thames, G.; Zerlin, A. Pomegranate juice and extracts provide similar levels of plasma and urinary ellagitannin metabolites in human subjects. *J. Med. Food* **2008**, *11*, 390–394. [CrossRef]

3. González-Sarrías, A.; García-Villalba, R.; Núñez-Sánchez, M.Á.; Tomé-Carneiro, J.; Zafrilla, P.; Mulero, J.; Tomás-Barberán, F.A.; Espín, J.C. Identifying the limits for ellagic acid bioavailability: A crossover pharmacokinetic study in healthy volunteers after consumption of pomegranate extracts. *J. Funct. Foods* **2015**, *19*, 225–235. [CrossRef]
4. Alfei, S.; Marengo, B.; Zuccari, G. Oxidative stress, antioxidant capabilities, and bioavailability: Ellagic acid or urolithins? *Antioxidants* **2020**, *9*, 707. [CrossRef]
5. Djedjibegovic, J.; Marjanovic, A.; Panieri, E.; Saso, L. Ellagic acid-derived urolithins as modulators of oxidative stress. *Oxid. Med. Cell. Longev.* **2020**, *2020*, 5194508. [CrossRef]
6. Hussein, M.Z.; Al Ali, S.H.; Zainal, Z.; Hakim, M.N. Development of antiproliferative nanohybrid compound with controlled release property using ellagic acid as the active agent. *Int. J. Nanomed.* **2011**, *6*, 1373–1383. [CrossRef] [PubMed]
7. Wang, H.; Zhang, Y.; Tian, Z.; Ma, J.; Kang, M.; Ding, C.; Ming, D. Preparation of β-CD-ellagic acid microspheres and their effects on HepG2 cell proliferation. *Molecules* **2017**, *22*, 2175. [CrossRef] [PubMed]
8. Avachat, A.M.; Patel, V.G. Self nanoemulsifying drug delivery system of stabilized ellagic acid–phospholipid complex with improved dissolution and permeability. *Saudi Pharm. J.* **2015**, *23*, 276–289. [CrossRef]
9. Arulmozhi, V.; Pandian, K.; Mirunalini, S. Ellagic acid encapsulated chitosan nanoparticles for drug delivery system in human oral cancer cell line (KB). *Colloids Surf. B Biointerfaces* **2013**, *110*, 313–320. [CrossRef]
10. Sampaio, A.D.G.; Gontijo, A.V.L.; Lima, G.D.M.G.; de Oliveira, M.A.C.; Lepesqueur, L.S.S.; Koga-Ito, C.Y. Ellagic acid–cyclodextrin complexes for the treatment of oral candidiasis. *Molecules* **2021**, *26*, 505. [CrossRef]
11. Liu, Z.; Ye, L.; Xi, J.; Wang, J.; Feng, Z.-G. Cyclodextrin polymers: Structure, synthesis, and use as drug carriers. *Prog. Polym. Sci.* **2021**, *118*, 101408. [CrossRef]
12. Carneiro, S.B.; Costa Duarte, F.Í.; Heimfarth, L.; Siqueira Quintans, J.D.S.; Quintans-Júnior, L.J.; Veiga Júnior, V.F.D.; Neves de Lima, Á.A. Cyclodextrin–drug inclusion complexes: In vivo and in vitro approaches. *Int. J. Mol. Sci.* **2019**, *20*, 642. [CrossRef] [PubMed]
13. Kim, D.-H.; Lee, S.-E.; Pyo, Y.-C.; Tran, P.; Park, J.-S. Solubility enhancement and application of cyclodextrins in local drug delivery. *J. Pharm. Investig.* **2020**, *50*, 17–27. [CrossRef]
14. Ding, S.; Khan, A.I.; Cai, X.; Song, Y.; Lyu, Z.; Du, D.; Dutta, P.; Lin, Y. Overcoming blood–brain barrier transport: Advances in nanoparticle-based drug delivery strategies. *Mater. Today* **2020**, *37*, 112–125. [CrossRef] [PubMed]
15. Sabbagh, F.; Kim, B.S. Recent advances in polymeric transdermal drug delivery systems. *J. Control. Release* **2022**, *341*, 132–146. [CrossRef] [PubMed]
16. Li, Y.; Yang, H.Y.; Lee, D.S. Advances in biodegradable and injectable hydrogels for biomedical applications. *J. Control. Release* **2021**, *330*, 151–160. [CrossRef]
17. Mahmood, A.; Patel, D.; Hickson, B.; DesRochers, J.; Hu, X. Recent progress in biopolymer-based hydrogel materials for biomedical applications. *Int. J. Mol. Sci.* **2022**, *23*, 1415. [CrossRef]
18. Dreiss, C.A. Hydrogel design strategies for drug delivery. *Curr. Opin. Colloid Interface Sci.* **2020**, *48*, 1–17. [CrossRef]
19. Acharya, S.; Patra, S.; Pani, N.R. Optimization of HPMC and carbopol concentrations in non-effervescent floating tablet through factorial design. *Carbohydr. Polym.* **2014**, *102*, 360–368. [CrossRef]
20. Safitri, F.I.; Nawangsari, D.; Febrina, D. Overview: Application of carbopol 940 in gel. In Proceedings of the International Conference on Health and Medical Sciences (AHMS 2020); Atlantis Press: Amsterdam, Netherlands, 2021; pp. 80–84.
21. Seo, H.-S.; Bae, J.-Y.; Kwon, K.; Shin, S. Synthesis and assessment of amps-based copolymers prepared via electron-beam irradiation for ionic conductive hydrogels. *Polymers* **2022**, *14*, 2547. [CrossRef]
22. Naeem, A.; Yu, C.; Zhu, W.; Zang, Z.; Guan, Y. Study of Hydroxypropyl β-Cyclodextrin and Puerarin Inclusion Complexes Encapsulated in Sodium Alginate-Grafted 2-Acrylamido-2-Methyl-1-Propane Sulfonic Acid Hydrogels for Oral Controlled Drug Delivery. *Gels* **2023**, *9*, 246. [CrossRef] [PubMed]
23. Krstic, M.; Miladinovic, Z.R.; Barudzija, T.; Mladenovic, A.; Suljovrujic, E. Stimuli-responsive copolymeric hydrogels based on oligo (ethylene glycol) dimethacrylate for biomedical applications: An optimisation study of pH and thermoresponsive behaviour. *React. Funct. Polym.* **2022**, *170*, 105140. [CrossRef]
24. Savic, I.M.; Jocic, E.; Nikolic, V.D.; Popsavin, M.M.; Rakic, S.J.; Savic-Gajic, I.M. The effect of complexation with cyclodextrins on the antioxidant and antimicrobial activity of ellagic acid. *Pharm. Dev. Technol.* **2019**, *24*, 410–418. [CrossRef] [PubMed]
25. Naeem, A.; Yu, C.; Zang, Z.; Zhu, W.; Deng, X.; Guan, Y. Synthesis and Evaluation of Rutin–Hydroxypropyl β-Cyclodextrin Inclusion Complexes Embedded in Xanthan Gum-Based (HPMC-g-AMPS) Hydrogels for Oral Controlled Drug Delivery. *Antioxidants* **2023**, *12*, 552. [CrossRef]
26. Li, Z.; Jiang, X.; Huang, H.; Liu, A.; Liu, H.; Abid, N.; Ming, L. Chitosan/zein films incorporated with essential oil nanoparticles and nanoemulsions: Similarities and differences. *Int. J. Biol. Macromol.* **2022**, *208*, 983–994. [CrossRef] [PubMed]
27. Siddiqua, A.; Ranjha, N.M.; Rehman, S.; Shoukat, H.; Ramzan, N.; Sultana, H. Preparation and characterization of methylene bisacrylamide crosslinked pectin/acrylamide hydrogels. *Polym. Bull.* **2022**, *79*, 7655–7677. [CrossRef]
28. Ghumman, S.A.; Noreen, S.; Hameed, H.; Elsherif, M.A.; Shabbir, R.; Rana, M.; Junaid, K.; Bukhari, S.N.A. Synthesis of pH-Sensitive Cross-Linked Basil Seed Gum/Acrylic Acid Hydrogels by Free Radical Copolymerization Technique for Sustained Delivery of Captopril. *Gels* **2022**, *8*, 291. [CrossRef]
29. Chang, A.; Ye, Z.; Ye, Z.; Deng, J.; Lin, J.; Wu, C.; Zhu, H. Citric acid crosslinked sphingan WL gum hydrogel films supported ciprofloxacin for potential wound dressing application. *Carbohydr. Polym.* **2022**, *291*, 119520. [CrossRef]

30. Guan, Y.; Yu, C.; Zang, Z.; Wan, X.; Naeem, A.; Zhang, R.; Zhu, W. Chitosan/xanthan gum-based (Hydroxypropyl methylcellulose-co-2-Acrylamido-2-methylpropane sulfonic acid) interpenetrating hydrogels for controlled release of amorphous solid dispersion of bioactive constituents of Pueraria lobatae. *Int. J. Biol. Macromol.* **2023**, *224*, 380–395. [CrossRef] [PubMed]
31. Jozaghkar, M.R.; Sepehrian Azar, A.; Ziaee, F. Preparation, Characterization, and swelling study of N, N′-dimethylacrylamide/acrylic acid amphiphilic hydrogels in different conditions. *Polym. Bull.* **2022**, *79*, 5183–5195. [CrossRef]
32. Khan, M.A.; Azad, A.K.; Safdar, M.; Nawaz, A.; Akhlaq, M.; Paul, P.; Hossain, M.K.; Rahman, M.H.; Baty, R.S.; El-Kott, A.F. Synthesis and Characterization of Acrylamide/Acrylic Acid Co-Polymers and Glutaraldehyde Crosslinked pH-Sensitive Hydrogels. *Gels* **2022**, *8*, 47. [CrossRef]
33. Naeem, A.; Yu, C.; Zhu, W.; Chen, X.; Wu, X.; Chen, L.; Zang, Z.; Guan, Y. Gallic Acid-Loaded Sodium Alginate-Based (Polyvinyl Alcohol-Co-Acrylic Acid) Hydrogel Membranes for Cutaneous Wound Healing: Synthesis and Characterization. *Molecules* **2022**, *27*, 8397. [CrossRef] [PubMed]
34. Tapdiqov, S.; Tagiyev, D.; Zeynalov, N.; Safaraliyeva, S.; Fatullayeva, S.; Hummetov, A.; Raucci, M.; Mustafayev, M.; Jafarova, R.; Shirinova, K. Cumulative release kinetics of levothyroxine-Na pentahydrate from chitosan/arabinogalactane based pH sensitive hydrogel and it's toxicology. *React. Funct. Polym.* **2022**, *178*, 105334. [CrossRef]
35. Xu, Z.; Liu, G.; Li, Q.; Wu, J. A novel hydrogel with glucose-responsive hyperglycemia regulation and antioxidant activity for enhanced diabetic wound repair. *Nano Res.* **2022**, *15*, 5305–5315. [CrossRef]
36. Lorz, L.R.; Yoo, B.C.; Kim, M.-Y.; Cho, J.Y. Anti-wrinkling and anti-melanogenic effect of Pradosia mutisii methanol extract. *Int. J. Mol. Sci.* **2019**, *20*, 1043. [CrossRef] [PubMed]
37. Abbasi, A.R.; Sohail, M.; Minhas, M.U.; Khaliq, T.; Kousar, M.; Khan, S.; Hussain, Z.; Munir, A. Bioinspired sodium alginate based thermosensitive hydrogel membranes for accelerated wound healing. *Int. J. Biol. Macromol.* **2020**, *155*, 751–765. [CrossRef] [PubMed]
38. Mady, F.M.; Shaker, M.A. Enhanced anticancer activity and oral bioavailability of ellagic acid through encapsulation in biodegradable polymeric nanoparticles. *Int. J. Nanomed.* **2017**, *12*, 7405. [CrossRef]
39. Ali, A.; Khalid, I.; Minhas, M.U.; Barkat, K.; Khan, I.U.; Syed, H.K.; Umar, A. Preparation and in vitro evaluation of Chondroitin sulfate and carbopol based mucoadhesive controlled release polymeric composites of Loxoprofen using factorial design. *Eur. Polym. J.* **2019**, *121*, 109312. [CrossRef]
40. Yu, C.; Chen, X.; Zhu, W.; Li, L.; Peng, M.; Zhong, Y.; Naeem, A.; Zang, Z.; Guan, Y. Synthesis of Gallic Acid-Loaded Chitosan-Grafted-2-Acrylamido-2-Methylpropane Sulfonic Acid Hydrogels for Oral Controlled Drug Delivery: In Vitro Biodegradation, Antioxidant, and Antibacterial Effects. *Gels* **2022**, *8*, 806. [CrossRef] [PubMed]
41. Maciejewska, M.; Rogulska, M.; Józwicki, M.; Głodowska, N. Synthesis and characterization of porous copolymers of 2-hydroxyethyl methacrylate with ethylene glycol dimethacrylate. *Polym. Adv. Technol.* **2021**, *32*, 2566–2575. [CrossRef]
42. Sarfraz, M.; Iqbal, R.; Khan, K.U.; Minhas, M.U. Carbopol Based Hydrogels for ITOPRIDE Hydrochloride Delivery; Synthesis, Characterization and Comparative Assessment with Various Monomers. *J. Funct. Biomater.* **2022**, *13*, 295. [CrossRef] [PubMed]
43. Hussein-Al-Ali, S.H.; Abudoleh, S.M.; Hussein, M.Z.; Bullo, S.; Palanisamy, A. Graphene oxide-ellagic acid nanocomposite as effective anticancer and antimicrobial agent. *IET Nanobiotechnol.* **2021**, *15*, 79–89. [CrossRef] [PubMed]
44. Khan, S.A.; Azam, W.; Ashames, A.; Fahelelbom, K.M.; Ullah, K.; Mannan, A.; Murtaza, G. β-Cyclodextrin-based (IA-co-AMPS) Semi-IPNs as smart biomaterials for oral delivery of hydrophilic drugs: Synthesis, characterization, in-Vitro and in-Vivo evaluation. *J. Drug Deliv. Sci. Technol.* **2020**, *60*, 101970. [CrossRef]
45. Sun, C.; Cao, J.; Wang, Y.; Chen, J.; Huang, L.; Zhang, H.; Wu, J.; Sun, C. Ultrasound-mediated molecular self-assemble of thymol with 2-hydroxypropyl-β-cyclodextrin for fruit preservation. *Food Chem.* **2021**, *363*, 130327. [CrossRef]
46. Abarca, R.L.; Rodriguez, F.J.; Guarda, A.; Galotto, M.J.; Bruna, J.E. Characterization of beta-cyclodextrin inclusion complexes containing an essential oil component. *Food Chem.* **2016**, *196*, 968–975. [CrossRef] [PubMed]
47. Sakurai, H.; Suzuki, M.; Itakura, S.; Todo, H.; Arce, F., Jr.; See, G.L.; Tanikawa, T.; Inoue, Y. Preparation, characterization, solubility, and antioxidant capacity of ellagic acid-urea complex. *Materials* **2022**, *15*, 2836. [CrossRef]
48. Dudhipala, N.; Ettireddy, S.; Youssef, A.A.A.; Puchchakayala, G. Cyclodextrin complexed lipid nanoparticles of irbesartan for oral applications: Design, development, and in vitro characterization. *Molecules* **2021**, *26*, 7538. [CrossRef]
49. Suhail, M.; Fang, C.-W.; Khan, A.; Minhas, M.U.; Wu, P.-C. Fabrication and in vitro evaluation of pH-sensitive polymeric hydrogels as controlled release carriers. *Gels* **2021**, *7*, 110. [CrossRef]
50. Wang, J.; Yang, F. Preparation of 2-hydroxypropyl-β-cyclodextrin polymers crosslinked by poly(acrylic acid) for efficient removal of ibuprofen. *Mater. Lett.* **2021**, *284*, 128882. [CrossRef]
51. Li, Y.; Mei, L.; Guan, X.; Hu, Y. Ellagic acid solid dispersion: Characterization and bioactivity in the hydroxyl radical oxidation system. *Food Res. Int.* **2021**, *142*, 110184. [CrossRef] [PubMed]
52. Khan, S.; Anwar, N. Gelatin/carboxymethyl cellulose based stimuli-responsive hydrogels for controlled delivery of 5-fluorouracil, development, in vitro characterization, in vivo safety and bioavailability evaluation. *Carbohydr. Polym.* **2021**, *257*, 117617. [CrossRef]
53. Park, D.W.; Haam, S.; Lee, T.G.; Kim, H.S.; Kim, W.S. Chemoenzymatic synthesis of sugar-containing biocompatible hydrogels: Crosslinked poly(β-methylglucoside acrylate) and poly(β-methylglucoside methacrylate). *J. Biomed. Mater. Res. Part A* **2004**, *71*, 497–507. [CrossRef]

54. Liu, C.; Tripathi, A.K.; Gao, W.; Tsavalas, J.G. Crosslinking in Semi-Batch Seeded Emulsion Polymerization: Effect of Linear and Non-Linear Monomer Feeding Rate Profiles on Gel Formation. *Polymers* **2021**, *13*, 596. [CrossRef] [PubMed]
55. Tabassum, M.; Pervaiz, F.; Shoukat, H. Fabrication and evaluation of gelatin-PVA-co-poly(2-acrylamido-2-methylpropane sulfonic acid)-based hydrogels for extended-release of sitagliptin and metformin by employing response surface methodology. *Chem. Pap.* **2022**, *76*, 4081–4097. [CrossRef]
56. Khanum, H.; Ullah, K.; Murtaza, G.; Khan, S.A. Fabrication and in vitro characterization of HPMC-g-poly (AMPS) hydrogels loaded with loxoprofen sodium. *Int. J. Biol. Macromol.* **2018**, *120*, 1624–1631. [CrossRef]
57. Suhail, M.; Liu, J.-Y.; Hung, M.-C.; Chiu, I.-H.; Minhas, M.U.; Wu, P.-C. Preparation, In Vitro Characterization, and Cytotoxicity Evaluation of Polymeric pH-Responsive Hydrogels for Controlled Drug Release. *Pharmaceutics* **2022**, *14*, 1864. [CrossRef] [PubMed]
58. Jalil, A.; Khan, S.; Naeem, F.; Haider, M.S.; Sarwar, S.; Riaz, A.; Ranjha, N.M. The structural, morphological and thermal properties of grafted pH-sensitive interpenetrating highly porous polymeric composites of sodium alginate/acrylic acid copolymers for controlled delivery of diclofenac potassium. *Des. Monomers Polym.* **2017**, *20*, 308–324. [CrossRef] [PubMed]
59. Singh, B.; Sharma, V. Influence of polymer network parameters of tragacanth gum-based pH responsive hydrogels on drug delivery. *Carbohydr. Polym.* **2014**, *101*, 928–940. [CrossRef]
60. Wang, W.; Wang, A. Synthesis and swelling properties of pH-sensitive semi-IPN superabsorbent hydrogels based on sodium alginate-g-poly(sodium acrylate) and polyvinylpyrrolidone. *Carbohydr. Polym.* **2010**, *80*, 1028–1036. [CrossRef]
61. Richbourg, N.; Wancura, M.; Gilchrist, A.; Toubbeh, S.; Harley, B.; Cosgriff-Hernandez, E.; Peppas, N. Precise control of synthetic hydrogel network structure via linear, independent synthesis-swelling relationships. *Sci. Adv.* **2021**, *7*, eabe3245. [CrossRef]
62. Khalid, I.; Ahmad, M.; Minhas, M.U.; Barkat, K. Synthesis and evaluation of chondroitin sulfate based hydrogels of loxoprofen with adjustable properties as controlled release carriers. *Carbohydr. Polym.* **2018**, *181*, 1169–1179. [CrossRef] [PubMed]
63. Suhail, M.; Shih, C.-M.; Liu, J.-Y.; Hsieh, W.-C.; Lin, Y.-W.; Minhas, M.U.; Wu, P.-C. Synthesis, Characterization, In-Vitro and In-Vivo Evaluation of Ketorolac Tromethamine-Loaded Hydrogels of Glutamic Acid as Controlled Release Carrier. *Polymers* **2021**, *13*, 3541. [CrossRef] [PubMed]
64. Li, D.-Q.; Wang, S.-Y.; Meng, Y.-J.; Guo, Z.-W.; Cheng, M.-M.; Li, J. Fabrication of self-healing pectin/chitosan hybrid hydrogel via Diels-Alder reactions for drug delivery with high swelling property, pH-responsiveness, and cytocompatibility. *Carbohydr. Polym.* **2021**, *268*, 118244. [CrossRef]
65. Khan, M.U.A.; Yaqoob, Z.; Ansari, M.N.M.; Razak, S.I.A.; Raza, M.A.; Sajjad, A.; Haider, S.; Busra, F.M. Chitosan/poly vinyl alcohol/graphene oxide based pH-responsive composite hydrogel films: Drug release, anti-microbial and cell viability studies. *Polymers* **2021**, *13*, 3124. [CrossRef] [PubMed]
66. Hanna, D.H.; Lotfy, V.F.; Basta, A.H.; Saad, G.R. Comparative evaluation for controlling release of niacin from protein-and cellulose-chitosan based hydrogels. *Int. J. Biol. Macromol.* **2020**, *150*, 228–237. [CrossRef]
67. Ritger, P.L.; Peppas, N.A. A simple equation for description of solute release I. Fickian and non-fickian release from non-swellable devices in the form of slabs, spheres, cylinders or discs. *J. Control. Release* **1987**, *5*, 23–36. [CrossRef]
68. Derosa, G.; Maffioli, P.; Sahebkar, A. Ellagic acid and its role in chronic diseases. In *Anti-Nutraceuticals and Chronic Diseases*; Springer: Cham, Switzerland, 2016; pp. 473–479.
69. Yayan, J.; Ghebremedhin, B.; Rasche, K. Cefepime shows good efficacy and no antibiotic resistance in pneumonia caused by Serratia marcescens and Proteus mirabilis–An observational study. *BMC Pharmacol. Toxicol.* **2016**, *17*, 1–9. [CrossRef] [PubMed]
70. Kamaci, M.; Kaya, I. Melamine-based poly(azomethine) hydrogels: Mechanical, biodegradability, drug loading and antibacterial properties. *Eur. Polym. J.* **2018**, *108*, 107–115. [CrossRef]

Journal of
Functional
Biomaterials

MDPI

Article

Biological Activity and Thrombogenic Properties of Oxide Nanotubes on the Ti-13Nb-13Zr Biomedical Alloy

Agnieszka Stróż [1], Maciej Gawlikowski [2,3], Katarzyna Balin [4], Patrycja Osak [1], Julian Kubisztal [1], Maciej Zubko [5], Joanna Maszybrocka [1], Karolina Dudek [6] and Bożena Łosiewicz [1,*]

1 Institute of Materials Engineering, Faculty of Science and Technology, University of Silesia in Katowice, 75 Pułku Piechoty 1A, 41-500 Chorzów, Poland; agnieszka.stroz@us.edu.pl (A.S.); patrycja.osak@us.edu.pl (P.O.); julian.kubisztal@us.edu.pl (J.K.); joanna.maszybrocka@us.edu.pl (J.M.)
2 Faculty of Biomedical Engineering, Silesian University of Technology, 40 Roosevelt, 41-800 Zabrze, Poland; maciej.gawlikowski@polsl.pl
3 Artificial Heart Laboratory, Professor Zbigniew Religa Foundation of Cardiac Surgery Development, 345a Wolności, 41-800 Zabrze, Poland
4 August Chełkowski Institute of Physics, Faculty of Science and Technology, University of Silesia in Katowice, 75 Pułku Piechoty 1A, 41-500 Chorzów, Poland; katarzyn.balin@us.edu.pl
5 Department of Physics, Faculty of Science, University of Hradec Králové, Rokitanského 62, 500 03 Hradec Králové, Czech Republic; maciej.zubko@us.edu.pl
6 Institute of Ceramics and Building Materials, Refractory Materials Center, Łukasiewicz Research Network, Toszecka 99, 44-100 Gliwice, Poland; karolina.dudek@icimb.lukasiewicz.gov.pl
* Correspondence: bozena.losiewicz@us.edu.pl; Tel.: +48-32-3497527

Abstract: The success of implant treatment is dependent on the osseointegration of the implant. The main goal of this work was to improve the biofunctionality of the Ti-13Nb-13Zr implant alloy by the production of oxide nanotubes (ONTs) layers for better anchoring in the bone and use as an intelligent carrier in drug delivery systems. Anodization of the Ti-13Nb-13Zr alloy was carried out in 0.5% HF, 1 M $(NH_4)_2SO_4$ + 2% NH_4F, and 1 M ethylene glycol + 4 wt.% NH_4F electrolytes. Physicochemical characteristics of ONTs were performed by high-resolution electron microscopy (HREM), X-ray photoelectron spectroscopy (XPS), and scanning Kelvin probe (SKP). Water contact angle studies were conducted using the sitting airdrop method. In vitro biological properties and release kinetics of ibuprofen were investigated. The results of TEM and XPS studies confirmed the formation of the single-walled ONTs of three generations on the bi-phase ($\alpha + \beta$) Ti-13Nb-13Zr alloy. The ONTs were composed of oxides of the alloying elements. The proposed surface modification method ensured good hemolytic properties, no cytotoxity for L-929 mouse cells, good adhesion, increased surface wettability, and improved athrombogenic properties of the Ti-13Nb-13Zr alloy. Nanotubular surfaces allowed ibuprofen to be released from the polymer matrix according to the Gallagher–Corrigan model.

Keywords: anodization; biological activity; biomaterials; drug delivery system; oxide nanotubes; Ti-13Nb-13Zr alloy; athrombogenity

1. Introduction

Each implant introduced into a living organism is initially treated as a foreign body and causes a defensive reaction of the immune system in the form of allergy or inflammation. The material that is to be used to produce a biomedical implant should have many features that will prove high biocompatibility, called biotolerance. It should show very good corrosion resistance and no adverse impact of degradation on the surrounding body cells. Ensuring high biocompatibility has become the reason for a far-reaching reduction of the content of harmful elements in metallic biomaterials [1–7]. The literature discusses in detail the influence of the excess of some biocompatible elements in the human body on human organs and tissues, such as DNA damage and mutations, carcinogenicity, and metal sensitivity [8].

Currently, the most common titanium alloys for biomedical applications include the Ti-13Nb-13Zr alloy [9–14]. The superiority of the willingness to use Ti-13Nb-13Zr alloy includes the fact that there is less release of metal ions during the spontaneous passivation of Ti-13Nb-13Zr because the corrosion products of the smaller alloy elements Nb and Zr are less soluble than Al and V. In addition, the native oxide layer on the alloy surface reveals higher resistance to corrosion and provides better protection for the underlying alloy [4,13–17]. The combination of the three most biocompatible elements, i.e., titanium, niobium, and zirconium, that do not show toxic or carcinogenic reactions with tissue and cells, allowed this alloy to be classified as the most promising material for bone implants [8,18].

Titanium and its alloys are used as implants for the osteosynthesis of the limbs and the skull and face, dental implants, some elements for contact joints, implants for cardiac surgery, implants for laryngology, elements for reconstruction, knee and hip endoprosthesis and bone implants. Implants are artificial bodies implanted in the body to recreate the natural function or aesthetics of the damaged organ. Implants replacing hard tissues are most commonly used [1,2,7,8]. The success of implant treatment is mainly dependent on the osseointegration of the implant [2,19–21]. It is clinically confirmed by the lack of mobility of the implant and no signs of inflammation. The process of structural and functional connection between the tissue and the implant is influenced by many factors, like the technique of inserting the implant, its stabilization, bone quality, physical properties of the bioimplant, and its shape and surface [2,5,22,23]. The first condition necessary for the correct course of the osseointegration process is to ensure the primary stabilization of the implant. The stabilization is influenced by the surface structure, bone density at the site of implementation, and the shape and size of the biomaterial. It has been proven that the denser the bone in which the implant is implanted then, the better the primary stabilization. The surface of the bone and implant materials play an important role in osteoblast adhesion and bone growth. Many factors affect the quality of the connection between bone and implant, including the chemical composition as well as the morphology of the implant surface [2,24]. Appropriate development of the implant surface seems to be an important factor for determining the level of interaction between tissues and biomaterials; therefore, the modification methods used are aimed at obtaining the appropriate surface roughness, both at the micro- and nano-scale. In vivo studies demonstrate smooth predisposing surfaces for fibrous tissue formation and rough surfaces at a microscale lead to more favorable bone formation. The rough surface, due to the presence of micro-latches, affects better anchoring but also the distribution of pressure on the surrounding environment between the implant and human tissue. Moreover, the mentioned implants, compared to those with a smooth surface, show better contact with the bone, provide greater mechanical support, and result in faster integration of osseointegration compared to implants with a smooth surface [2,25,26].

Nano-engineered surfaces have the unique ability to directly interact with cells on the overall biological response of implanted biomaterial. Therefore, various nanotechnology-based techniques have been developed to produce nano-scale surfaces on existing biocompatible implant materials. Porous nanostructured titanium alloy oxide layers in the form of nanotubes make them more suitable surgical materials for implantation. Based on numerous studies, it has been proven that implants covered with a layer of oxide nanostructures have the ability to exhibit antibody properties and thus inhibit microbial infections. Titanium nanotube materials can provide a continuous drug delivery system of the pharmacological agent to the specific place in the body where it is needed, ensuring adequate treatment over a longer period [4,27–31].

Anodizing is one of the techniques for modifying the surface of titanium and titanium-based biomaterials [32–37]. Electrochemical oxidation of biomedical Ti-13Nb-13Zr alloy in aqueous solutions containing fluoride ions allows obtaining an anodic nanotubes layer protecting against corrosion and the passage of metal ions, as well as improves the bioactivity of the implant [13,32,33]. The electrolyte selection for electrochemical oxidation allows assigning the obtained layers of nanotubes to one of several generations [13,34–37].

Due to our interest in the modification of the surface of the newest group of titanium alloys, this research was undertaken to study the effect of anodizing conditions on various biological properties of three generations of oxide nanotubes (ONTs) obtained on the Ti-13Nb-13Zr alloy surface. The aim of the research was to produce first-generation (1G), second-generation (2G), and third-generation (3G) ONTs and investigate their influence on biological properties such as cytotoxity and adhesion, thrombogenic, hemocompatibility, wettability and how they act as drug delivery system.

2. Materials and Methods

2.1. Preparation of Research Material

The investigated disc-shape samples of the Ti-13Nb-13Zr (wt.%) alloy were prepared by cutting the rod with a diameter of 0.9 mm. Samples after grinding with abrasive paper with a gradation of 1200 and 2500# were polished using the OP-S suspension and next washed in an ultrasonic washer in ultrapure water (Milli-Q, 18.2 MΩ cm^2) for 20 min. Electrochemical production of 1G ONTs was carried out at room temperature at the voltage 20 V for 2 h in 0.5% HF solution. Moreover, 2G ONTs were obtained at room temperature in 1M $(NH_4)_2SO_4$ solution with 2 wt.% of NH_4F addition at the voltage 20 V for 120 min. Also, 3G ONTs were produced at room temperature in 1M $C_2H_6O_2$ solution with 4 wt.% content of NH_4F. The time of anodizing was 80 min at the voltage of 50 V. Hydrofluoric acid (48% HF), ammonium sulfate (≥98.5% trace metals basis), ethylene glycol (anhydrous, 99.8%), and ammonium fluoride (≥99.99% trace metals basis) were used (Avantor Performance Materials Poland S.A., Gliwice, Poland). Anodizing was conducted using a Kikusui PWR800H Regulated DC Power Supply (Kikusui Electronics Corporation, Yokohama, Japan).

2.2. Material Characterization

The structure of formed ONTs layers was examined using high-resolution electron microscopy (HREM) technique using a JEOL JEM-3010 Transmission Electron Microscope (TEM, JEOL Ltd., Tokyo, Japan) operating at 30 kV equipped with 2k × 2k Orius TM 833 SC200D Gatan CCD camera. To produce TEM samples, the anodized alloy under investigation was suspended in isopropanol and sonicated for 60 min in an ultrasonic bath. The resulting liquid was dropped on standardized Cu grid with an amorphous carbon film, and after evaporation under normal conditions, samples were studied using TEM. The bright field images were recorded. Chemical states of the Ti-13Nb-13Zr alloy surface in the initial state and after anodizing were studied using X-ray photoelectron spectroscopy (XPS) by means of a Prevac photoelectron spectrometer with a VG SCIENTA R3000 hemispherical analyzer (Pleasanton, CA, USA). Monochromatic X-rays, characterized by energy of 1486.74 eV and power of 400 W, were applied.

2.3. Scanning Kelvin Probe Measurements

Contact potential difference (*CPD*) maps of the Ti-13Nb-13Zr alloy surface covered with ONTs layers were registered using SEW-PAR Model 370 device (Princeton Applied Research, Oak Ridge, TN, USA). A tungsten Kelvin probe was used (KP, ø150 μm, Princeton Applied Research, Oak Ridge, TN, USA). The surface area of 1 × 1 mm^2 was scanned. The sample was placed at a distance of ca. 80 μm from the micro-probe. Statistical analysis of the *CPD* maps allowed us to determine histograms as well as the height and spatial parameters that quantitatively characterized *CPD* magnitudes and their distribution on the surface of tested material. The arithmetic average (CPD_{av}), the root mean square deviation (CPD_{rms}), the skewness (CPD_{sk}), the excess kurtosis (CPD_{ku}), and the autocorrelation length (CPD_{al}) parameters were determined.

2.4. Wettability Measurements

Water contact angle measurements were carried out using an OCA 15EC goniometer (Future Digital Scientific Corp., Westbury, NY, USA) with an accuracy of ±0.01° by the sitting airdrop method. Moreover, 10 images of water drops with a volume of about 5 µL placed on the tested surface were recorded within 10 s. On the basis of the received images, the mean values of the contact angle (Θ) were determined. The average of five measurements conducted in different parts of the tested surface was taken as the final values of the Θ.

2.5. In Vitro Hemocompatibility Test

Hemocompatibility of the ONTs layers on the Ti-13Nb-13Zr alloy substrate was investigated in accordance with the ASTM F756-17 [38]. Healthy human volunteers were donors of blood (Regional Blood Donation and Blood Treatment Center, Katowice, Poland). Based on the International Committee for Standardization in Hematology (ICSH), the hemoglobin (Hb) calibration curve meeting the requirements was prepared. Phosphate buffered saline (PBS) was used for preparation of dilutions to the Hb concentration of 10(1) g L^{-1}. Specimens with the determined surface area were applied at a ratio of 3 cm^2 surface area to 1 mL of test blood solution. In case of samples with produced ONTs layers, 0.57(02) ml human blood was applied. Exposition of the final samples in human blood lasted for 4 h at 37(1) °C. After incubation for 4 h, the fluid was transferred to the test tubes and centrifuged at 3000 rpm for 15 min in a standard clinical centrifuge. The supernatant was removed, being careful not to disturb any button of erythrocytes in the test tube. Then, the solution absorbance was investigated using a spectrophotometer at a wavelength of 540 nm. Calculation of % hemolysis was based on the following Formula (1):

$$\%\ \text{hemolysis} = \frac{\text{concentration of hemoglobin released in supernatant} \cdot 100\%}{\text{total hemoglobin concentration in tube}}. \quad (1)$$

2.6. Cell Culture and Cytotoxicity Assays

Cytotoxicity tests were performed in accordance with ISO 10993-5:2009 [39]. Mammalian cell culture monolayer consisting of L-929 mouse Fibroblast cells (Sigma-Aldrich, St. Louis, MO, USA, Lot: 10i019) was used. Extraction of the test material was performed by incubating the material with MEM supplemented with 10% FBS, Penicillin/Streptomycin, and GlutaMAX at 37(1) °C (humidified) in 5(1)% CO_2 for 24(2) h. Quadruplicate monolayers of L-929 mouse fibroblast (passage no.: 15) cells were dose with 1×, 2×, 3× and 4× dilutions of the extract and incubated at 37(1) °C in the presence of 5(1) % CO_2 for 24(1) h. Following the incubation, 50 µL of the MTT solution, prepared just before use, was dispended in each well and incubated for 120(15) min at 37(1) °C (humidified) in 5(1) % CO_2. Following the incubation, the MTT solution was replaced with 100 µL isopropanol and incubated for 10 min at 37(1) °C (humidified) in presence of 5(1) % CO_2. The percent viability for the test article and control article were determined from the blanks. Reduction of the number of living cells caused a decrease in the metabolic activity in the sample. That decrease was directly connected with the amount of blue-violet formazan, whose presence was confirmed by the optical density at 570 nm with differential filter of 650 nm.

Negative Control was HDPE (Granulat G. Motloch, LOT: C7260) extract with MEM supplemented with 10% FBS, Penicillin/Streptomycin, and GlutaMAX. Positive Control was MEM supplemented with 10% FBS, Penicillin/Streptomycin, GlutaMAX, and 30% DMSO. Blank Control was MEM supplemented with 10% FBS, Penicillin/Streptomycin, and GlutaMAX.

2.7. Qualitative In Vitro Cell Adhesion Assay

Duplicated test articles, with the indicated side up, were placed individually in a well of a six-well plate. The L929 mouse Fibroblast cells (Sigma-Aldrich, St. Louis, MO, USA, Lot: 10i019, passage no.:8) were harvested using trypsin and counted. To each well, 80,000 cells were added with enough MEM (supplemented with 10% FBS, Penicillin/Streptomycin, and GlutaMAX) to cover the discs. The plates were incubated at 37(1) °C (humidified) in 5(1) % CO_2 for 24(2) h. After the incubation period, the cells were fixed in 10% PFA for 15 min, followed by the Hematoxylin and Eosin staining. PFA was replaced with Hematoxylin and incubated at room temperature for 5 min. Each well was washed 3 times with tap water. Then, Eosin was added, and plates were incubated for 5 min at room temperature, followed by 3 washes with tap water. The stained cells were visualized using Delta Optical stereomicroscope SZ-630T. The photos were captured using ScopeImage 9 software and HDCE-X5 camera.

2.8. *Thrombogenity Test*

2.8.1. Blood Donation and Platelet-Reach Plasma Preparation

Blood was collected for the anticoagulant CPDA-1 from healthy human volunteers after making sure that they did not take any anticoagulants, including acetylsalicylic acid, clopidogrel, or warfarin/acenocumarol over 14 days. Storing the collected blood lasted up to 24 h at 2–7 °C. Blood count (hematology automaton BC 2800 VET, Mindray, Shenzhen, China), platelets aggregation under the adenosine diphosphate (ADP) and arachidonic acid (impedance aggregometer Multiplate, Roche, Switzerland, with ADPtest and ASPItest tests) and concentration of plasma-free hemoglobin fHB (spectrophotometer Plasma/Low Hb, Hemocue AB, Ängelholm, Sweden), were controlled before starting further measurements. Blood was qualified for further tests, provided that the blood count was normal, the platelet count was higher than 1.2×10^5 L μL^{-1}, the ADP test result was above 122 AUC, the ASPItest result was higher than 136 AUC, and the fHB below 0.2 g dL^{-1}. Platelet-rich plasma (PRP) [40] was prepared directly before the tests by centrifugation of whole blood at 100 G for 10 min at room temperature. Plasma morphology was investigated before the use of PRP in the test. Examined samples were put into polypropylene test tubes with a flat bottom of Falcon type with a volume of 50 mL and a diameter of 30 mm. Each sample was put into a separate test tube so that the sample area, which was not subjected to final processing and polishing, was at the bottom. Test tubes were filled with 10 mL of PRP, and the studied samples were incubated with PRP for 60 min at the temperature of 37(1) °C. The test tubes used for the incubation were placed on the hematology cradle at deflection $\pm 5^\circ$ and frequency 10 cycles/minute, ensuring even coverage of the samples with platelets and their aggregates. Before the incubation ended, the examined samples were withdrawn from the test tubes and carefully washed with PBS, and next fixed in 4% buffered formalin. The material prepared in such a way was then the subject of imaging tests.

2.8.2. Qualitative Thrombogenicity Scale

The analysis of thrombogenicity test was carried out on 39 specimens, including 12 specimens of the 1G ONTs, 9 specimens of the 2G ONTs, 9 specimens of the 3G ONTs, and 9 specimens of the non-anodized Ti-13Nb-13Zr alloy. Neither literature data nor standards (e.g., ISO 10993-5:2009 [39]) give quantitative method of measurement thrombogenicity of biomaterials. Therefore, in the studies described in this paper, a qualitative method was used. In order to make the measurement more reliable, the assessment was performed by two experts who used a six-level ordinal scale (Table 1) [41]. As the experts, a biologist with 25 years of experience in cell testing and a bioengineer with 20 years of experience in thrombogenicity and medical statistics were chosen.

Table 1. Ordinal thrombogenicity scale together with description and exemplary images of surface of the sample belonging to a given class [41].

Class	Description	Example
0	contains samples characterized by minimal thrombogenicity: separated platelets of low diverse level, no platelet aggregates	
1	contains samples characterized by very low-degree thrombogenicity: a dozen or so adhered blood platelets not creating aggregates	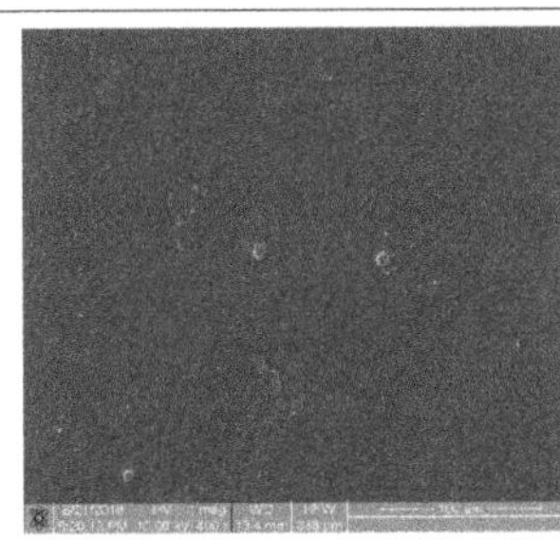
2	contains samples characterized by very low-degree thrombogenicity: several dozen of visible platelets which can be present as single, separated aggregates with a small area	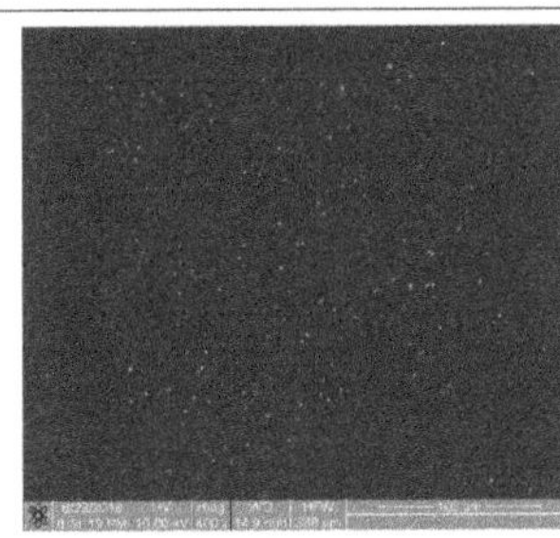
3	contains samples characterized by average-degree thrombogenicity: biological material mainly comprises aggregates larger than individual blood platelets	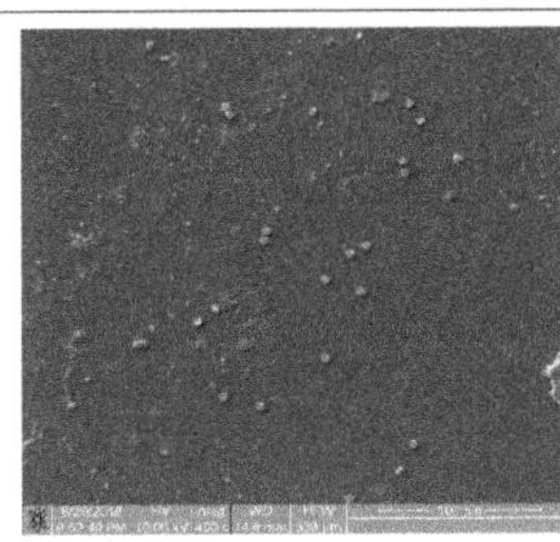

Table 1. *Cont.*

Class	Description	Example
4	contains samples characterized by high-degree thrombogenicity: sample is covered with highly differentiated biological material, and the individual objects are connected with each other without possibility of separating them	
5	contains samples characterized by very high-degree thrombogenicity: platelets are highly differentiated and form numerous aggregates, which are connected with each other without possibility of separating and counting objects	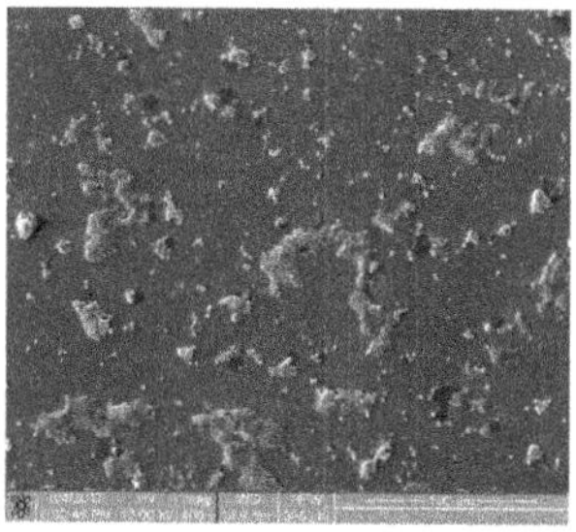

The class 0 constituted negative control. As a reference material, polyurethane based on polyesters Bionate 55D (DSM Biomedical Inc., Geleen, The Netherlands) was chosen. This material is used in medical devices devoted to long-term contact with blood. The material samples were prepared in the form of disks of 8 mm diameter and 0.8 mm thickness by high-pressure injection. The surface roughness described by an arithmetic mean deviation of the roughness profile was $Ra = 0.16$.

Class 5 constituted positive control. As a reference material, glass disks covered by collagen (Neuvitro Corporation, Vancouver, WA, USA) were chosen. Collagen is a natural fibrous protein that exists in extracellular matrix and has strong ability to activate platelets.

2.8.3. Statistical Analysis Methods

Both experts evaluated the same material in six-level ordinal scale. In order to study the degree of compliance of the two experts the alpha–Krippendorf coefficient was used. The coefficient has values from 0 to 1. It is agreed that if its value is >0.80, the compliance of assessments is very good. The Kruskal–Wallis test was used for that data analysis because the number of classes was higher than 2, variable describing thrombogenicity was on ordinal scale, and the experimental model was independent. The Kruskal–Wallis test is nonparametric equivalent of variance analysis. Multiple comparison test was applied for post-hoc analysis.

2.9. Drug Delivery System

The Ti-13Nb-13Zr samples with ONTs layers were subjected to surface functionalization heparine–dopamine (Hep-DOPA) conjugate by mixing 40 mg mL^{-1} heparin, 19.06 mg mL^{-1} EDAC (*N*-(3-Dimethylaminopropyl)-*N'*-ethylcarbodiimide, hydrochloride) and 11.5 mg mL^{-1} NHS (*N*-Hydroxysuccinimide) and reacted with 10 mL of MES buffer pH = 4.5 for 10 min (solution 1). Then, 102.2 mg mL^{-1} dopamine was mixed with 1 mL MES buffer pH = 4.5 (solution 2). Solution 1 and solution 2 were mixed and reacted for 12 h in the dark. The Ti-13Nb-13Zr alloy with ONTs layers was placed into the mixture prepared for 12 h. The material obtained in this way was dried, then ibuprofen was immobilized on the surface of the heparinized melt by adding 10 mg mL^{-1} of ibuprofen to 10 mL of Tris-HCl at pH = 8. The reaction was conducted for 24 h at room temperature with gentle shaking. The release kinetics of ibuprofen from the nanotubular layer was investigated by immersing the sample in 15 mL PBS with pH = 7.45 at 37(1) °C for 24 h. The kinetics of the released drug was studied for 60 min, taking the solution for analysis every 10 min. Each time 1 mL of the solution was withdrawn by adding fresh solution. Using UV-VIS spectroscopy, the amount of substance released from the nanotubular oxide layer was determined. The absorbance value was measured at the wavelength λ = 257 nm, determining the absorbance value of the PBS in the first step and then the absorbed solution. Based on the following Formula (2), the percentage amount of released drug was calculated:

$$\%\ \text{drug release} = \frac{\text{actual absorbance} - \text{absorbance 0 h}}{\text{actual absorbance}}. \quad (2)$$

3. Results and Discussion

3.1. FE-SEM and TEM Characterization

The selected Ti-13Nb-13Zr alloy to obtain 1G, 2G, and 3G ONTs layers is a new type of vital titanium alloy. The addition of Nb and Zr in the amount of 13 wt.% provides appropriate properties for application in regenerative medicine. Additionally, it ensures better biocompatibility and higher corrosion resistance compared to titanium [11–14]. Anodization of the Ti-13Nb-13Zr alloy was conducted using the anode made of the tested sample and the Pt cathode at a distance of 25 mm in a face-to-face position (Figure 1).

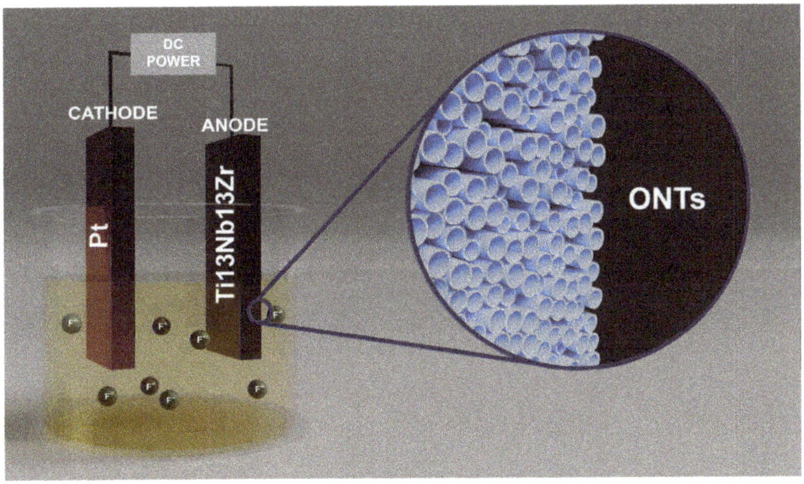

Figure 1. Scheme of the set-up for anodizing the Ti-13Nb-13Zr alloy in aqueous solution with fluoride ions.

The obtained FE-SEM images of surface morphology for 1G, 2G, and 3G ONTs layers on the Ti-13Nb-13Zr substrate with corresponding TEM images are presented in Figure 2. From the observed regions, the selected area electron diffraction (SAED) patterns were recorded. SAED patterns (see insight in Figure 2) clearly indicate that all layers of 1G, 2G, and 3G ONTs exhibit amorphous structures. From selected areas of the FE-SEM images of three generations of ONTs layers obtained via anodization, the morphological parameters of the nanotubes were determined and summed up in Table 2.

Based on the results shown in Table 2, it can be seen that each generation of ONTs is characterized by different morphological parameters. For 1G ONTs, the smallest diameter of the nanotubes is obtained. In the case of 2G ONTs, an increase of 20% in the length of the outer diameter compared to 1G ONTs is observed. More than four and a half times larger outer diameters of 3G ONTs compared to 1G ONTs is confirmed. The longest oxide nanotubes are obtained for 3G ONTs of the order of almost 10 μm. The shortest ones are observed for 1G ONTs. The proposed anodic oxidation conditions for 2G ONTs allow to obtain nanotubes almost 4 μm long.

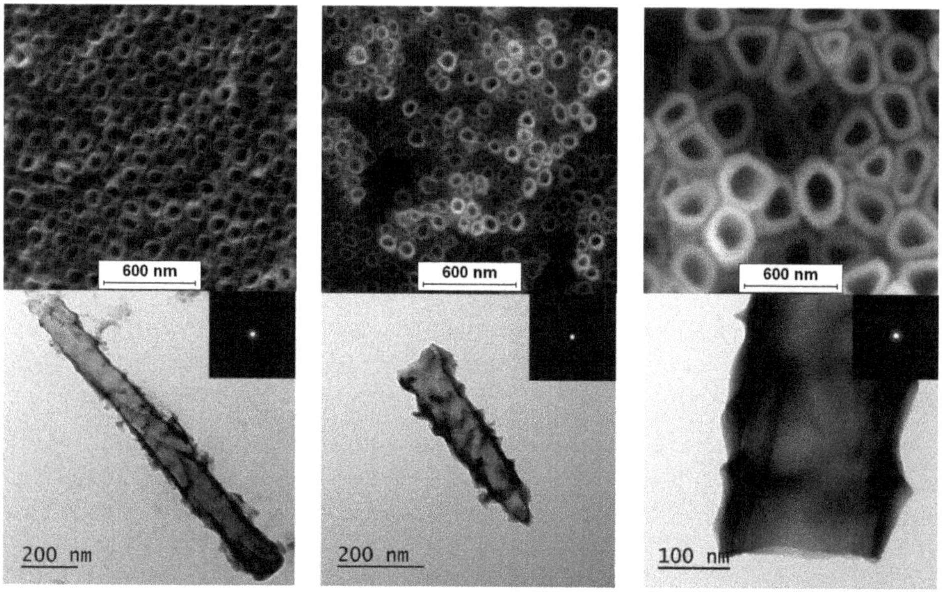

(**a**) (**b**) (**c**)

Figure 2. FE-SEM and corresponding below TEM images of the oxide nanotubes obtained on the Ti-13Nb-13Zr alloy: (**a**) 1G ONTs produced in 0.5% HF solution [10]; (**b**) 2G ONTs produced in 1M $NH_4(SO_4)_2$ + 2% NH_4F solution; (**c**) 3G ONTs produced in 1M $C_2H_6O_2$ + 4% NH_4F solution [13].

Table 2. Morphological parameters of 1G [10], 2G, and 3G [13] ONTs produced on the Ti-13Nb-13Zr alloy via anodization.

Electrolyte	**Anodization Parameters**	**ONT Internal Diameter (nm)**	**ONT Outer Diameter (nm)**	**ONTs Length (μm)**
0.5% HF	E = 20 V, t = 120 min	71(7)	87(10)	0.94(9)
1M $(NH_4)_2SO_4$ +2% NH_4F	E = 20 V, t = 120 min	61(6)	103(10)	3.9(4)
1M $C_2H_6O_2$ +4% NH_4F	E = 50 V, t = 80 min	169(17)	342(34)	9.7(9)

Based on the literature, the influence of anodizing conditions on the diameters and lengths of oxide nanotubes obtained for different generations on the Ti-13Nb-13Zr alloy can be confirmed. The influence of voltage change on the diameter of 2G ONTs on the Ti-13Nb-13Zr alloy is presented in the paper [42]. In the voltage range of 10–45 V, an increase in nanotube diameter from 55 to 250 nm can be seen. For 3G ONTs on the same substrate at the voltage of 15–35 V, the outer diameter of the nanotube increased from 104(13) to 230(30) nm [43].

3.2. Roughness Profile Measurements

Since the roughness of the contact surface affects the adhesion and, thus, the strength of the connection, an important element for obtaining a good adhesive connection is the proper development of the contact surface of biomaterials. For titanium implants such as orthopedic and dental, it is advisable to obtain a permanent connection between the tissue and the material; therefore, the aim is to obtain an optimum surface roughness of *Ra* between 1 and 3 μm, while in the case of surgical tools and implants intended, among others, for implants prepared for contact with blood surfaces with as little roughness as possible them [43–45].

The geometric structure of the surface (GSS) of the Ti-13Nb-13Zr alloy without and with ONTs layers of three generations was characterized by surface micro-geometry measurements in a two-dimensional (2D) system. The discussion of the influence of anodizing conditions on the GSS was based on the selected profile height parameter *Ra*. Figure 3 presents the exemplary roughness profiles after alignment for the 1G, 2G, and 3G ONTs layers on the Ti13-Nb-13Zr alloy. All obtained surface profiles were symmetrical. A similar value of *Ra* = 0.16(01) and *Ra* = 0.13(01) parameters for the 1G and 2G ONTs layers was determined, respectively. The 3G ONTs were characterized by the highest *Ra* parameter of 1.34(04).

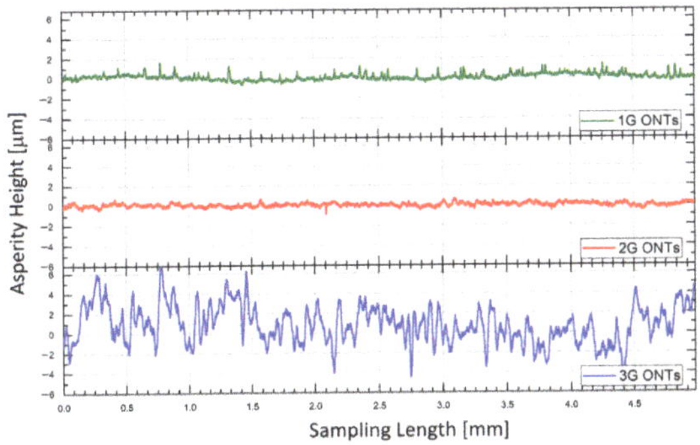

Figure 3. Roughness profile for the 1G, 2G, and 3G ONTs layers obtained on the Ti13-Nb-13Zr alloy via anodization.

The *Ra* for the 3G ONTs increased over 8 times in comparison with the 1G ONTs and 10 times in relation to the 2G ONTs due to the differences in the morphological parameters of the obtained nanotubes on the Ti-13Nb-13Zr alloy. It can be seen that the most developed surface and the thickest layer of nanotubes were obtained for the 3G ONTs layer (Table 2). Based on the obtained results, it can be expected that the 3G ONTs layers will allow for better stability at the implant–bone interface, improved osseointegration, and reduced risk of metal ion release as products of corrosion processes and biotribological wear. In our earlier work [43], it was reported that deviations of the roughness profile from the mean line at the micro-scale were not observed for the smooth surface of the Ti-13Zr-13Nb alloy before anodizing, for which *Ra* was only 0.10 μm. The positive role of surface roughness was reported in studies on stainless steel, Co-Cr alloy, titanium, Ti-6Al-4V, and Ti-6Al-7Nb alloys using human osteoblasts [46,47]. The authors studied the activity of bone tissue after implanting titanium implants with a smooth and rough surface on rabbits. Better contact of the implant with the bone and a larger volume of bone tissue was obtained for rough surfaces compared to smooth surfaces.

3.3. XPS Study of Chemical States

The XPS studies concerned the determination of atomic concentration, and chemical states analysis of the obtained ONTs components. Detailed analysis of the shape and position of Ti2p, Nb3d, and Zr3d photoemission lines for the 1G and 2G ONTs in Figure 4 a–f was conducted and compared with the results of our previous XPS research on the Ti-13Nb-13Zr alloy reported in the earlier work [13].

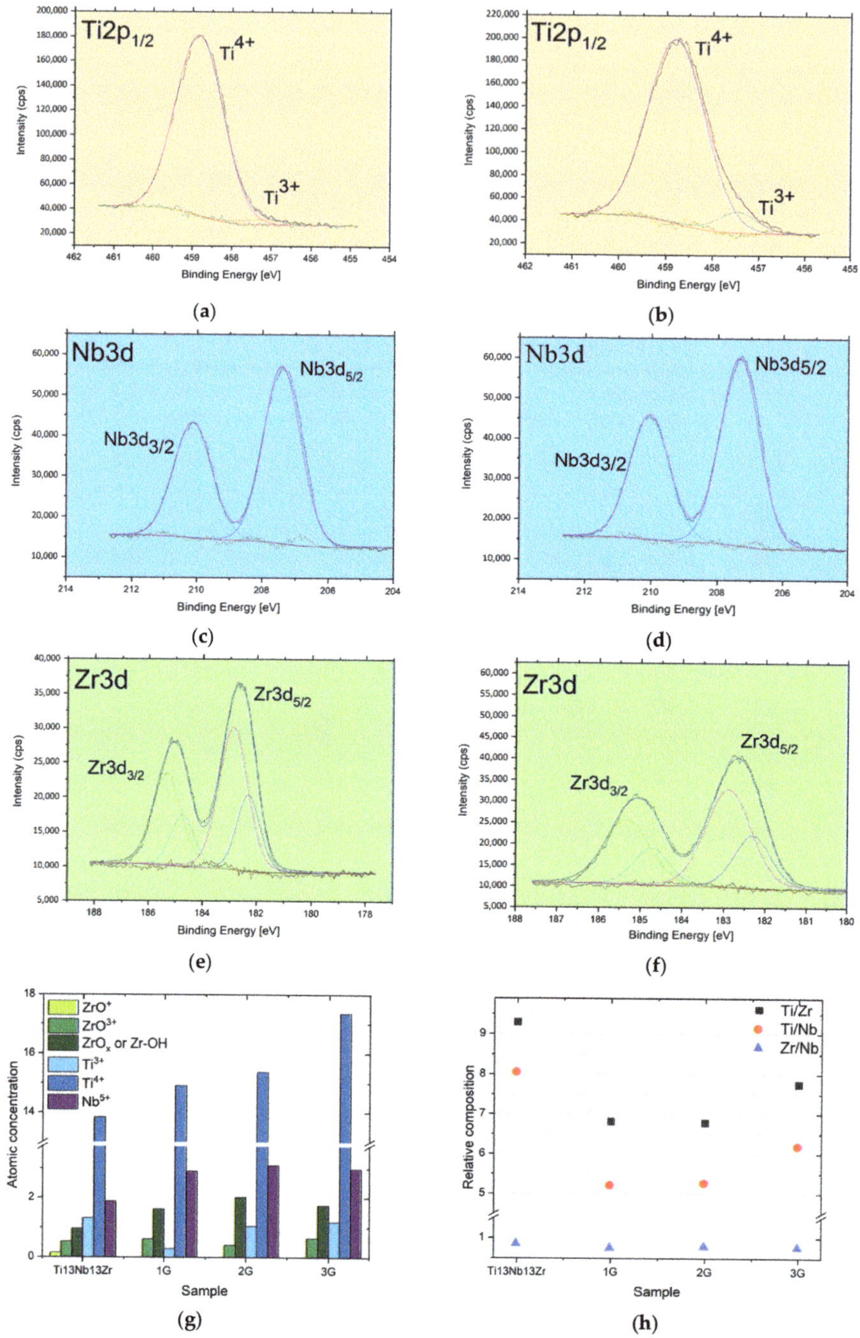

Figure 4. XPS high-resolution spectra for $Ti2p_{7/2}$: **(a)** 1G ONTs, $Ti2p_{1/2}$; **(b)** 2G ONTs, $Ti2p_{1/2}$; **(c)** 1G ONTs, Nb3d; **(d)** 2G ONTs, Nb3d; **(e)** 1G ONTs, Zr3d; **(f)** 2G ONTs, Zr3d; **(g)** Sample-dependent atomic concentration; **(h)** Relative composition elements dependent on the sample.

The titanium in electrochemically obtained 1G and 2G ONTs occurs mainly as the TiO_2. The binding energy of the prominent peak (Figure 4a) is located at 458.8 eV and is characteristic of the Ti^{4+} oxidation state as observed in anatase [48]. A weak contribution of oxidized titanium characteristic for trivalent titanium is visible at binding energy 457.2 eV [49]. Both chemical states were previously observed in the Ti-13Nb-13Zr alloy, for which 91.64% of titanium atoms were in the 4^+ valence state and 8.36% in the 3^+ [13]. The amount of the trivalent titanium in the 1G and 2G ONTs is lower than in mentioned reference sample; for the 1G ONTs, Ti^{3+} atoms account for only 1.81% of all titanium atoms, whereas for the 2G ONTs, it is only 6.35%.

The deconvolution of the lines Nb3d of the 1G and 2G ONTs indicates the presence of Nb in one chemical state—the position of the $Nb3d_{5/2}$ at about 207.4 eV (Figure 4c,d) is characteristic of the Nb_2O_5 oxide [50]. The same result for niobium was observed in 3G ONTs in our previous studies [13]. Analysis of the zirconium lines in Figure 4e,f revealed some similarities between the surfaces of the 1G and 2G ONTs and previously reported electrochemically modified Ti-13Nb-13Zr. The positions of deconvoluted peaks indicate the presence of ZrO_2 with a peak at 182.3 eV and Zr in another oxidation state with a peak at 182.9 eV or Zr(OH) [51]. The amount of Zr in a particular chemical state is different for 1G and 2G ONTs and differs even more when compared with the previously analyzed 3G ONTs sample [13].

The results of the contribution of the particular chemical state for the electrochemically obtained 1G, 2G, G3 ONTs layers, and reference alloy are summarized in Figure 4g. The data points represent the calculated atomic concentration for each atom in each chemical state. The general observation suggests that Nb and Zr bonded with oxygen or OH group in anodic ONTs layers are relatively stable—their amount does not depend on the applied procedure of electrochemical modification. In the case of Ti, applied anodization generally influences the amount of titanium but also titanium chemical states. This is worth noting that applied procedures for electrochemical oxidation of Ti-13Nb-13Zr in all three generations lead to changes in the relative ratios of the elements under consideration (Figure 4h). Those changes are related to titanium as only the relative ratios of Ti/Zr and Ti/Nb are changed when compared with the reference sample. Based on the 1G and 2G ONTs layers studies, it can also be observed that even if the relative amount of sample constituents are almost identical, as observed for the 1G and 3G [13] ONTs layers, their chemical composition is different.

3.4. Electronic Properties

Statistical analysis of the contact potential difference maps in Figure 5 allowed us to determine the arithmetic average (CPD_{av}), the root mean square deviation (CPD_{rms}), the skewness (CPD_{sk}), the excess kurtosis (CPD_{ku}), and the autocorrelation length (CPD_{al}), i.e., parameters that quantitatively describe electronic properties of the Ti-13Nb-13Zr alloy surface covered with ONTs. The values of the above parameters are presented in Table 3.

Table 3. Statistical parameters calculated using *CPD* maps of the Ti-13Nb-13Zr substrate and for the 1G, 2G, and 3G ONTs; CPD_{av} is the arithmetic average, CPD_{rms} is the root mean square deviation, CPD_{al} is the autocorrelation length, CPD_{sk} is the skewness, and CPD_{ku} is the excess kurtosis; V_{KP} is the voltage measured versus Kelvin probe.

Parameter	Ti-13Nb-13Zr	1G ONTs	2G ONTs	3G ONTs
CPD_{av} (mV_{KP})	−634.2	−566.5	−480.4	−386.7
CPD_{rms} (mV_{KP})	17.8	19.1	23.7	24.7
CPD_{al} (μm)	63.61	31.37	43.12	52.29
CPD_{sk}	−0.20	0.06	−0.15	0.07
CPD_{ku}	−0.09	0.05	0.28	−0.02

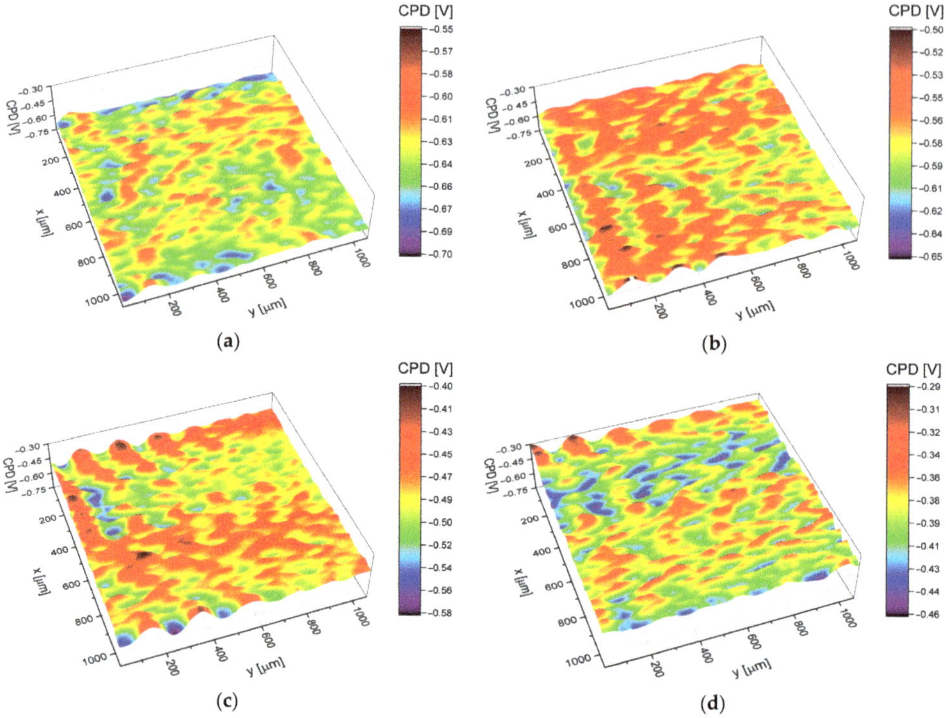

Figure 5. *CPD* maps determined for (**a**) Ti-13Nb-13Zr alloy; (**b**) 1G ONTs; (**c**) 2G ONTs; (**d**) 3G ONTs.

It was found that the substrate surface covered with ONTs is characterized by the higher value of the CPD_{av} in comparison with the biomedical Ti-13Nb-13Zr alloy, regardless of the solution composition from which nanotubes were obtained. Moreover, it was stated that the 3G ONTs are characterized by the highest CPD_{av} value (ca. -387 mV_{KP}) among all the investigated biomaterials. This result may be related to the different chemical compositions of solutions and hence different concentrations of fluorine ions in electrolytes (Table 2), from 0.5% F^- for the 1G ONTs, 2% for the 2G ONTs, and 4% for the 3G ONTs.

The root mean square deviation (CPD_{rms}) determines the deviation of *CPD* heights in relation to the arithmetic average, whereas autocorrelation length (CPD_{al}) characterizes the spatial distribution of *CPD* heights on the material surface. In other words, CPD_{al} is a measure of the distance over the surface by which one would find a surface feature (*CPD* in this case) that is statistically different from the one that can be found in the original location. The CPD_{rms} parameters obtained for the investigated surfaces indicate increasing heights of *CPD* in the order Ti-13Nb-13Zr, 1G ONTs, 2G ONTs, and 3G ONTs. Simultaneously values of the CPD_{al} parameter show that the correlation length is the highest for the Ti-13Nb-13Zr substrate and decreases for surfaces covered with the nanotubes. Generally, both parameters i.e., CPD_{rms} and CPD_{al} indicate that the Ti-13Nb-13Zr substrate is characterized by the most uniform surface of all the samples tested and also that the production of nanotubes on the Ti-13Nb-13Zr surface increases its electrical heterogeneity. The increase in CPD_{rms} and CPD_{al} determined for the surfaces covered with ONTs can be explained by increasing the dimensions of outer diameters of the nanotubes from 87(10) nm for the 1G ONTs, 103(10) nm for the 2G ONTs, and 342(34) nm for the 3G ONTs. Skewness (CPD_{sk}) and excess kurtosis (CPD_{ku}) describe the shape of the *CPD* distribution and give additional information on the *CPD* peaks/valleys profile. It was found that for all investigated samples CPD_{sk} and CPD_{ku} parameters change in the range ± 0.3 (see Table 3); thus, one can state that for each material tested, the *CPD* distribution follows a Gaussian (normal) distribution.

Histograms of the *CPD* values with fitted Gaussian distributions are shown in Figure 6. The comprehensive description of the histogram preparation and the determination of the parameters can be found elsewhere [52–54].

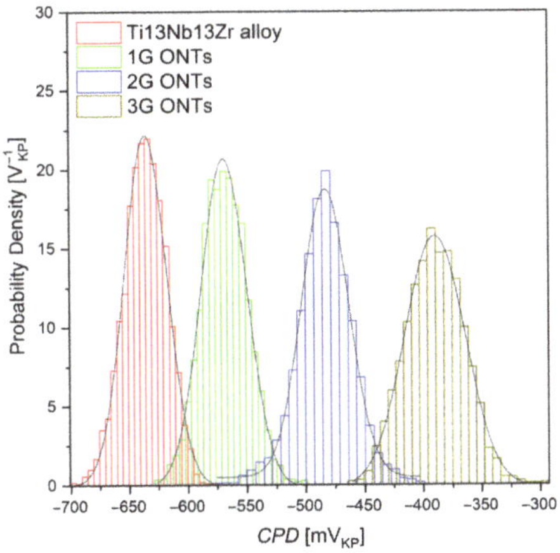

Figure 6. *CPD* histograms determined for the Ti-13Nb-13Zr alloy and for the 1G, 2G, and 3G ONTs; solid lines—fit of the Gaussian function.

Approximation of the histograms using the Gaussian function allows determining the arithmetic average CPD_{av} and the standard deviation, which in this case corresponds to the CPD_{rms} parameter. Values of CPD_{sk} and CPD_{ku} also indicate that the *CPD* heights are symmetrically distributed around the average as well as that the investigated surfaces do not show inordinately high peaks/deep valleys. Generally, one can state that the entire surface of the Ti-13Nb-13Zr alloy is evenly covered with ONTs irrespective of the different production processes (solution composition, anodization parameters).

3.5. Surface Wettability

The nature of the interaction of the biomaterial with the tissue, related to each of the key properties of the surface layer mentioned above, is also determined by surface wettability. It determines protein adsorption, blood coagulation, and biological response. Most of the commonly used biomaterials are hydrophobic and have a high affinity for many proteins. Immediately after implantation, the biomaterial is covered with a layer of proteins. These are mainly albumin, fibrinogen, fibronectin, immunoglobulins, and von Willebrand factors. In shaping the surface properties of implants, wettability should also be taken into account, which is important for the osetoinduction process preceding osseointegration and affects the absorption of molecules favoring the adhesion of fibroblasts and/or bacteria [55,56]. Hydrophilic surfaces have better biological activity in contact with body fluids and, thus, provide better osseointegration [57]. The surface wettability tests of the produced ONTs layers showed that the contact angle measured for the Ti-13Nb-13Zr alloy without and with vertically oriented 1G, 2G, and 3G ONTs took the following Θ values in sequence: 62.9(9) °, 25.3(5) °, 11.9(1) °, and 14.7(2) °, respectively (Figure 7).

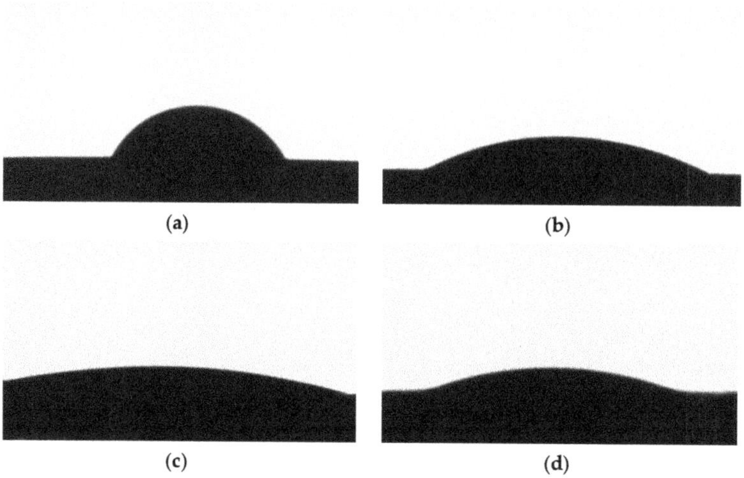

Figure 7. Image of a water drop on the surface of the Ti-13Nb-13Zr alloy: (**a**) Non-anodized; (**b**) Anodized in 0.5% HF; (**c**) Anodized in 1 M $(NH_4)_2SO_4$ + 2% NH_4F; (**d**) Anodized in 1 M $C_2H_6O_2$ + 4% NH_4F.

The tests performed confirmed the favorable hydrophilic nature of the produced ONTs layers. Investigation of the contact angle of the individual sample surface showed that they were hydrophilic in nature both before and after anodization (Figure 7a–d). A reduction in Θ value was observed for the samples after anodization, which indicates an increase in hydrophilicity. The most advantageous hydrophilic properties showed the 2G ONTs, then 3G ONTs, 1G ONTs, and the smallest Ti-13Nb-13Zr alloy. The obtained wettability results of nanotubular surfaces on titanium are similar [58]. Using anodization as a method of electrochemical modification enhances the surface wettability of titanium and its alloys.

3.6. *In Vitro Hemocompatibility Study*

Currently, the most popular method of determining hemocompatibility is the hemolysis test. The process of hemolysis is based on the transition of hemoglobin into the cytoplasma due to the rupture of erythrocytes. According to the ASTM F756-17 standard [38], the biocompatibility of the 1G and 2G ONTs examinations were performed (Figure 8).

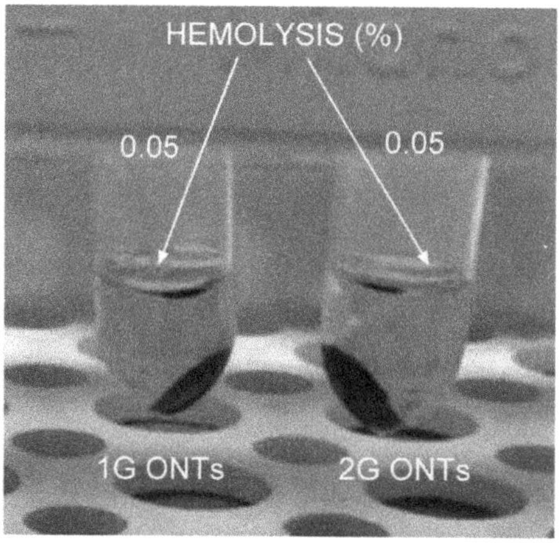

Figure 8. Anti-hemolytic activity of the 1G and 2G ONTs on the Ti-13Nb-13Zr alloy.

The value of the hemolytic index lower than 2 indicates that the biomaterial is non-hemolytic. The obtained results of in vitro hemocompatibility study shown in Figure 8 revealed the value of the hemolytic index of 0.05 for both the 1G and 2G ONTs. We found the hemolytic index for the 3G ONTs to be 0.00 [13]. The highest hemolytic index of 0.30 was reported for the non-anodized Ti-13Nb-13Zr alloy [13]. The obtained values prove that the proposed electrochemical modification ensures outstanding hemocompatibility. In the case of the 3G ONTs, it is even possible to completely eliminate hemolysis.

3.7. Cytotoxity and Cell Adhesion Assay

The interaction of the substrate material with a nanotubular structure with the biological environment can also be assessed during the use of cell cultures and cellular response on the surface prepared in this way. In the past, in order to evaluate the cytotoxicity of biomaterials for medicine, in vitro mammalian cell culture tests were used. At present, morphology, chemistry surface, and type of cells, especially concentration and time of exposure, determine the cytotoxicity of nanomaterials. The test article showed no cytotoxic potential to L-929 mouse fibroblast cells for the non-anodized Ti-13Nb-13Zr alloy and with the obtained 1G, 2G, and 3G ONTs layers (Table 4). In the case of oxide nanotubes produced on the vital Ti-13Nb-13Zr alloy by the anodizing method, the obtained cytotoxicity for mouse fibroblast cells is similar. The adhesion, proliferation, and migration of cells forming bone tissue are related to the diameters of nanotubes. This is confirmed by numerous studies showing that the ONTs surface is conducive to the growth of cells. It should be noted that different research groups used different cell colonies, which affected the results of the study [59–61].

Table 4. Cell response for the Ti-13Nb-13Zr alloy before and after formation of 1G, 2G, and 3G ONTs.

Material	Percent Viability (%)	System Suitability
Positive control	0.54	No Cytotoxic Potential
Negative control	98.33	No Cytotoxic Potential
Ti-13Nb-13Zr (1×)	92.26	No Cytotoxic Potential
Ti-13Nb-13Zr (2×)	97.18	No Cytotoxic Potential
Ti-13Nb-13Zr (3×)	97.49	No Cytotoxic Potential
Ti-13Nb-13Zr (4×)	99.63	No Cytotoxic Potential
1G ONTs (1×)	100.6	No Cytotoxic Potential
1G ONTs (2×)	85.29	No Cytotoxic Potential
1G ONTs (3×)	103.8	No Cytotoxic Potential
1G ONTs (4×)	98.67	No Cytotoxic Potential
2G ONTs (1×)	87.91	No Cytotoxic Potential
2G ONTs (2×)	99.59	No Cytotoxic Potential
2G ONTs (3×)	106.3	No Cytotoxic Potential
2G ONTs (4×)	106.2	No Cytotoxic Potential
3G ONTs (1×)	88.45	No Cytotoxic Potential
3G ONTs (2×)	89.97	No Cytotoxic Potential
3G ONTs (3×)	95.02	No Cytotoxic Potential
3G ONTs (4×)	96.63	No Cytotoxic Potential

Based on the prepared samples for cytotoxicity testing, cell adhesion to layers obtained via anodization and to the starting material was also tested. The cells adhere with different efficiency, which can be seen in Table 5. The obtained results of the adhesion test showed a different degree of adhesion depending on the tested oxide layer. For the self-passive oxide layer present on the Ti-13Nb-13Zr alloy and for the 1G ONTs, high cell adhesion was obtained. For the 2G and 3G ONTs, the medium adhesion was revealed. It can be correlated with the diameter and length of the obtained nanotubes in dependence of generation. Cell adhesion decreased with the growth and length of the ONTs.

Table 5. Estimated cell adherence to the Ti-13Nb-13Zr alloy before and after formation of 1G, 2G, and 3G ONTs.

Material	Level of Adhesion
Ti-13Nb-13Zr	High
1G ONTs	High
2G ONTs	Medium
3G ONTs	Medium

ONTs layers are able to increase the bioactivity of the implant surface. First of all, they increase the surface roughness at the nano-scale, forming a biomimetic nanostructure, which is similar to natural rough bone tissue. Bone-forming cells (osteoblasts) have been proven in numerous studies [62,63] to adhere to a surface that is morphologically and chemically similar to natural bone tissue. The interaction of the nanotube-structured substrate material with the biological environment can also be assessed during the use of cell culture. Cell adhesion is related to the diameter of the nanotubes; research is shown in [64]. The authors showed that oxide nanotubes with a smaller diameter had a more stimulating effect on cell growth and differentiation.

3.8. Thrombogenicity Test

The alpha Kappendorf coefficient was 0.88, which proved very good compatibility with the thrombogenicity assessment carried out by the two experts. The relationship between the evaluations is shown in Table 6. Numbers in the table cells represent the number of samples.

Table 6. Number of samples assigned to each expert.

		Expert 2				
		Class 1	Class 2	Class 3	Class 4	Class 5
Expert 1	Class 1	5	0	0	0	0
	Class 2	1	4	0	0	0
	Class 3	0	1	8	1	0
	Class 4	0	0	1	9	1
	Class 5	0	0	0	0	7

The result of the Kruskal–Wallis test was significant ($p = 0.0000$), which means that at least one group differs from the rest. Results of the post-hoc test are shown in Table 7 and Figure 9.

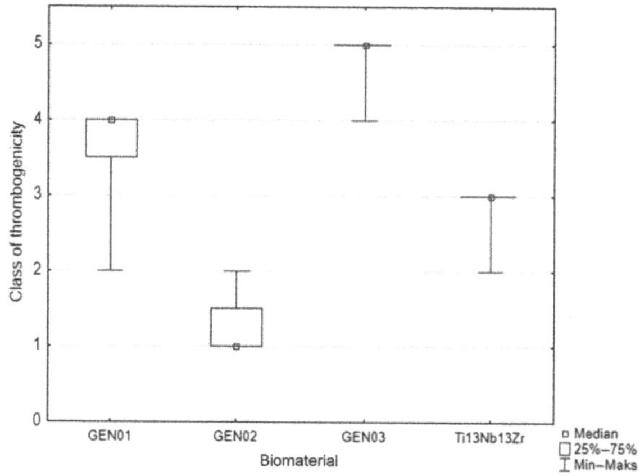

Figure 9. Thrombogenicity of the studied Ti-13Nb-13Zr alloy before and after formation of 1G, 2G, and 3G ONTs (in six-level ordinal scale).

Table 7. Results of the post-hoc test.

	1G ONTs	2G ONTs	3G ONTs	Ti-13Nb-13Zr
1G ONTs		0.0030	0.1520	0.5908
2G ONTs	0.0030		0.0000	0.4582
3G ONTs	0.1520	0.0000		0.0017
Ti-13Nb-13Zr	0.5908	0.4582	0.0017	

Class 0 meant very small thrombogenicity comparable with negative control. Class 5 meant very high thrombogenicity comparable with positive control. The meaning of a given class is described in Table 1, and each description was exemplified by images of the biomaterial surfaces (Bionate 55D polymer, PEEK, Ti6Al7Nb alloy with a layer of TiN, PEEK polymer, ZrO_2+Y_2O_3 ceramics, and oraz glass covered by collagen) dotted by thrombocytes and their aggregates. Usage of the interval scale limited the possibility of applying advanced statistical methods and made worse the quality of inference but, on the other hand, made carrying out a statistical proof possible.

In order to study how the expert assessments differ, the alfa Kappenrorf coefficient was used. Taken values from 0 to 1 where 0 means total discrepancy of the expert assessments and 1 means their total agreement. It is accepted in the literature data that a coefficient value larger than 0.8 means a very good agreement in the assessments. The alpha Kappendorf coefficient for the presented studies was 0.88; thus, the expert's opinions were practically equal. Further analysis was carried out with the use of the Kruskal–Wallis tests with the post-hoc multiple comparison method.

Thrombogenicity of the 1G and 3G ONTs layers is practically the same, and those biomaterials strongly unfavorably influence the activation of coagulation factors. They were classified into classes 4 and 5, respectively. Class 5 contains samples of positive control, so the 3G ONTs biomaterial activates the coagulation system to the same degree as strongly thrombogenic collagen. Athorombogenic properties of the 1G ONTs biomaterial are only slightly better than these of the 3G ONTs, but one should remember that there are no statistically important differences between those two materials (p = 0.1520—see Table 4). Thrombogenicity of the 2G ONTs and Ti-13Nb-13Zr does not differ; however, these biomaterials show much better athrombogenic properties than the 1G and 3G ONTs. The 2G ONTs and Ti-13Nb-13Zr were classified into classes 1 and 3, respectively. Class 1 contained biomaterials slightly worse than the positive control (Table 1). Thus, the 2G ONTs biomaterial has a small effect on the coagulation system. The Ti-13Nb-13Zr alloy is situated in class 3; however, there is no statistical proof that it differs from the 2G ONTs (p = 0.4582, compared to Table 4).

3.9. Drug Release Kinetics

To check the possibility of the potential use of ibuprofen-loaded Hep-DOPA/ONTs as carriers for the controlled release of the drug was compared the ibuprofen release profiles for three generations of oxide nanotubes on the Ti-13Nb-13Zr alloy obtained via anodization. The analysis of the obtained results showed a rapid increase in the released ibuprofen in the first 10 min for the 1G ONTs (Figure 10). A continuous increase in drug content is observed for up to 30 min. After this time, the ibuprofen content began to decrease, and after 60 min, the drug content dropped to 0. In the first 10 min, ibuprofen is released from 16.25% for the 2G ONTs and 10.96% for the 3G ONTs. Between 20 and 30 min, there is an increase in drug release to about 35 and 36%. From 40 min, the release of the drug decreases to less than 10% at 60 min. The high dose released from the 1G ONTs in the first minutes proves the possibility of rapid anti-inflammatory and analgesic effects by releasing the substance from the nanotubular coating, which is necessary to relieve pain in peri-implantation tissues and reduce inflammation without using oral analgesic therapy [65].

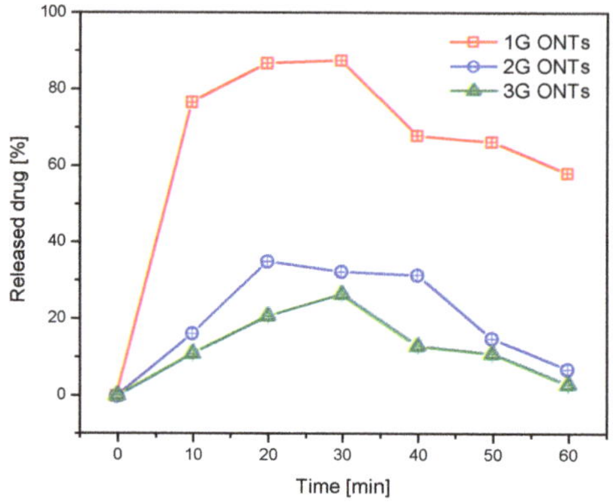

Figure 10. Ibuprofen release profile from the 1G, 2G, and 3G ONTs on the Ti-13Nb-13Zr alloy in function of the time.

Ibuprofen ($C_{16}H_{18}O_2$) is a non-steroidal anti-inflammatory drug, a derivative of propionic acid [66]. It has anti-inflammatory, analgesic, and antipyretic properties. It inhibits platelet aggregation. The action mechanism of ibuprofen is based on the inhibition of the activity of the COX-1 and COX-2 cyclooxygenase enzymes [66]. COX-2 enzyme activity increases rapidly in inflamed tissues. The inhibition of this enzyme by ibuprofen reduces the inflammatory process from the first moments of action. Orally administered ibuprofen has a number of side effects. Therefore, the administration of ibuprofen in the form of a drug release system reduces the risk of side effects without irritating the gastrointestinal mucosa, which is especially important in ulceration and bleeding from the stomach and duodenum [67]. Ibuprofen is a drug that cannot be used long-term, like antibiotics [67]. Therefore, the rapid release of a dose of ibuprofen in the first moment after implantation can effectively inhibit the action of the COX-2 enzyme and thus limit the development of the first inflammation in the tissues surrounding the implant. Orally administered ibuprofen disintegrates very rapidly. The disintegration time of ibuprofen in the liver is about 2 h; therefore, ibuprofen is an excellent substance for application in controlled drug release systems [68–70]. The drug immobilized inside the nanotubes must be soluble in water environments so that they dissolve in body fluids, in particular in blood. This condition must be met to achieve full biodistribution in the human body. The advantage of using ibuprofen is that it is 90% bound to plasma proteins [70].

In addition, the material to which the drug is applied must be biocompatible. Oxide nanotubes belong to a group of materials characterized by a developed and diversified surface, and thus a greater possibility of application of therapeutics [71]. In the case of ONTs of the 1G, 2G, and 3G with a single-walled structure, the drug is applied to the inside of the nanotube by attaching the drug to the surface with covalent amide or ester bonds [72,73]. Ibuprofen from the nanotubes is released through the so-called "burst effect", i.e., a rapid release of the drug within the first 15 min [71,74]. The primary mechanism of drug release is the Gallagher–Corrigan model. This model describes a two-stage drug release kinetics. According to the Gallagher–Corrigan model, the first phase of drug release is its burst from the polymer Hep-DOPA matrix. The second stage is slow release, determined by matrix degradation. The rate of the drug release process in this type of drug delivery system is high in the initial period, then it decreases [71].

4. Conclusions

The obtained FE-SEM and TEM results confirmed the presence of the 1G, 2G, and 3G oxide nanotubes on the Ti-13Nb-13Zr alloy surface obtained via anodization in different conditions. The morphological parameters of the obtained oxide nanotubes increased with the increase in the fluorine ions content in the solution causing the increase in the surface roughness. The *Ra* parameter for the 3G ONTs was over 8 times higher in comparison with the 1G ONTs and 10 times higher in relation to the 2G ONTs. XPS studies showed that these nanotubular layers of three generations were composed of TiO_2, Nb_2O_5, ZrO_2, and ZrO_x. The electronic properties of the 1G, 2G, and 3G ONTs tested by the SKP method depended on the content of F^- ions. Statistical analysis of the contact potential difference maps showed that the quantitative parameters in the form of the arithmetic mean and the square root of the height irregularity increased with the increase in the content of fluorine ions in the solution from 0.5% to 4%. The 2G nanotubular oxide layers show the best hydrophilic properties. Biological assessment of hemocompatibility of the obtained ONTs revealed no hemolytic effects confirming the fulfillment of the requirements for clinical use. The best adhesion was shown by the 1G ONTs and the alloy before surface modification. The thrombogenicity of the 2G ONTs and Ti-13Nb-13Zr alloy does not differ from each other, but they have much better athrombogenic properties than the 1G and 3G ONTs. The ibuprofen release profile from the Hep-DOPA matrix from three types of oxide nanotube generation was investigated. A two-stage Gallagher–Corrigan model was selected to describe the kinetics of the ibuprofen release mechanism.

Author Contributions: Conceptualization, B.Ł.; methodology, A.S. and M.G.; software, J.K.; validation, A.S. and M.G.; formal analysis, M.G., K.B., P.O., J.K., M.Z., J.M. and K.D.; investigation, A.S., M.G., K.B., P.O., J.K., M.Z., J.M. and K.D.; resources, A.S.; data curation, A.S.; writing—original draft preparation, A.S.; writing—review and editing, B.Ł., M.G., K.B., P.O. and J.K.; visualization, A.S., M.G., K.B., P.O., J.K., M.Z., J.M. and K.D.; investigation, A.S., M.G., K.B., P.O., J.K., M.Z., J.M. and K.D.; supervision, B.Ł.; project administration, A.S.; funding acquisition, B.Ł. All authors have read and agreed to the published version of the manuscript.

Funding: This research received no external funding.

Data Availability Statement: MDPI Research Data Policies.

Conflicts of Interest: The authors declare no conflict of interest.

References

1. Davis, R.; Singh, A.; Jackson, M.J.; Coelho, R.T.; Prakash, D.; Charalambous, C.P.; Ahmed, W.; da Silva, L.R.R.; Lawrence, A.A. A comprehensive review on metallic implant biomaterials and their subtractive manufacturing. *Int. J. Adv. Manuf. Technol.* **2022**, *120*, 1473–1530. [CrossRef]
2. Branemark, P.I. *The Osseointegration Book: From Calvarium to Calcaneus*, 1st ed.; Quintessence: Berlin, Germany, 2007; ISBN 1850970904/978-1850970903.
3. Dudek, K.; Dulski, M.; Łosiewicz, B. Functionalization of the NiTi Shape Memory Alloy Surface by HAp/SiO_2/Ag Hybrid Coatings Formed on SiO_2-TiO_2 Glass Interlayer. *Materials* **2020**, *13*, 1648. [CrossRef] [PubMed]
4. Stróż, A.; Maszybrocka, J.; Goryczka, T.; Dudek, K.; Osak, P.; Łosiewicz, B. Influence of Anodizing Conditions on Biotribological and Micromechanical Properties of Ti–13Zr–13Nb Alloy. *Materials* **2023**, *16*, 1237. [CrossRef] [PubMed]
5. Łosiewicz, B.; Stróż, A.; Osak, P.; Maszybrocka, J.; Gerle, A.; Dudek, K.; Balin, K.; Łukowiec, D.; Gawlikowski, M.; Bogunia, S. Production, Characterization and Application of Oxide Nanotubes on Ti–6Al–7Nb Alloy as a Potential Drug Carrier. *Materials* **2021**, *14*, 6142. [CrossRef] [PubMed]
6. Aniołek, K.; Łosiewicz, B.; Kubisztal, J.; Osak, P.; Stróż, A.; Barylski, A.; Kaptacz, S. Mechanical properties, corrosion resistance and bioactivity of oxide layers formed by isothermal oxidation of Ti-6Al-7Nb alloy. *Coatings* **2021**, *11*, 505. [CrossRef]
7. Wang, W.; Yeung, K.W.K. Bone grafts and biomaterials substitutes for bone defect repair: A review. *Bioact. Mater.* **2017**, *2*, 224–247. [CrossRef]
8. Jakubowicz, J. (Ed.) Ti-Based Biomaterials. In *Ti-Based Biomaterials*; MDPI: Basel, Switzerland, 2020. [CrossRef]
9. Stróż, A.; Goryczka, T.; Łosiewicz, B. Electrochemical formation of self-organized nanotubular oxide layers on niobium (Review). *Curr. Nanosci.* **2019**, *15*, 42–48. [CrossRef]
10. Stróż, A.; Dercz, G.; Chmiela, B.; Łosiewicz, B. Electrochemical synthesis of oxide nanotubes on biomedical Ti13Nb13Zr alloy with potential use as bone implant. *AIP Conf. Proc.* **2019**, *2083*, 030004. [CrossRef]
11. Szklarska, M.; Dercz, G.; Simka, W.; Łosiewicz, B. Ac impedance study on the interfacial properties of passivated Ti13Zr13Nb alloy in physiological saline solution. *Surf. Interface Anal.* **2014**, *46*, 698–701. [CrossRef]
12. Stróż, A.; Luxbacher, T.; Dudek, K.; Chmiela, B.; Osak, P.; Łosiewicz, B. In Vitro Bioelectrochemical Properties of Second-Generation Oxide Nanotubes on Ti–13Zr–13Nb Biomedical Alloy. *Materials* **2023**, *16*, 1408. [CrossRef]

13. Stróż, A.; Łosiewicz, B.; Zubko, M.; Chmiela, B.; Balin, K.; Dercz, G.; Gawlikowski, M.; Goryczka, T. Production, structure and biocompatible properties of oxide nanotubes on Ti13Nb13Zr alloy for medical applications. *Mater. Charact.* **2017**, *132*, 363–372. [CrossRef]
14. Łosiewicz, B.; Stróż, A.; Kubisztal, J.; Osak, P.; Zubko, M. EIS and LEIS Study on In Vitro Corrosion Resistance of Anodic Oxide Nanotubes on Ti–13Zr–13Nb Alloy in Saline Solution. *Coatings* **2023**, *13*, 875. [CrossRef]
15. Sowa, M.; Piotrowska, M.; Widziołek, M.; Dercz, G.; Tylko, G.; Gorewoda, T.; Osyczka, A.M.; Simka, W. Bioactivity of coatings formed on Ti-13Nb-13Zr alloy using plasma electrolytic oxidation. *Mater. Sci. Eng. C Mater. Biol. Appl.* **2015**, *49*, 159–173. [CrossRef] [PubMed]
16. Levin, M.; Spiro, R.C.; Jain, H.; Falk, M.M. Effects of Titanium Implant Surface Topology on Bone Cell Attachment and Proliferation in vitro. *Med. Devices* **2022**, *15*, 103–119. [CrossRef] [PubMed]
17. Seramak, T.; Zieliński, A.; Serbiński, W.; Zasińska, K. Powder metallurgy of the porous Ti-13Nb-13Zr alloy of different powder grain size. *Mater. Manuf.* **2019**, *34*, 915–920. [CrossRef]
18. Eisenbarth, E.; Velten, D.; Müller, M.; Thull, R.; Breme, J. Biocompatibility of β-stabilizing elements of titanium alloys. *Biomaterials* **2004**, *25*, 5705–5713. [CrossRef]
19. Albrektsson, T.; Brånemark, P.I.; Hansson, H.A.; Lindström, J. Osseointegrated titanium implants: Requirements for ensuring a long-lasting, direct bone-to-implant anchorage in man. *Acta Orthop. Scand.* **1981**, *52*, 155–170. [CrossRef]
20. Shivaram, A.; Bose, S.; Bandyopadhyay, A. Mechanical degradation of TiO_2 nanotubes with and without nanoparticulate silver coating. *J. Mech. Behav. Biomed. Mater.* **2016**, *59*, 508–518. [CrossRef]
21. Williams, D.F. On the mechanisms of biocompatibility. *Biomaterials* **2008**, *29*, 2941–2953. [CrossRef]
22. Schenk, R.K.; Buser, D. Osseointegration: A reality. *Periodontology 2000* **1998**, *17*, 22–35. [CrossRef]
23. Gulati, K.; Maher, S.; Findlay, D.M.; Losic, D. Titania nanotubes for orchestrating osteogenesis at the bone–implant interface. *Nanomedicine* **2016**, *11*, 1847–1864. [CrossRef] [PubMed]
24. Kulkarni, M.; Mazare, A.; Gongadze, E.; Perutkova, Š.; Kralj-Iglič, V.; Milošev, I.; Schmuki, P.; Iglič, A.; Mozetič, M. Titanium nanostructures for biomedical applications. *Nanotechnology* **2015**, *26*, 062002. [CrossRef]
25. Hanawa, T. Titanium–Tissue Interface Reaction and Its Control With Surface Treatment. *Front. Bioeng. Biotechnol.* **2019**, *7*, 170. [CrossRef]
26. Awad, N.K.; Edwards, S.L.; Morsi, Y.S. A review of TiO_2 NTs on Ti metal: Electrochemical synthesis, functionalization and potential use as bone implants. *Mater. Sci. Eng. C Mater. Biol. Appl.* **2017**, *76*, 1401–1412. [CrossRef]
27. Li, Y.; Yang, Y.; Li, R.; Tang, X.; Guo, D.; Qing, Y.; Qin, Y. Enhanced antibacterial properties of orthopedic implants by titanium nanotube surface modification: A review of current techniques. *Int. J. Nanomed.* **2019**, *14*, 7217–7236. [CrossRef]
28. Rani, S.; Roy, S.C.; Paulose, M.; Varghese, O.K.; Mor, G.K.; Kim, S.; Yoriya, S.; LaTempa, T.J.; Grimes, C.A. Synthesis and applications of electrochemically self-assembled titania nanotube arrays. *Phys. Chem. Chem. Phys.* **2010**, *12*, 2780–2800. [CrossRef]
29. Lyndon, J.A.; Boyd, B.J.; Birbilis, N. Metallic implant drug/device combinations for controlled drug release in orthopaedic applications. *J. Control. Release* **2014**, *179*, 63–75. [CrossRef]
30. Al-Dubai, H.; Pittner, G.; Pittner, F.; Gabor, F. Biocompatible medical implant materials with binding sites for a biodegradable drug-delivery system. *Nanotechnol. Sci. Appl.* **2011**, *4*, 87–94. [CrossRef]
31. Wu, B.; Tang, Y.; Wang, K.; Zhou, X.; Xiang, L. Nanostructured Titanium Implant Surface Facilitating Osseointegration from Protein Adsorption to Osteogenesis: The Example of TiO_2 NTAs. *Int. J. Nanomed.* **2022**, *17*, 1865–1879. [CrossRef] [PubMed]
32. Roy, P.; Berger, S.; Schmuki, P. TiO_2 Nanotubes: Synthesis and Applications. *Angew. Chem. Int. Ed.* **2011**, *50*, 2904–2939. [CrossRef] [PubMed]
33. Smołka, A.; Rodak, K.; Dercz, G.; Dudek, K.; Łosiewicz, B. Electrochemical Formation of Self-Organized Nanotubular Oxide Layers on Ti13Zr13Nb Alloy for Biomedical Applications. *Acta Phys. Pol. A* **2014**, *125*, 932–935. [CrossRef]
34. Smołka, A.; Dercz, G.; Rodak, K.; Łosiewicz, B. Evaluation of Corrosion Resistance of Nanotubular Oxide Layers on the Ti13Zr13Nb Alloy in Physiological Saline Solution. *Arch. Metall. Mater.* **2015**, *60*, 2681–2686. [CrossRef]
35. Stróż, A.; Dercz, G.; Chmiela, B.; Stróż, D.; Łosiewicz, B. Electrochemical Formation of Second Generation TiO_2 Nanotubes on Ti13Nb13Zr Alloy for Biomedical Applications. *Acta Phys. Pol. A* **2016**, *130*, 1079–1080. [CrossRef]
36. Aïnouche, L.; Hamadou, L.; Kadri, A.; Benbrahim, N.; Bradai, D. Interfacial Barrier Layer Properties of Three Generations of TiO_2 Nanotube Arrays. *Electrochim. Acta* **2014**, *133*, 597–609. [CrossRef]
37. Panaitescu, E.; Richter, C.; Menon, L. A Study of Titania Nanotube Synthesis in Chloride-Ion-Containing Media. *J. Electrochem. Soc.* **2008**, *155*, E7. [CrossRef]
38. *ASTM F756-17*; Standard Practice For Assessment Of Hemolytic Properties Of Materials. ASTM International: West Conshohocken, PA, USA, 2017.
39. *ISO 10993-5:2009*; Biological Evaluation of Medical Devices-Part 5: Tests for In Vitro Cytotoxicity. ISO: Geneva, Switzerland, 2009.
40. Dhurat, R.; Sukesh, M. Principles and Methods of Preparation of Platelet-Rich Plasma: A Review and Author's Perspective. *J. Cutan. Aesthet. Surg.* **2014**, *7*, 189–197. [CrossRef]
41. Gawlikowski, M.; Major, R.; Mika, B.; Komorowski, D.; Janiczak, K.; Tkacz, E.; Tamulewicz, A.; Piaseczna, N. Semi-Quantitative Method of Assessing the Thrombogenicity of Biomaterials Intended for Long-Term Blood Contact. *Materials* **2023**, *16*, 38. [CrossRef] [PubMed]

42. Handzlik, P.; Gutkowski, K. Synthesis of oxide nanotubes on Ti13Nb13Zr alloy by the electrochemical method. *J. Porous Mater.* **2019**, *26*, 1631–1637. [CrossRef]
43. Łosiewicz, B.; Skwarek, S.; Stróż, A.; Osak, P.; Dudek, K.; Kubisztal, J.; Maszybrocka, J. Production and Characterization of the Third-Generation Oxide Nanotubes on Ti-13Zr-13Nb Alloy. *Materials* **2022**, *15*, 2321. [CrossRef]
44. Łosiewicz, B.; Osak, P.; Maszybrocka, J.; Kubisztal, J.; Stach, S. Effect of Autoclaving Time on Corrosion Resistance of Sandblasted Ti G4 in Artificial Saliva. *Materials* **2020**, *13*, 4154. [CrossRef] [PubMed]
45. Ossowska, A.; Sobieszczyk, S.; Supernak, M.; Zielinski, A. Morphology and properties of nanotubular oxide layer on the "Ti–13Zr–13Nb" alloy. *Surf. Coat. Technol.* **2014**, *258*, 1239–1248. [CrossRef]
46. Suzuki, K.; Aoki, K.; Ohya, K. Effects of surface roughness of titanium implants on bone remodeling activity of femur in rabbits. *Bone* **1997**, *21*, 507–514. [CrossRef]
47. Schmidt, C.; Kaspar, D.; Sarkar, M.R.; Claes, L.E.; Ignatius, A.A. A scanning electron microscopy study of human osteoblast morphology on five orthopedic metals. *J. Biomed. Mater.* **2002**, *63*, 252–261. [CrossRef]
48. Biesinger, M.C.; Lau, L.W.M.; Gerson, A.R.; Smart, R.S.C. Resolving surface chemical states in XPS analysis of first row transition metals, oxides and hydroxides: Sc, Ti, V, Cu and Zn. *Appl. Surf. Sci.* **2010**, *257*, 887–898. [CrossRef]
49. Vikulova, E.S.; Karakovskaya, K.I.; Korolkov, I.V.; Koretskaya, T.P.; Chepeleva, E.V.; Kuz'min, N.B.; Fedorenko, A.D.; Pischur, D.P.; Guselnikova, T.Y.; Maksimovskii, E.A.; et al. Application of Biocompatible Noble Metal Film Materials to Medical Implants: TiNi Surface Modification. *Coatings* **2023**, *13*, 222. [CrossRef]
50. Naumkin, A.V.; Kraut-Vass, A.; Gaarenstroom, S.W.; Powell, C.J. *NIST X-ray Photoelectron Spectroscopy Database*; NIST Standard Reference Database 20, Version 4.1; National Institute of Standards and Technology: Gaithersburg, MD, USA, 2000.
51. Gondal, M.A.; Fasasi, T.A.; Baig, U.; Mekki, A. Effects of Oxidizing Media on the Composition, Morphology and Optical Properties of Colloidal Zirconium Oxide Nanoparticles Synthesized via Pulsed Laser Ablation in Liquid Technique. *J. Nanosci. Nanotechnol.* **2018**, *18*, 4030–4039. [CrossRef] [PubMed]
52. Kubisztal, J.; Łosiewicz, B.; Dybał, P.; Kozik, V.; Bąk, A. Water-Induced Corrosion Damage of Carbon Steel in Sulfolane. *Energies* **2020**, *13*, 4580. [CrossRef]
53. Łosiewicz, B.; Osak, P.; Maszybrocka, J.; Kubisztal, J.; Bogunia, S.; Ratajczak, P.; Aniołek, K. Effect of Temperature on Electrochemically Assisted Deposition and Bioactivity of CaP Coatings on CpTi Grade 4. *Materials* **2021**, *14*, 5081. [CrossRef] [PubMed]
54. Kubisztal, J.; Łosiewicz, B.; Dybal, P.; Kozik, V.; Bak, A. Temperature-Related Corrosion Resistance of AISI 1010 Carbon Steel in Sulfolane. *Materials* **2020**, *13*, 2563. [CrossRef]
55. Grigorescu, S.; Pruna, V.; Titorencu, I.; Jinga, V.V.; Mazare, A.; Schmuki, P.; Demetrescu, I. The two step nanotube formation on TiZr as scaffolds for cell growth. *Bioelectrochemistry* **2014**, *98*, 39–45. [CrossRef] [PubMed]
56. Grigorescu, S.; Ungureanu, C.; Kirchgeorg, R.; Schmuki, P.; Demetrescu, I. Various sized nanotubes on TiZr for antibacterial surfaces. *Appl. Surf. Sci.* **2013**, *270*, 190–196. [CrossRef]
57. Kulkarni, M.; Patil-Sen, Y.; Junkar, I.; Kulkarni, C.V.; Lorenzetti, M.; Iglič, A. Wettability studies of topologically distinct titanium surfaces. *Colloids Surf. B Biointerfaces* **2015**, *129*, 47–53. [CrossRef]
58. Shin, D.H.; Shokuhfar, T.; Choi, C.K.; Lee, S.H.; Friedrich, C. Wettability changes of TiO_2 nanotube surfaces. *Nanotechnology* **2011**, *22*, 315704. [CrossRef]
59. Brammer, K.S.; Oh, S.; Cobb, C.J.; Bjursten, L.M.; Heyde, H.; van der Jin, S. Improved bone-forming functionality on diameter-controlled TiO_2 nanotube surface. *Acta Biomater.* **2009**, *5*, 3215–3223. [CrossRef] [PubMed]
60. Citeau, A.; Guicheux, J.; Vinatier, C.; Layrolle, P.; Nguyen, T.P.; Pilet, P.; Daculsi, G. In vitro biological effects of titanium rough surface obtained by calcium phosphate grid blasting. *Biomaterials* **2005**, *26*, 157–165. [CrossRef] [PubMed]
61. Wang, N.; Li, H.; Lü, W.; Li, J.; Wang, J.; Zhang, Z.; Liu, Y. Effects of TiO_2 nanotubes with different diameters on gene expression and osseointegration of implants in minipigs. *Biomaterials* **2011**, *32*, 6900–6911. [CrossRef] [PubMed]
62. Aninwene, G.E.I.; Yao, C.; Webster, T.J. Enhanced osteoblast adhesion to drug-coated anodized nanotubular titanium surfaces. *Int. J. Nanomed.* **2008**, *3*, 257–264. [CrossRef]
63. Oh, S.; Daraio, C.; Chen, L.H.; Pisanic, T.R.; Fiñones, R.R.; Jin, S. Significantly accelerated osteoblast cell growth on aligned TiO_2 nanotubes. *J. Biomed. Mater. Res. A* **2006**, *78A*, 97–103. [CrossRef]
64. Bauer, S.; Pittrof, A.; Tsuchiya, H.; Schmuki, P. Size-effects in TiO_2 nanotubes: Diameter dependent anatase/rutile stabilization. *Electrochem. Commun.* **2011**, *13*, 538–541. [CrossRef]
65. Shankland, N.; Wilson, C.C.; Florence, A.J.; Cox, P.J. Refinement of Ibuprofen at 100 K by Single-Crystal Pulsed Neutron Diffraction Conmaent. *Acta Cryst.* **1997**, *C53*, 951–954. [CrossRef]
66. Bushra, R.; Aslam, N. An Overview of Clinical Pharmacology of Ibuprofen. *Oman Med. J.* **2010**, *25*, 155–161. [CrossRef]
67. Al-Janabi, A.A. In vitro antibacterial activity of Ibuprofen and acetaminophen. *J. Glob. Infect. Dis.* **2010**, *2*, 105–108. [CrossRef]
68. Zhao, P.; Liu, H.; Deng, H.; Xiao, L.; Qin, C.; Du, Y.; Shi, X. A study of chitosan hydrogel with embedded mesoporous silica nanoparticles loaded by ibuprofen as a dual stimuli-responsive drug release system for surface coating of titanium implants. *Colloids Surf. B Biointerfaces* **2014**, *123*, 657–663. [CrossRef]
69. Ren, Z.; Romar, H.; Varila, T.; Xu, X.; Wang, Z.; Sillanpää, M.; Leiviskä, T. Ibuprofen degradation using a Co-doped carbon matrix derived from peat as a peroxymonosulphate activator. *Environ. Res.* **2021**, *193*, 110564. [CrossRef]

70. Jia, H.; Kerr, L.L. Sustained ibuprofen release using composite poly(lactic-co-glycolic acid)/titanium dioxide nanotubes from Ti implant surface. *J. Pharm. Sci.* **2013**, *102*, 2341–2348. [CrossRef]
71. Jarosz, M.; Pawlik, A.; Szuwarzyński, M.; Jaskuła, M.; Sulka, G.D. Nanoporous anodic titanium dioxide layers as potential drug delivery systems: Drug release kinetics and mechanism. *Colloids Surf. B Biointerfaces* **2016**, *143*, 447–454. [CrossRef] [PubMed]
72. Oyetade, O.A.; Martincigh, B.S.; Skelton, A.A. The Interplay between Electrostatic and Hydrophobic Interactions in the pH-Dependent Adsorption of Ibuprofen onto Acid-Functionalized Multiwalled Carbon Nanotubes. *J. Phys. Chem. C* **2018**, *122*, 22556–22568. [CrossRef]
73. Kurtoglu, Y.E.; Mishra, M.K.; Kannan, S.; Kannan, R.M. Drug release characteristics of PAMAM dendrimer-drug conjugates with different linkers. *Int. J. Pharm.* **2010**, *384*, 189–194. [CrossRef] [PubMed]
74. Saravanan, M.; Bhaskar, K.; Srinivasa Rao, G.; Dhanaraju, M.D. Ibuprofen-loaded ethylcellulose/polystyrene microspheres: An approach to get prolonged drug release with reduced burst effect and low ethylcellulose content. *J. Microencapsul.* **2003**, *20*, 289–302. [CrossRef]

Journal of
Functional
Biomaterials

MDPI

Review

Drug Delivery Application of Functional Nanomaterials Synthesized Using Natural Sources

Mekala Veerapandian [1,†], Subramaniyan Ramasundaram [2,†], Peter Jerome [2], Gayathri Chellasamy [1], Saravanan Govindaraju [1], Kyusik Yun [1,*] and Tae Hwan Oh [2,*]

[1] Department of Bionanotechnology, Gachon University, Soengnam 13120, Republic of Korea; mekalaveerapandian@gmail.com (M.V.); gayathri.chellasamy@gmail.com (G.C.); biovijaysaran@gmail.com (S.G.)
[2] School of Chemical Engineering, Yeungnam University, Gyeongsan 38436, Republic of Korea; ramasundaram79@hotmail.com (S.R.); jeromepeter7688@gmail.com (P.J.)
* Correspondence: ykyusik@gachon.ac.kr (K.Y.); taehwanoh@ynu.ac.kr (T.H.O.)
† These authors contributed equally to this work.

Abstract: Nanomaterials (NMs) synthesized from natural sources have been attracting greater attention, due to their intrinsic advantages including biocompatibility, stimuli-responsive property, nontoxicity, cost-effectiveness, and non-immunogenic characteristics in the biological environment. Among various biomedical applications, a breakthrough has been achieved in the development of drug delivery systems (DDS). Biocompatibility is necessary for treating a disease safely without any adverse effects. Some components in DDS respond to the physiological environment, such as pH, temperature, and functional group at the target, which facilitates targeted drug release. NM-based DDS is being applied for treating cancer, arthritis, cardiovascular diseases, and dermal and ophthalmic diseases. Metal nanomaterials and carbon quantum dots are synthesized and stabilized using functional molecules extracted from natural sources. Polymers, mucilage and gums, exosomes, and molecules with biological activities are directly derived from natural sources. In DDS, these functional components have been used as drug carriers, imaging agents, targeting moieties, and super disintegrants. Plant extracts, biowaste, biomass, and microorganisms have been used as the natural source for obtaining these NMs. This review highlights the natural sources, synthesis, and application of metallic materials, polymeric materials, carbon dots, mucilage and gums, and exosomes in DDS. Aside from that, challenges and future perspectives on using natural resources for DDS are also discussed.

Keywords: natural sources; drug delivery system: metallic nanoparticles; polymeric nanomaterials; carbon dots; mucilage and gums; exosomes

1. Introduction

Nano drug carriers are important for addressing the delivery of drugs with poor solubility, high toxicity, and less bioavailability. Various nanocarriers synthesized from natural resources such as organic, metallic, and polymeric NMs, including liposomes, exomes, dendrimers, and micelles, are formulated for target DDS. A depiction of the different shapes and types of the natural sources of NMs toward DDS is shown in Figure 1. As synthesized nanomaterials have different shapes such as nanosheets, nanopins, nanotubes, etc., and different sizes, they are being used as DDS for various diseases like cancer, brain, heart, skin, and bone diseases. Their properties, such as size, surface charge, shape, and hydrophobicity, also enhance the bioactivity of nanomaterials. As a substitute for synthetic materials, NMs prepared using natural sources can be incorporated in DDS for performing various functions such as carrier, imaging, stimuli responsive moiety, and super disintegrant. The natural resource-based synthesis of NMs started from the 1900s [1–3]. Mostly, phenols, alcohols, saponins, alkaloids, and terpenes containing natural resources have been used. Various types of natural sources such as plant extracts, roots, stems, flowers, and microorganisms have been used for the synthesis of the above-mentioned nanomaterials [4]. In particular, the plant extracts, activated carbon, biomass, biowaste, fungi, algae, bacteria, chitosan, gelatin, fibrin, cellulose, and chitin are some of the natural sources used for obtaining these NMs. The natural resources used for the synthesis and morphology of NMs for various biomedical applications is presented in Figure 2. The use of natural resources improves the safety of the final product. The use of natural resources for the synthesis offers renewable materials based on green technology and reduces the hazardous components, such as toxic chemicals as reducing agents, surfactants, and the risks in post effluent treatments.

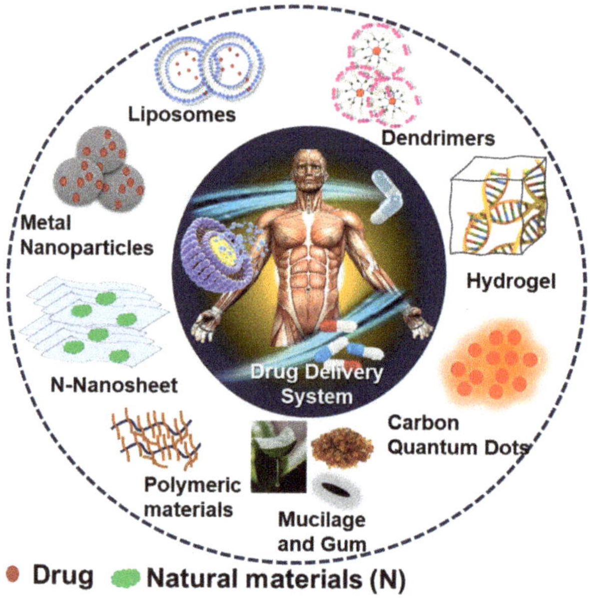

Figure 1. Depiction of the different shapes and structural NMs toward drug delivery systems.

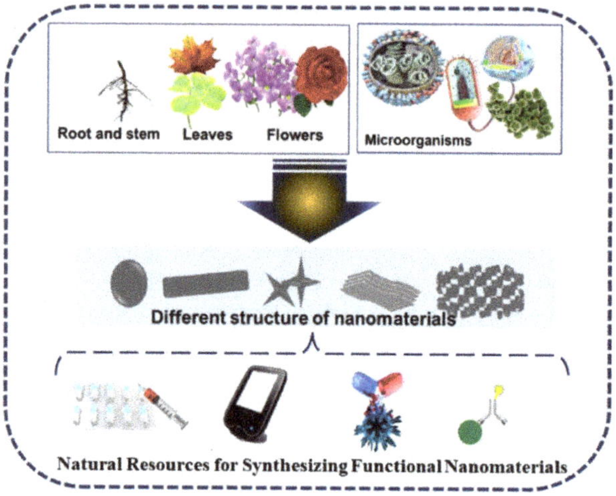

Figure 2. Plant parts and microorganisms used in the synthesis of functional nanomaterials toward biomedical application.

Unlike synthetic materials, the components derived from natural resources or sustainable biological systems do not possess potential side effects or inherent toxicity. The functional NMs from renewable natural resources offer biocompatibility, versatile surface functionalities, and biodegradability. The improvement in biocompatibility increases the safety margin of drugs as they prevent side effects and drug rejection [5]. Biocompatible and biodegradable functional components can minimize the toxicity of nonbiodegradable residual parts used in DDS. DDS based on natural anticancer agents exhibits improved bioavailability, biodistribution, therapeutic activity, and stability [6,7]. For example, naturally derived tricalcium phosphate (TCP) shows high protein encapsulation efficiency than synthetic TCP with an identical Ca/P ratio [8]. These green drug carriers were found to increase the therapeutic activity of anticancer drugs by facilitating the controlled release and increasing the extent of targeting [9].

The naturally derived molecules have been used in the synthesis of metal-based NMs due to their reducing and stabilizing properties. The molecules with reducing and capping properties are used for the single-step synthesis of metal- and metal oxide-based NMs, especially nanoparticles (NPs). Gold (Ag), copper (Cu), silver (Ag), and iron oxide (Fe_2O_3) are used in typical DDS. The metal-based NMs are widely used in DDS as a therapeutic agent and imaging agent for diagnosis. Certain phytoconstituents, phenolics, enzymes, vitamins, proteins, polysaccharides, and other biomolecules possess the natural behavior of reduction and capping. Once the stock of natural extract is obtained, the natural resource-based synthesis can be completed in a single step that is economic and consumes less time than the chemical methods [3,10]. Bottom-up and top-down synthesis methodologies based on the natural sources are depicted in Figure 3.

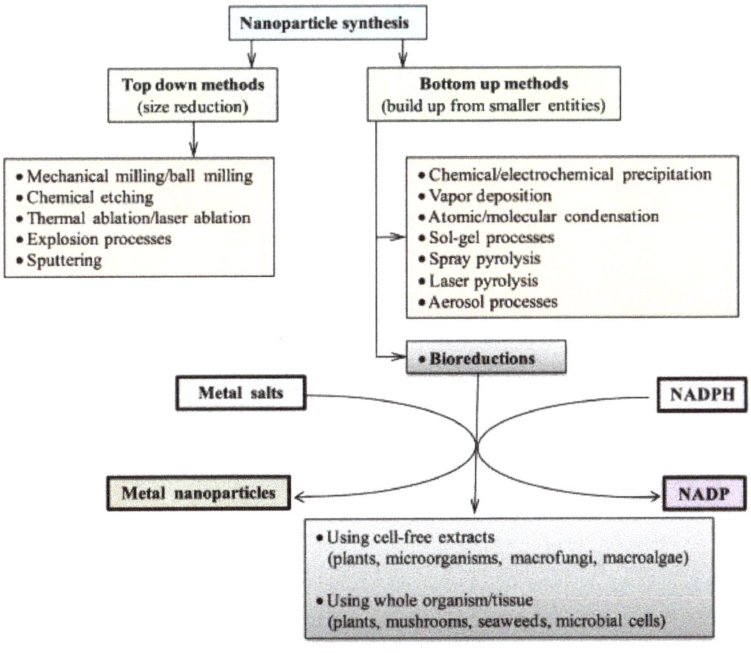

Figure 3. Bottom-up and top-down synthesis methodologies used in natural source-based functional nanomaterials synthesis (adopted with permission from Ref. [3]).

In DDS, naturally obtained polymers are used as a carrier, stimuli responsive moiety, target specific biding interface, and stealth coating. The molecules with biological activity, such as anticancer, antimicrobial, and anticoagulant activity, was used as therapeutic agents or natural drugs. Plant- or microbe-derived poly(saccharides) and poly(phenols) can act as a mechanical support ligand for linking and delivering the drug [11]. Natural polymers are ecofriendly, nonirritant, biodegradable, biocompatible, cheap, and easily available. Chitosan acquired from animals, plants, seaweed, and microorganisms is an excellent example of a naturally derived biopolymeric drug carrier. In addition to that, chitosan can reduce and stabilize metal salts. The amino group in chitosan can bind the drugs and biological molecules via a non-covalent interaction sensitive to pH, temperature, and molecules using competitive interactions [12–14].

Carbon quantum dots (CDs) have functional groups such as hydroxyl, epoxy, carboxyl, and amino on their surface and these surface moieties can bind with inorganic or organic functional groups endowing both covalent and non-covalent interactions. CDs are capable of molecular recognition. When irradiated under ultraviolet radiation (UV, λ = 370 nm), CDs exhibit fluorescence. In DDS, CDs function as performance components for imaging, targeting, drug delivery, and photodynamic therapy. The hydrothermal carbonization of natural resources and waste spanning from rice husk to food waste have been used as the raw materials for preparing natural carbon-based CDs (NCDs) [15,16]. The plant-derived mucilage and gums (MGs) are also used as the drug encapsulation matrix and environment-responsive drug release agents. MGs are a bio macromolecular assembly. MGs have been traditionally used as the excipient and bioadhesive in drug formulations. Excipients are the non-active constituents in the drug formulation, such as the protective coating, bulking agent, binders, diluents, coloring material, and flavoring agents. MGs exhibit mucoadhesive behavior and are stable, non-toxic, naturally available in abundance, and undergoes less regulatory issues than the synthetic polymers [17,18].

Exosomes are small endosomal, naturally nanosized (30–150 nm) extracellular vesicular structures that are enclosed by a lipid bilayer membrane. Exosomes are mostly present in eukaryotic cells and released from the cells during several physiological processes. Despite their early discovery in 1980 [19], most often, due to its secretion from the cells via several metabolic processes resulting from cell damage, cellular homeostasis, etc., they were initially distinguished as "cellular wastes" [20]. Later, exosomes emerged as "superior functional nanovehicles" due to reasons such as the significance of these membrane-enclosed extracellular vehicles (EVs) in establishing intercellular communication, their ability to penetrate the bio membranes and escape during metabolic destruction, the lack of undesired accumulation, and their innate biocompatibility [21,22]. As far as DDS is concerned, the source, processing, synthesizing methodology, and functionalization of the above functional NMs are the most important. This review discusses the important efforts taken towards the development of DDS based on metallic materials, polymeric materials, NCDs, MGs, and exosomes derived or synthesized using natural resources.

2. Natural Source-Synthesized Au and Ag NPs in Drug Delivery Systems

Flavonoids also play a main role in the NMs' synthesis as a reducing agent and in the chelation of metal ions. Flavonoids from the *Ocimum basilicum* and *Mangifera indica* leaf were used for the synthesis of Ag NPs and plays a main role in the reduction in Ag ions to Ag NPs. The other most potential flavonoid, quercetin, also acts as a strong chelating agent due to its carbonyl and hydroxyl groups. These kinds of biological molecules have important roles in the synthesis of NMs to inhibit its aggregation and enhance the stability and solubility in biomedical applications. Vitamin C is also a well-known reducing agent, as it can reduce the metal ions into metal NPs in an aqueous medium. Vitamin C is used to reduce the iron hydroxide into iron NPs during the hydrothermal process. The other vitamins, like B and E, are also used to reduce the metal ions into metal NPs [23–27]. Biosynthesized metallic NPs possess various biological activities such as anti-cancer, anti-inflammatory, and antimicrobial activities. When combined with drugs, these biological activities are used for addressing drug resistance.

The surface plasmonic properties of metallic NPs are useful for tracking the biodistribution of drugs via imaging, photothermal therapy, and theranostic applications. Au and Ag NPs have been widely used, as they can be conjugated with various biologically relevant molecules including oligosaccharides and proteins. These molecules are useful for receptor-sensitive targeting of the pathobiological site to be treated. The use of chemical reducing agents such as sodium borohydride, hydrazine hydrate, phenyl hydrazine, and sodium citrate are considered as toxic to humans. These reducing agents require the use of surfactants for stabilization. In order to combat the issues affecting the environment and addressing the toxicity to human health posed by biomedically relevant metallic NPs, biosynthesis methodologies capable of yielding eco-friendly and biocompatible products have been preferred to use in DDS [10]. During biosynthesis, the plant- and microorganism-derived reducing agents have also been used as stabilizing/capping agents. Au and Ag NPs synthesized using plant extract and microbe-derived proteins were reported as efficient to be used in DDS. The selection of natural resource with a high abundance of constituents capable of reducing/capping metallic NPs assures the stability required during their application in DDS.

Kim et al. reported a strategy for preparing NPs of Au, Ag, cadmium selenide (CdSe), and europium selenide (EuSe) inside an alginate gel matrix by using the cell lysate obtained from a recombinant Escherichia coli strain. The alginate gel is used as a bioreactor. The cell lysate contains metal binding proteins, Rabidopsis thaliana phytochelatin synthase (AtPCS), and *Pseudomonas putida* metallothionein (PpMT). When exposed to UV irradiation, the metal precursor reduces to form metal nanoparticles due to the photochemical catalyzing agent and sensitization of the metal precursor. The thiol groups present in the proteins play a pivotal role in the synthesis of metallic NPs. While the metal NPs are used as an imaging agent, the alginate gel is used as a bioreactor as well as a carrier for encapsulating dual drugs, doxorubicin (DOX), and Rifampicin (RIF). The drug release was pH dependent. RIF, encapsulated with CdSe@gel and EuSe@gel, was not released under acidic pH and the release was increased above pH 7.4. The release of RIF was completed within ~250 min. At pH 7.4, DOX release continued up to $\sim$400 min. The electrostatic interaction between alginate and drugs played a decisive role in the drug release [28].

Au NPs (43.0 $\pm$ 2.2 nm) synthesized using the aqueous extract of walnut tree (Juglans regia) bark was used for the controlled release of zonisamide (ZNS, 1,2-benzisoxazole-3-methanesulfonamide). ZNS is an antiepileptic drug used for treating psychiatric and neurological diseases (Parkinson's disease and epilepsy). The polyphenolic compounds present in walnut bark can reduce and cap the metal salts in metal NPs. The ZNM-Au NP complex was prepared via simple solution blending of ZNS and Au NPs. When tested in vitro, ZNS-Au NPs exhibited a controlled release of ZNS. After 10 days, 31% of ZSM was released, whereas an 81% release was noticed when free ZNS was used. The ZNS-Au NP complex also hindered the growth of CTX TNA2 cells. Au NPs were used as a carrier for ZNS, and this complex was proposed as useful in treating acute spinal cord injury [29].

The magnetic, anti-oxidant, antibacterial, and anticandidal properties of Fe_3O_4 NPs (37.8 nm) are widely utilized in theranostic imaging and antibiotic and anticandidal drugs formulations. Patra et al. synthesized Fe_3O_4 NPs using the aqueous extract of corn ear leaves. The major chemical constituent (37 to 64%) present in corn leaves is phytol (3,7,11,15-tetramethyl2-hexadecen-1-ol). The Fe_3O_4 NPs exhibited proteasome inhibitory, antioxidant, and anticandidal activities. Proteasome inhibitory activity was expected useful in cancer treatment and drug delivery. The Fe_3O_4 NPs were considered useful in drug delivery systems meant for addressing the drug resistance and toxicity [30]. Epigallocatechin gallate (EGCG), the polyphenol-type compound found in green tea, was used for synthesizing the flower-shaped Au nanoclusters (50 nm, Au NCs). EGCG is most abundant in green tea and used as both a reducing and capping agent. Au NCs were stable for 6 weeks and used as a carrier for methotrexate and DOX. These drugs were conjugated with Au NCs via a cysteine bridge. This dual drug conjugate was used for tumor-targeted drug delivery. When tested with HeLa cells in both in vivo and in vitro conditions, these conjugates were entered into the cell. The folic acid receptor's overexpressed tumor cells can be targeted by this conjugate. The efficient cellular uptake and sustained drug release increased the bioavailability (acting time) of the drugs [31].

Inorganic NPs can also be synthesized via the metabolism of living microbes, including bacteria, fungi, and yeast. When the metal ions were taken by these organisms, insoluble precipitates were formed via bioreduction caused by the metal-binding protein secreted by this microbe when maintaining homeostasis. Similar to Kim et al., PpMT and AtPCS were used for the in vitro biosynthesis of FeSe NPs under UV irradiation. The FeSe NPs were conjugated with poly-γ-glutamic acid (PGA). This conjugate was used as a carrier for encapsulating DOX, a nonselective anti-cancer drug whose continuous consumption leads to the inherent risk of long-term side effects in the heart, kidney, liver, and brain. So, the targeted and controlled release of DOX is necessary to prevent any side effects. PGA is a non-toxic and naturally occurring peptide capable of exhibiting pH-dependent conformational change. Under acidic pH, PGA can retain the drugs loaded inside the conjugate and quickly releases the drug at pH 6–7. The use of FeSe NPs allowed for the mapping of the biodistribution of the FeSe NPs-PGA-DOX conjugate over time in mice, and also confirmed the delivery of drugs to the target [32].

An aqueous extract of meadow grass, *Poe annua* (*P. annua*), was used for the synthesis of Ag NPs (36 to 43 nm). The flavonoids in *P. annua* can be used as a non-toxic, eco-friendly, and cost-effective reducing agent for the synthesis of Ag NPs. The Ag NPs were coated with flavonoids, phenols, and alkaloids present in *P. annua*. These Ag NPs were used as a carrier for delivering anticancer biomedicine derived from Euphorbia dracunculiodes Lam (EDL). EDL is a medicinal plant used in Indian and Chinese traditional medicine and applied for treating neurodegenerative diseases, cardiovascular diseases, and diabetes mellitus. EDL is a source of phenolic compounds and triterpenoids. The conjugate of Ag NPs and EDL were prepared and stabilized with starch coating. When orally administered to Sprague Dawley rats, there was no significant cytotoxicity found even after 7 days. This conjugate exhibited a good biocompatibility to healthy cells but targeted cancer cells. The combination of biosynthesized Ag NPs and plant-derived anticancer medicine has proven to be a promising anti-cancer nanomedicine [33]. Furthermore, the green-synthesized metal-based NPs have a certain limitation in the parameters (temperature and pH) and stability. The obtained NPs are less stable in nature as compared to chemically-synthesized NPs. NPs ensure stabilization in two ways: electrostatic repulsion and steric stabilization. For the electrostatic repulsion, the extract should have low ionic strength, which results in a more dispersed double layer. In the case of high ionic strength, which leads to the van der Waals interaction. Secondly, the steric stabilization provides the surface barrier [34,35]. For large scale productions, it is necessary to overcome these types of limitations and develop the green synthesis of metal-based nanoparticles.

3. Natural Source-Derived Polymeric Nanomaterials in Drug Delivery Systems

The surface of NMs incorporated with DDS is very important as they directly contact the body fluids and organs. The hydrophilic polymer-coated NMs stay a long time in blood circulation and performs site-specific delivery upon rupture in their interactions with drugs by surrounding the pH and enzymes. Typically, naturally occurring polymers such as poly(peptides), poly (amino acids), poly(saccharides), starch, collagen, alginate, gelatin, elastin, chitosan, and cellulose are known to be degraded under enzymatic conditions. These natural polymers can be obtained from both animal and plant sources. For example, cellulose can be derived from both plants and bacteria. Plants derivatives or bacteria are the main sources for the nanocellulose materials (Nanosize cellulose fibers or nanocrystal). The bacteria species, such as *Gluconacetobacter*, *Agrobacter*. and *Sarcina*, are known to be capable of producing highly pure and water-retaining cellulose. Due to the difficulties in preparing NMs, these natural polymers were cross-linked at the surface of nanosized drugs and imaging agents. A schematic illustration of the application of biopolymer modified with nanoparticles in DDS is shown in Figure 4. The natural polymer-modified surface is used for forming protective, biocompatible, stimuli responsive surfaces [36].

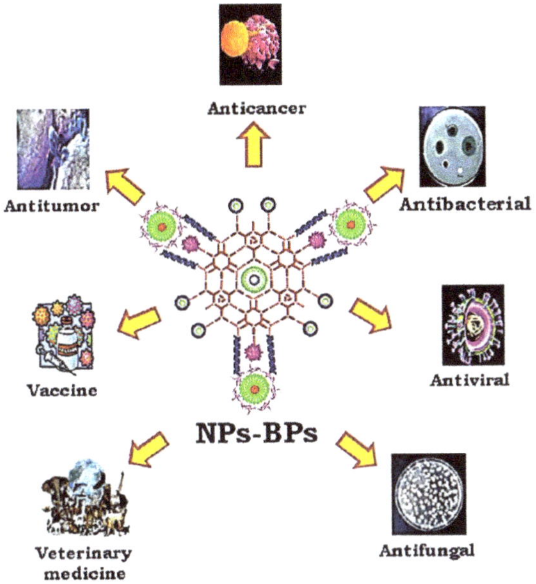

Figure 4. Drug delivery applications of biopolymer modified with nanoparticles (adopted with permission from Ref. [6]).

The biopolymer, Kappa carrageenan (KC), extracted from microalgae was conjugated with ZnO NPs and used as a biofilm-based drug carrier. KC is water soluble and contains sulfated D-galactan. The KC-ZnO conjugate is a non-toxic and eco-friendly "nano-anti super bug drug", used as a nano-antibiotic for treating disease infections caused by Methicillin-resistant Staphylococcus aureus (MRSA). KC functions as a capping agent and plays a major role in inhibiting bacterial cell growth. KC also reduces the hydrophobicity of the bacterial cell surface. As a result, the KC-ZnO nonocomposite was applied to the in vitro anti-inflammatory using the embryonic fibroblast cell line derived from the NIH3T3 mouse. About 82% of anti-inflammatory activity was noticed [37]. Green synthesis of the hydrolyzed starch–chitoson (HS-C-NC) composite were applied as DDS against the Gram-negative bacteria. This combination of two biopolymers loaded with the antibiotic exhibited good results than the individual biopolymer. Ciprofloxacin loaded with HS-C-NC was prepared via an ionic exchange method. The studies carried out in the Gram-negative bacterial strains, *Enterobactor aerogenes* and *Pseudomonas aeruginosa*, demonstrated that the minimum inhibition concentration (MIC) of the Ciprofloxacin-loaded HS-C-NC were 62.5 and 125 μg/mL, respectively. The in vitro drug release study showed a 86% drug release was attained after 20 h at pH 1.5, and it was 33% at pH-7.5. The intact structure and high inhibition activity were considered as the reason for the good performance of HS-C-NC [38].

Almaida, et al. investigated DDS based on the natural rubber latex (NRL) membrane with various pore sizes such as 2000, 6000, and 10,000 pore/cm^2. The drug loading capacity of NRL was evaluated via swelling studies, where the swelling rate of NRL reached its maximum (1.07 ± 0.03 g/g). NRL is used as a solid matrix drug delivery as it enhances the wound healing process. The NRL membrane loaded with ciprofloxacin showed the kinetics of drug release dependence on the pore size linearly increasing at the final concentration. There was an interaction between ciprofloxacin and NRL via hydrogen bonding. The drug release was determined using an ultrafast laser micromachining process [39]. Molecularly-imprinted polymer (Chitosan) (MIP) was also used in DDS. MIP has high chemical and mechanical strength, high absorption, selectivity, and storage capability of a prolonged lifetime without loss of the target molecule. MIP was used as a carrier for riboflavin, a drug used for stabilizing the vitamin B_2 in our body. The drug release was determined via the Higuchi model. Riboflavin loaded in the polymer showed a good drug releasing efficiency (55.07%), with a 1:20 ratio of the NaCl media. This amount is equal to the vitamin B_2 requirement in humans for 5 days [40].

Chitosan is majorly used in DDS because it is a cationic biopolymer, so the drug was easily loaded and served as a good carrier. The functionalization of NPs derived from ginger-derived chitosan (C-GDNC) was used for the controlled release of 5-amino salicylic acid (5-ASA), the drug used for treating inflammatory bowel diseases (IBD). They observed that the controlled release of the drug was more than 50% at pH 6.8. The polysaccharides play a vital role in drug delivery as well as has a self-healing potential against IBD [41]. Lignin-based hallow nanospheres were synthesized using the efficient fast vacuum evaporation process and are used as a carrier for Ibuprofen. This DDS exhibited excellent pH responsive drug delivery because of the repulsive force generated by the deprotonated carboxyl and hydroxyl groups present in lignin. At a neutral pH, a 90% drug release was noticed within 2–3 h, and at pH 1.8, only 18% of drug was released [42].

The biopolymer, pectin, was synthesized from plant cells consisting of rhamnogalacturonan I (RG-I), galacturonan, and rhamnogalacturonan II (RG-II) proanthocyanidine. Gunter et al. green-synthesized pectin from a callus culture encapsulated with ZnO hydrogel beads and used it for developing and delivering drugs in the gastrointestinal tract. The grape seed extract (GSE) delivery system consists of proanthocyanidines and phenol hydroxyl groups, where both have great potential for treating colon inflammation. But, the phenol group present in the GSE has poor stability when it reaches the gastrointestinal tract. When combined with hydrogels, the controlled release of GSE was achieved at pH 2.3 and 5.3. GSE-ZnO hydrogel was found to be promising in DDS for treating colon inflammation [43]. Hyaluronic acid (HA) is anionic polymer and also known as polysaccharides. HA, when combined with polyethyleneimine (PEI) to form nanogels (HA-PEI- NG), is applied for the controlled drug delivery in cancer treatment. In this mechanism, the hyaluronan receptor was involved in the binding process of nanogel, and there was no other surfactant used for drug binding with HA-PEI-NG. The NG was loaded with DOX. The high DOX encapsulation efficiency (83.4%) was noticed. The controlled drug release at the targeting site of the CD44 cell rendered a good therapeutic effect. The drug releasing efficiency in three different media (acidic, neutral, and alkaline) was determined via a drug diffusion mechanism, where the drug releasing efficiencies were 85%, 93%, and 97%, respectively [44]. Based on the literature survey, chitosan played a vital role in DDS due to being less toxic in nature compared to the synthetic polymers. Finally, the biopolymers provided good biomedical application especially in DDS because of their loading and nontoxic behavior. But, it is still necessary to investigate issues associated with stability and long-term-effect-related clinical studies.

4. Natural Source-Derived Carbon Dots in Drug Delivery Systems

NCDs derived from natural sources have gained immense attention for developing DDS. NCDs are synthesized from natural products such as plant extracts, fruit juice, spices, milk, egg yolk oil, lotus root, honey, and food waste. NCDs are eco-friendly, water soluble, biocompatible, and available with diverse functional groups on the surfaces of hydroxyl, carboxyl, and thiol groups. The functional groups of NCDs can easily bind to the surface of metallic, polymeric, and biological molecules. Naturally synthesized CDs have good fluorescent properties and are used for drug delivery and bioimaging applications. NCDs have been used as a tracing probe, photo-activated antioxidant, and therapeutic and neurodegenerative agents [45,46]. Figure 5 depicts the application of NCDs in DDS. Iqra et al. developed an NCD-capped AgO/ZnO nanocomposite using banana juice as source for NCDs and the AgO/ZnO NPs were synthesized from *Fiscus carica* leaf extracts as a reducing agent to carry epirubicin for the chemotherapeutic drug delivery system to the breast cancer cells. This composite DDS inhibited 80% of cell viability, and 90% of cell viability was inhibited at a concentration of 50.0 μM, due to the electron acceptor and transporter property of NCD. When the nanocarrier is used in the acidic medium for the drug release, the cell viability decreased by 54.64% [47]. The nitrogen-functionalized NCD was used as a drug nanocarrier, as Morteza et al. prepared nitrogen-doped NCD and loaded the drug, gemcitabine (GC). The size of the nanocarrier is small, so it can easily enter and penetrate the cell membrane. When compared with a prepared NCD, the nitrogen-doped NCD exhibited a better anticancer effect [48]. NCD synthesized from pasteurized milk via the hydrothermal method served as a multi-functionalized hetero atom CD. These NCDs were used for encapsulating Lisionopril. When tested with HeLa cells, a controlled drug release was noticed at pH 5.2, 6.2, and 7.4. This composite shows as non-toxic to the Hela cells and can be used as effective DDS for treating hypertension and renal diseases [49]. Fluorescent quantum dots were synthesized via the hydrothermal synthesis method from mulberry leaves (*Morus alpha* L.). These NCDs were encapsulated with Lycorine, the anticancer drug, and the cytotoxicity study was performed with LX-2 and HepG2 cell lines. The cell biocompatibility study was performed with LX-2 cell lines. With a concentration up to 500 μg/, the NCDs showed good compatibility, whereas free drug biocompatibility was only up to 12 μg/mL. The NCD-Lycorine composite exhibited high anticancer activity to the HepG2 cell lines than the free drug. Lycorine-CDs can be useful to apply to intracellular imaging and target drug delivery to the cancer cells simultaneously. [50]. Hydroxyapatite-based NCDs (CD-HAP) were hydrothermally synthesized using a biowaste precursor under four different heating temperatures, 150, 170, 190, and 210 °C. The NCDs synthesized at 190 °C delivered high fluorescence and were used as a carrier for Acetaminophen, a common antibiotic. It has the highest loading capacity of 48.5% to the CD-HAP-40 and the drug releases slowed in CD-HAP-40 composite [51]. An aqueous root extract from Korean red ginseng was also used as a natural source for obtaining NCDs via microwave heating and were loaded with the drug, rutin (Ru-CDs). These NCDs were useful as both a drug carrier and imaging agent, emitting multicolor fluorescence and exhibiting reactive oxygen species scavenging in both an extra- and intra-cellular environment. The cytotoxicity study was performed with the NKE cell lines, and the Ru-CDs showed less toxicity at 100 μg/mL. Antibacterial activity was also performed against both the Gram-negative and Gram-positive bacteria under the light expose. It damaged produced more reactive oxygen species and also damaged the DNA in the bacteria [52]. To this extent, the QDs contain only carbon on one hand, and on the other hand, it did not have any toxic or heavy metals. Due to this property, it would be applied in DDS, imaging, and also in cancer therapy. But, there are still some issues related to reproducibility and clinical usage. The issues related to reproducibility should be rectified and more studies are needed that are related to QDs with cells and in vivo studies.

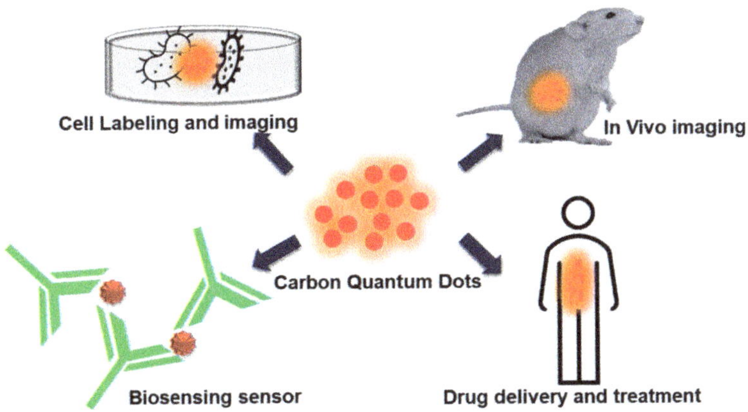

Figure 5. Drug delivery applications of natural resource-derived carbon quantum dots.

5. Natural Source-Derived Mucilage and Gums in Drug Delivery Systems

MGs are naturally occurring, high molecular weight (~200,000) polyuronides with the units of sugar and uronic acid. They are the physiological product of plant metabolism. MGs are produced within the cell, deposited on its walls, and serve as a food reserve and membrane thickener. MGs function as a medium of water storage and aid in the germination of seeds. Figure 6 illustrates the various MGs derived from plant sources. Mucilage and gums (MGs) have been derived from animals, plants, microorganisms, and seaweed. MGs are more abundant in plants than in animals. The gums derived from herbal plants were applied as emulsifying, binding, thickening, suspending, stabilizing, and binding agents and sustained the drug release. Non-ionic (amylose, arabinans, and cellulose) and anionic (arabic, agar, algin, and pectic acid) MGs are available. MGs were extracted via heating and solvent extraction methods. Due to its sticky and mucoadhesive nature, MGs found an application in DDS. Additionally, the compounds present in the gums, named resins and tannins, provide a controlled drug release and inhibitory properties. The highly viscous and gradual swelling-induced slow aqueous solubility behavior of MGS increases the residence time of drug loading on the biological surface, such as ocular and gastrointestinal tracts; thereby, MGs are considered as the suitable carrier matrix for prolonged or sustained drug release. The constant contact established between the biological surface and DDS minimizes the drug resistance. Some of the important DDS-based MGs are discussed in this section [18,53].

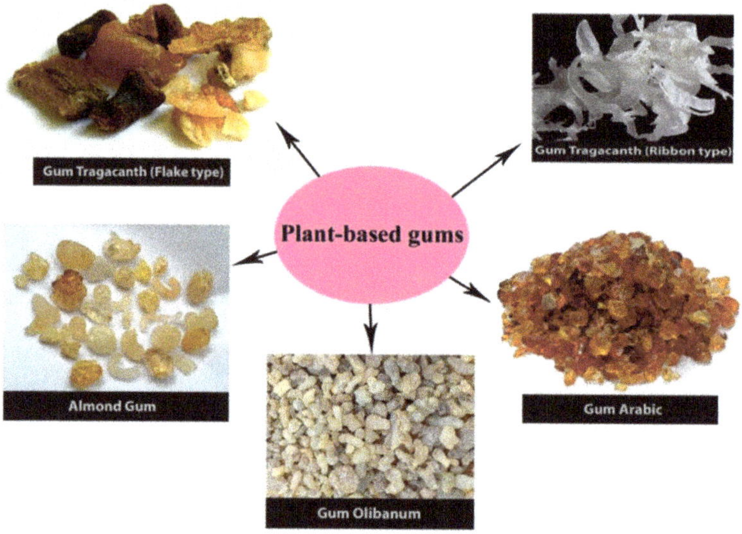

Figure 6. Mucilage and gums derived from various plant sources (adopted with permission from Ref. [54]).

The gum obtained from *Hakea gibbosa* (HG) was used for formulating mucoadhesive and sustained the release Buccal tablets. The chlorpheniramine maleate (CPM) was used as a model drug. The tablets without HG gum released 90% CPM within 14 min, whereas the tablets with 2, 12, 22, and 32 mg of HG gum exhibited a 90% CPM release after 48, 120, 330, and 405 min, respectively. The slow relaxation of the hydrated HG gum resulted in a sustained drug release. Aside from that, the excellent mucoadhesive properties for HG gum formulation and its mucoadhesive strength can be modulated by varying its quantity [54]. Galactomannan gum, derived from the seeds of *Mimosa scabrella*, was used for the controlled release of theophylline. This drug is used for treating asthma and chronic obstructive pulmonary disease. The in vitro drug release studies indicated the decrease in drug release in response to the increase in gum concentration. The formulation with 25% w/w of the gums exhibited an excessive sustained release. An erosion-type drug release was noticed with the tablets with lower gum concentration while high gum content led to fast hydration and swelling [55].

The combination of xanthan and locust bean gum (XlBG) was used for the controlled delivery of Metoprolol tartrate (MPT). Metoprolol tartrate is a nonselective beta-adrenergic blocking agent used for angina pectoris and treating hypertension and cardiovascular disorders. The drug MPT has a limitation related to bioavailability (30%) and drug releasing properties. The drug was suitable for a controlled drug release because it has a very short half-life of about 2–5 h. The rate of drug release was normal with zero-order kinetics and there is no chemical interaction between the drug and the used gum confirmed by DSC thermogram studies. The tablets formulated with xanthan and locust bean gum exhibited a sustained drug release due to the strong and elastic gel formed via the synergistic interaction between these two materials. The swelling and erosion studies revealed that the high ability to swell and the weight loss from the tablet was around 70% for 8 h [56]. *Konjac glucomannan* (KGM), isolated from the tubers of Amorphophallus konjac, was used for formulating sustained DDS with Xanthan. The small molecular drugs, theophylline and diltiazem, were used as the models. The KGM and Xanthan ratio of 1:1 was found to be suitable for obtaining formulation with physical integrity of the drugs and a sustained release of 8 h. In this, the diffusion coefficient value of KGM/XG was lower than individual KGMs, and the value close to XG indicates that the mobility of the drug is determined by the structure of XG. The synergistic interaction of KGM with Xanthan is responsible for the controlled drug release [57].

Mucilage from *Mimosa pudica* seeds contains d-xylose and d-glucuronic acid. These seeds are known to easily undergo hydration and swelling. Diclofenac was formulated with *Mimosa pudica* seeds and dibasic calcium phosphate (diluent). The resultant granules were studied for drug release in an aqueous dissolution media (pH 6.8, 37 °C) for 24 h. Additionally, the mucilage content and swelling property increased in the drug, and the erosion decreased. In response to the increase in the concentration of *Mimosa pudica* seeds, the drug release decreased. As a result, the drug release was dependent on the ratio of mucilage to drug. Granules with high mucilage content followed the diffusion type release while lower mucilage content led to a drug release via erosion and diffusion. Granules with a 1:40 mucilage to diclofenac ratio matches the commercially sustained release formulation [58]. Ganesh et al. used cashew nut tree gum for the sustained release of diclofenac Sodium. The tablets were formulated using cashew nut tree gum, hydroxypropyl methyl cellulose, and Carbopol. These tablets exhibited a sustained release. That is, the kinetics studies reveals that the drug releasing rate decreased as the CG content increased about 40% in the matrix. Since the gum content is too low, the formation of the gel layer did not occur on the surface. Higher amounts of CG lead to the prolonged drug release in a controlled manner. The advantages are lower dose intake, minimum blood level oscillations, low risk of adverse effects, and improved patient compliance [59].

When mixed with natural gums, the commercial xanthan gum proved to exhibit a synergistic effect for a colon-specific sustained release in a controlled drug delivery. The mixture of Xanthan and the natural gum galactomannan extracted from *Gleditsia sinensis Lam* was studied for the sustained release of theophylline. The formulation with 10% of each component released ~90% of the drug after 24 h. The synergistic interactions between these gums and the relaxational and diffusional drug release mechanism effectively controlled the drug release. The relation between hydration and drug release was characterized by the morphological changes and radial swelling behavior of the drug. Xanthan and galactomannan, with a ratio of 7:3, demonstrated a good performance in terms of the sustained release (75.5% after 24 h). These kinds of studies are evident for the potential of xanthan gum towards sustained and targeted DDS [60]. Mucoadhesive microspheres formulated with non-toxic and edible polysaccharide were extracted from the okra fruit (*Abelmoschus esculentus*). *A. esculentus* contains galacturonic acid, galctose, and rhamnose, where the components act as high absorbents due to its high-level polar groups. This leads to the formation complex with gel consistency and a bioadhesive compound. This formulation was studied for the nasal delivery of rizatriptan benzoate. This drug is used for narrowing brain blood vessels and treating severe headaches. Microspores were prepared via emulsification. Epichlorohydrin was used as the cross-linking agent. About 50% of the drug was released within 15 min and the remaining 50% was sustained for an hour. An increase in the polysaccharide concentration decreased the drug release. When administered to the nasal cavity of rabbits, the nasal retention of these microspheres was found to be better than the aqueous solution. The use of okra polysaccharides as a carrier for nasal delivery formulation improved the retention at the nasal surface and minimized the drainage via mucociliary clearance [61].

The mucoadhesive formulation-based oral DDS is suitable for sustained drug release. The good drug adhesion of DDS to the biological surface increases drug residence time and bioavailability. Mucoadhesive beads containing a glibenclamide *Plantago ovata F.* husk mucilage–alginate was prepared using a ionotropic gelation method and studied for sustained release. $CaCl_2$ was used as the cross-linker. The drug encapsulation efficiency of the mucoadhesive beads was $94.43 \pm 4.80\%$ w/w with a rate of zero-order kinetics. Good mucoadhesive with the biological membrane was observed, and drug release was sustained for 10 h. The adhesive nature of beads was different for different pHs, with the gastric pH (1.2) being $64.88 \pm 5.06\%$, but the intestinal pH was $30.47 \pm 3.86\%$. When orally administered to alloxan-induced diabetic rats, a significant antidiabetic effect was noticed for a prolonged period, with a rapid reduction in the blood glucose level within 2–3 h. Therefore, the glibenclamide-Plantago ovata F. husk mucilage–alginate formulation proved to be suitable for the sustained release of glibenclamide and for improving patient compliance in managing noninsulin-dependent diabetes [62]. With the objective of drug delivery to the colon, gum from *Grewia mollis Juss* stem bark was used to formulate Ibuprofen. Compression-coated Ibuprofen tablets were formed using powder and granules of this gum or hydroxypropyl methyl cellulose (HPMC). The drug release was studied under simulated gastro-intestinal fluids. The GC-coated tablets exhibited the prolonged half-life (8.66 h) and the oral relative bioavailability of GC was noted as 87.65%, which indicates the remarkable reduced side effects and considered colon delivery system. Ibuprofen remained for a longer time in the gum powder-coated tablets than in others. In the in vivo studies conducted with New Zealand rabbits, it was confirmed that the gum powder-coated formulation delivered the drug to the colon, and the release in the gastrolienal tract was minimized. Thus, the Grewia mollis stem bark gum–Ibuprofen formulation can be effectively used in colon-specific DDS [63].

Almond gum (prunus amygdalus exudes) was used for the colon-specific formulation of 5-aminosalicylic acid, an anti-inflammatory agent known to be degraded by gastric fluid in stomach. Microcrystalline cellulose was used as diluents. The developed matrix was evaluated by various studies concerning diameter, hardness, weight variation, friability, and in vitro drug release. The in vitro drug release studies confirmed that at pH 1.2, the drug release was controlled, and after 10 h, the drug release was 50% [64]. Chitosan extracted from discarded shells of Carinosquilla multicarinata was used for the sustained release of Diclofenac. The Chitosan and tripolyphosphate formulation with the ratio of 2.5:1 exhibited maximum drug encapsulation efficiency. When studied using simulated biological fluid (pH 7.4), 10 h was taken to observe an 80% drug release. The drug release profile suggests that chitosan NPs are stable enough to deliver a sustained drug release than the free drug. This work proves that the marine scrap from fisheries can be effectively used in DDS meant for curing anti–inflammatory diseases [65].

Aloe vera (AV) mucilage-polyacrylamide DDS was prepared by polymerizing acrylamide using the free radical polymerization of acrylamide in the presence of Aloe vera mucilage. An increase in the concentration of AV mucilage enhanced swelling, porosity, and drug release, and meanwhile, decreased gel formation. High hydroxyl group content made this DDS more hydrophilic. In the case of DDS with 2% AV mucilage, within 30 min, the drug release exceeded 85% at pH 1.2 and pH 7.4. Mixing with hydrophobic type MGs can render a prolonged drug release property [66]. The buoyancy and anti-ulcer activity of okra mucilage was utilized for gastro-retentive DDS formulations for delivering antacids. This formulation minimized the side effects. As it is an anti-diabetic food, the use of okra has an additional advantage. The use of food products for DDS purposes can be useful to avoid a series of complex medical trials [67].

The super disintegrant property of MGs can be used for developing rapid DDS. Mucilage extracted from *Plantago ovata* (PO) was used to develop fast disintegrating Diclofenac potassium tablets. *Plantago ovata* mucilage is known to be a natural super disintegrant. Diclofenac Potassium is a non-steroidal, anti-inflammatory, analgesic, and antipyretic drug. It is absorbed faster in the gastrointestinal tract than by the Diclofenac sodium salt. PO mucilage-containing tablets exhibited fast disintegration (18 s) than the commercial disintegrant-containing (Sodium Starch Glycolate = 39 s, and Ac-Di-Sol = 49 s) tablets [68]. Apart from PO, a large number of MGs are available and studied for super disintegrant application. MGs from fenugreek seeds, Lepidium sativum, karaya gum, Cassia fistula, guar gum, *Hibiscus rosa-sinensis* Linn, pectin from mango peel, soy polysaccharides, dehydrated banana powder, and locust beans have been explored as super disintegrants in DDS [69].

6. Natural Source-Derived Exosomes in Drug Delivery Systems

As an efficient drug cargo, exosomes can be diversely modified with therapeutic biomolecules, nucleic acids, proteins, etc., which are critical in the discovery of advanced clinical diagnostics predominantly as drug delivery agents and biomarkers. Apart from exosomes, more extensive research has been established in the development of polymeric nanoparticles and liposomes for their broad range of applicability for antifungal and anticancer drugs, analgesics, and biocompatibility with a long-circulating capability by evading the immune system [70,71]. However, the intrinsic targeting ability of exosomes with minimally invasive effects to the cells or tissues recognizes them as a protected natural carrier bypassing immune responses and engulfment by lysosomes and phagocytosis. Figure 7 depicts the application of exomes in DDS.

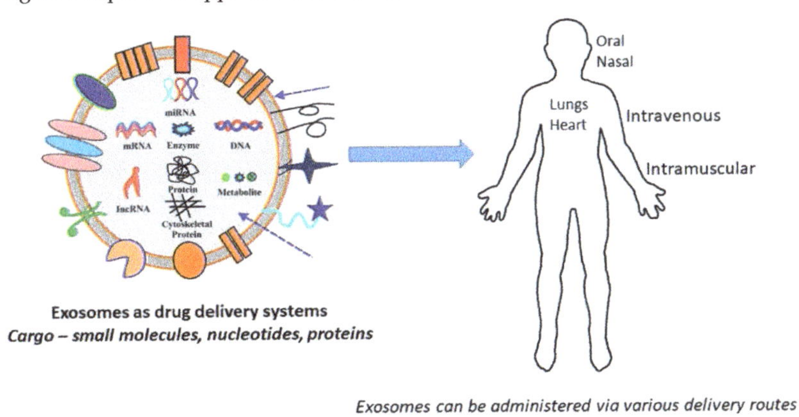

Figure 7. Application of Exosomes in DDS (adopted with permission from Ref. [72]).

Recently, exosomes have gained greater attention for their crucial role in bridging cell-to-cell communication during several pathophysiological processes. Although the exosomes were initially discovered in mammalian systems, its current spotlight as new biologically active substances in plants can extend their applicability as cargos for biomolecules that directly influences the growth of plants and develops protective mechanisms against pathogens [73]. Such plant exosomes are nanosized membrane-bound vesicles secreted by the plant cells, which serve as natural cargos for the transport of diverse biomolecules, including proteins, nucleic acids, lipids, and metabolites. To expand the scope of drug therapies, plant-derived exosome-like nanoparticles (PENs) are expected to boom as modern therapeutic modalities which are biocompatible, eco-friendly, and cost-effective with abundantly available nanoplatforms [72].

Generally, PENs undergo few common techniques such as biogenesis, isolation, sequential characterization, and other drug delivery methods that are necessary to enhance its stabilized utility, transport, and long-term circulation [74]. Based on the fundamental features and bioactivities of PENs, these exosomes and other secondary metabolites were widely extracted from diverse plant species including ginseng, grape, grapefruit, green tea, lemon, broccoli, etc., refs. [73,75]. Interestingly, plant exosomes are derived from the endosomal system through the biogenesis process involved in the formation of the intraluminal vesicles (ILVs) within the multivesicular bodies (MVBs) governed by endosomal sorting complex, which is required for transport (ESCRT) machinery. Two main pathways contribute to plant exosome biogenesis: the ESCRT-dependent pathway and the ESCRT-independent pathway. The ESCRT-dependent pathway facilitates the invagination of the endosomal membrane and cargo sorting, which plays a crucial role in the formation of ILVs and the subsequent exosome release. Meanwhile, the ESCRT-independent pathway involves lipid raft formation and exosome secretion (with the help of ESCRT-associated proteins) [76,77].

Intriguingly, the exosome release in certain plants, like grapefruit and tomato, are influenced by specific cargo compositions such as proteins, nucleic acids, lipids, and metabolites, which can be isolated from their flesh, juice extracts, and roots. Grapefruit and tomato exosome vesicles are known to contain diverse arrays of proteins, such as the enzymes that are involved in metabolic pathways (hydrolases, transferases, and oxidoreductases) the intercellular signaling molecules, including growth factors, cytokines, antioxidants (catalase and superoxide dismutase) protecting the cells from oxidative stress, and other flavor-related proteins [78,79]. Recently, natural exosome-like nanovesicles were designed (size: 131 nm) from edible tea flowers which remarkably triggered cellular apoptosis of breast tumors and inhibited lung metastasis conditions [80]. Such nanovehicles comprising large amounts of polyphenols, flavonoids, lipids, etc., exhibited strong cytotoxicity against the cancer cells, causing mitochondrial damage and arresting the cell cycle due to reactive oxygen species amplification. In addition, some reports utilized edible plant-derived exosomal NPs as potentially advanced therapeutic agents, such as ginger exosome-like NPs (GELNs) from the periodontal pathogen *Porphyromonas gingivalis*, for treating chronic periodontitis [70]; ginseng-derived exosomes (G-Exos) to effectively stimulate the neural differentiation of bone marrow-derived mesenchymal stem cells (BMSCs) by transferring the incorporated miRNAs to BMSCs [81]; and Beta vulgaris extract (BEX) for its anticancer and proangiogenic effects [82].

Some of the citrus fruit varieties, specifically under the Rutaceae family, have high therapeutic values due to the innate presence of flavanone hesperidin with exceptional hepatoprotective properties triggered via diverse cellular mechanisms, including improved activity of heme oxygenase 1, antioxidant response elements following enzymatic and non-enzymatic pathways, C-reactive proteins, etc., [83]. Such essential components obtained from citrus have also been used as anti-corpulence and anticancer drugs [84]. Furthermore, specific groups of secondary metabolites (furanocoumarins) isolated from grapefruits like *Citrus paradisi* possess superior anti-inflammatory and anti-cancerous properties promoting bone health and regeneration [85]. Mostly, these properties resulted from the specific functioning of flavonoids, phenolic acids, and polyphenols present in grapefruit extracts that can generate reactive oxygen species intrinsically and can eventually become beneficial in decreasing the risk factors associated in cardiovascular health issues and several other age-related neurodegenerative disorders [86–88]. Constructing unique designs of PENs can unravel the diverse functionalities of plant exosomes holding control over the cellular and metabolic activities, eventually driving the delivery of natural compounds to specific cell targets with enhanced efficacy. The ability to transversely penetrate through the bio membranes, have hyper compatibility, and be less prone to allergic natures is what makes plant-based exosomes more compact and prominent vehicles for drug delivery and targeted therapeutic treatments.

7. Other Natural Sources Derived Materials in Drug Delivery Systems

Other than metals, polymers, and quantum dots, various nanomaterials are also active in DDS, due to their versatile properties, such as cell targeting, good biocompatibility, and loading capacity. Bio-modified cell plasma membranes are applied to Nano vesicles in biomedical applications. Also, DNA-based hydrogels used in drug delivery has a property of bioactivity toward drug prevention from chemical and enzyme degradation. Highly programmable DNA hydrogels are potential carriers for various DDS, to achieve high performance systems for chemotherapy, immunotherapy, and gene therapy [89]. Like that, extra cellular vehicles (EVs) derived from milk has immunogenicity and are non-toxic, which is supported for use in drug carriers. It has the characteristics of prolonged drug releasing capacity and enhances the cellular and reducing toxic effect. Recently, researchers have reported that milk EVs have increased anti-proliferative activities, as to determine from milk EVs certain encapsulated drugs such as berry anthocyanidins, paclitaxel, and aglycons [90]. The anti-proliferative effects of exomes were analyzed in various cancer cell lines, namely lung (A549, H1299), breast cancer cells (MCF7, MDA-MB-231), pancreatic (Pancl, DU145), ovarian, and colon cell lines (OVCA432, HCT116). The results showed that the inhibition of cell growth recorded in a 4–60-fold decrease when treated with 50 μM of Exo-Anthose for 72 h [91].

Another main biosource is lipid-based nanoparticles (L-NPs), which serves as nano carriers for drug delivery. The special characteristics of L-NPs are its potential to cross the gastrointestinal barrier and its great lipophilicity. As a result, L-NPs acts as a nano vesicle for less soluble drugs. There are many sources for L-NPs, such as fatty acids, glycerides, and phospholipids [92]. Rahila et al. reported an embelin-loaded phospholipid complex (EPC) containing embelin, which is a drug naturally occurring from the fruit of Emblia ribes. This drug is used as an analgesic, antimicrobial, antioxidant, and antitumor agent. The poor water solubility of this drug can be increased by combining it with phospholipids. In a deionized water medium, after 2 h, the free embelin shows a 19% drug release, and EPC attained a 99.80% drug release [93]. To this extent, the ginger derived L-NPs (GDLNPs) applied as lipid vehicles for siRNA were achieved via GDLNPs loaded with siRNA-CD. GDLPs have certain components such as phosphatidic acid, monogalactosyldiacyglycerol, and digalactosyldiacyglycerol, with 41.9%, 18,9%, and 27.4% of total lipids, respectively. The mono and digalactosyldiacyglycerol played a major role as a stabilizer for drug-loaded LPNPs. In this, GDLNPs/siRNA efficiently and selectively act against the colonic CD98 cells and reduce the gene expression by 20.2 ± 5.1% for 24 h of colonic CD98 (Colon-26 tumors). These LNPs shows a potential delivery of siRNA, which is equivalent to the Lipofectamine 2000 commercial drug delivery system. As shown in the results, the naturally derived GDLNPs show effective transfection results determined by the in vitro studies on various cell lines [94]. Similarly, the GDLNPs are used as drug carriers for doxorubicin (Dox) to Colon-26 tumors. The viability and apoptosis assay of GDLNPs exhibit good biocompatibility, reduced cell proliferation, and increased apoptosis at a concentration of 200 μM/L. Additionally, it shows an excellent targeted pH-dependent drug release to colon-26 tumors and an enhanced inhibition of tumor growth as compared with the free drug [95]. Ginger-derived L-NPs are widely used in targeted DDS chemotherapeutic agents, as well as delivering proteins to various types of cells due to its biocompatibility and the fact that it did not generate immune toxicity [96,97].

Another emerging bio-based NMs are cell membrane derived cargos, which vide various advantages such as the functional proteins on their surface and the natural cell-to-cell interactions. For the improvement of the activity in the anti-cancer drug, gemcitabine and paclitaxel were encapsulated with components derived from a pancreatic tumor cell membrane (CMNP-GEM-PTX). This result shows that the CMNP-GEM-PTX has high stability and a greater cytotoxicity effect on tumor cells (PANC-1). The efficiency of encapsulation for GEM is about 50% with a drug release capacity of 25% for 48 h. It did not reveal any immune toxicity effect or reduced adverse effect of treatments, and it will need clinical trials for further improvement [98]. Various cell membrane-based DDS attracted scientific attention. Cell membranes, such as the erythrocyte membrane, platelet membrane, leukocyte membrane, stem cell membrane, and cancer cell membrane, provide the ability to penetrate into tumor sites. These exhibited cell membrane-derived NMs encapsulated with therapeutic agents are considered as promising DDS, specifically for cancer therapy [99]. In this way, the adipocyte mesenchymal stem cell membrane (ADSC) loaded with NPs are used for treatment for rheumatic arthritis (RA), which is a chronic and inflammatory autoimmune disease. The in vitro and in vivo studies revealed that pro-inflammatory factors, such as IL-1β, IL-6, and tumor necrosis factor-α decreased, and the anti-inflammatory factor (IL-10) increased without causes of any adverse effects [100].

Smart nanocarrier-derived from viruses and bacteria have been applied as targeted or personalized DDS. The different types of viruses, such as adeno-associated viruses, lentivirus, and other animal viruses used various drugs as well as gene carriers and controlled the releasing of the therapeutic agent in DDS. Due to the potential physical stability of the viral particles, no chemicals or conditions affected the drug delivery process. In some cases, the viral coating plays a role in recognizing specific disease biomarkers or receptors and functions as triggerable agents. Even though there are still several challenges in therapeutic gene delivery, like purity, low production yield, target specificity, they need to be addressed [101]. Distinct natural source-based NMs for DDS applications are tabulated and presented in Table 1.

Table 1. Natural source-mediated nano materials application in DDS.

Nanomaterials	Natural Sources	Shape/Size (nm)	Drug Delivery	Reference
AgNPs	Horse chestnut	50 ± 5	Resveratol	[27]
Au, Ag, CdSe, EuSe NPs	Aliginate gel	Spherical, 21.6 ± 1.8, 14.1 ± 3.4, 33.1 ± 7.0, 23.1 ± 7.3	Doxorubicin, Rifampicin	[29]
AuNPs	Walnut tree bark	43 ± 2.2	Zonisamide	[30]
AuNCs	Green tea	Flower shape, 50	Doxorubicin	[32]
FeSeNPs	Protein of *Peseudomonus pudida* metallothionin	Spherical, 201.8 ± 4.7	Doxorubicin	[33]
AgNPs	*Poe annua*	Spherical, 36–43	Anti-cancer drug	[34]
Biopolymer- ZnO	Kappa carrageenan	Hexagonal, 97.03 ± 9.05	Used as biofilm	[38]
Membrane	Natural rubber latex	Pore size 2000, 6000, 10,000 pore/cm^2	Ciprofloxacin	[40]
Molecularly Imprinted Polymer	Chitoson	-	Riboflavin	[41]
Carbon dots (CD)	Pasteurized milk	2.5 ± 1.0	LisinoPril	[50]
Quantum dots (QDs)	Mulberry leaves	2–4	Lycorine	[51]
N-CD	Korean Red Ginseng	13.94 ± 1.13	Rutin	[53]
Natural gum	*Geleditisia sinensis Lam*	-	Theophylline	[62]
Polysaccharide	Okra fruit	Microsphere	Rizhatriptan benzoate	[63]
Gum	Grewia mollis Juss stem bark		Ibuprofen	[64]
Chitosan	Shells of *Carinosquilla multicarniata*	-	5-amino salicylic acid	[66]
Exosome	Tea flower	131	Anti-cancer drug	[82]
Phospholipid	Soya	50–500	Embeline herbal drug	[95]
Polymer NPs	Cinnamon biopolymer	95.35 ± 10.25	Doxorubicin–Erlotinib	[102]

8. Conclusions and Outlook

The development of eco-friendly methodologies based on natural resources are inevitable for a sustainable future. The development of biomaterials has resulted in notable breakthroughs in the territory of medication delivery. These naturally sourced biomaterials provide generous benefits, including targeted medication delivery, controlled release, and improved therapeutic efficacy. Functional nanomaterials have changed drug administration using various methods, including nanoparticles, liposomes, dendrimers, and carbon-based nanomaterials, and they have the potential to overcome many of the drawbacks of traditional DDS. The functionalized NMs-enhanced solubility, stability, and enormous bioavailability makes them promising candidates for the therapeutic outcomes.

In addition, under certain circumstances, functional biomaterials can cross biological barriers, such as the blood–brain barrier, making it easier to distribute medication to previously inaccessible locations. The biocompatibility and safety profiles of these biomaterials are being worked on, along with ways to synthesize them more efficiently and upscale them for mass manufacturing. Efforts are also being made to deal with regulatory issues and guarantee the clinical application of these novel DDS. Natural resource-based DDS was found to be capable of improving treatment outcomes, lowering side effects, and enabling individualized medicine for effective healthcare.

The findings also indicate that the obstacles related to natural resource-based DDS need to be resolved. Microbes, plants extract, fruit, and other food source-based methods were developed for synthesizing NMs relevant to DDS. Food resource-based methods can create distress over the use of limited food resources for industrial purpose as it raises concern over the issue of feeding billions of people. The other issues of food-based materials are they are abundant in all seasons and require laborious extraction and purification processes. In countries like India, the annual vegetable and fruit wastage was estimated to be 18–40%. Therefore, the food waste-based method will be beneficial. Thus, in the future, agriculture and biowaste-based green synthesis methods must be given importance for developing on the industrial scale. The food waste biomass can also be converted into NCDs. The continuous availability of biowaste is useful for economic and large-scale production of NMs associated with DDS.

The synthesis of naturally derived NMs remains largely complicated, especially concerning the polymeric NPs. A detailed study may be required to address concerns about the allergens or toxic impurities found in the plant extracts. Moreover, there is no standard, optimized, and reproducible procedure established for the purpose of preparing the natural extract-based synthesis of metal NPs and NCDs. The addition of external pH stabilizing agents affects the eco-friendliness of the system, and the reaction control is often optimized by tuning the reaction temperature optimization, concentration, and extent of the bio-extract addition (volume/min). More attention needs to be made towards establishing a standard optimized procedure, at least for each type of plant extract meant to be used for the synthesis of metallic NMs. Though there is an endless source of natural resources, their performance largely remained inferior to their synthetic counterparts. The questions relevant to the manufacturing process and their actual impact on climate, human health, and the environment still need to be resolved. Aside from that, the entire life cycle of NMs, from biosynthesis to disposal, is not clearly established. Although there are still obstacles that need to be solved, the tremendous advancements in this area lay a solid groundwork for a next-generation drug delivery system.

Author Contributions: Writing—original draft preparation, M.V. and S.R.; visualization and revision, P.J.; writing and analysis, G.C. and S.G.; writing—revision, K.Y.; conceptualization, editing, supervision, project administration, and funding acquisition, T.H.O. All authors have read and agreed to the published version of the manuscript.

Funding: This work was supported by the National Research Foundation of Korea (NRF) grant funded by the Korean government (MSIT) (No. 2022R1A2C1004283). The authors would like to thank the Core Research Support Center for Natural Products and Medical Materials (CRCNM) in Yeungnam University. This work was supported by the Gachon University research fund of 2022 (GCU-202206070001).

Data Availability Statement: Data is contained within the article.

Conflicts of Interest: The authors declare no conflict of interest.

References

1. Afzal, O.; Altamimi, A.S.; Nadeem, M.S.; Alzarea, S.I.; Almalki, W.H.; Tariq, A.; Mubeen, B.; Murtaza, B.N.; Iftikhar, S.; Riaz, N.; et al. Nanoparticles in Drug Delivery: From History to Therapeutic Applications. *Nanomaterials* **2022**, *12*, 4494. [CrossRef]
2. Patra, J.K.; Das, G.; Fraceto, L.F.; Campos, E.V.R.; Rodriguez-Torres, M.D.P.; Acosta-Torres, L.S.; Diaz-Torres, L.A.; Grillo, R.; Swamy, M.K.; Sharma, S.; et al. Nano based drug delivery systems: Recent developments and future prospects. *J. Nanobiotechnol.* **2018**, *16*, 71. [CrossRef] [PubMed]
3. Mittal, A.K.; Chisti, Y.; Banerjee, U.C. Synthesis of metallic nanoparticles using plant extracts. *Biotechnol. Adv.* **2013**, *31*, 346–356. [CrossRef] [PubMed]
4. Noah, N.M.; Ndangili, P.M. Green synthesis of nanomaterials from sustainable materials for biosensors and drug delivery. *Sens. Int.* **2022**, *3*, 100166. [CrossRef]
5. Zhang, Y.; Poon, K.; Masonsong, G.S.P.; Ramaswamy, Y.; Singh, G. Sustainable Nanomaterials for Biomedical Applications. *Pharmaceutics* **2023**, *15*, 922. [CrossRef] [PubMed]
6. Gopi, S.; Amalraj, A.; Thomas, S. Effective drug delivery system of biopolymers based on nanomaterials and hydrogels—A review. *Drug Des.* **2016**, *5*, 1000129. [CrossRef]
7. Sousa, F.; Ferreira, D.; Reis, S.; Costa, P. Current insights on antifungal therapy: Novel nanotechnology approaches for drug delivery systems and new drugs from natural sources. *Pharmaceuticals* **2020**, *13*, 248. [CrossRef]
8. Kumar, T.S.; Madhumathi, K.; Rajkamal, B.; Zaheatha, S.; Malar, A.R.; Bai, S.A. Enhanced protein delivery by multi-ion containing eggshell derived apatitic-alginate composite nanocarriers. *Colloids Surf. B* **2014**, *123*, 542–548. [CrossRef]
9. Elbagory, A.M.; Marima, R.M.; Dlamini, Z. Role and merits of green based nanocarriers in cancer treatment. *Cancers* **2021**, *13*, 5686. [CrossRef]
10. Chandrakala, V.; Aruna, V.; Angajala, G. Review on metal nanoparticles as nanocarriers: Current challenges and perspectives in drug delivery systems. *Emergent Mater.* **2022**, *5*, 1593–1615. [CrossRef]
11. Barclay, T.G.; Day, C.M.; Petrovsky, N.; Garg, S. Review of polysaccharide particle-based functional drug delivery. *Carbohydr. Polym.* **2019**, *221*, 94–112. [CrossRef] [PubMed]
12. Li, J.; Xiang, H.; Zhang, Q.; Miao, X. Polysaccharide-Based Transdermal Drug Delivery. *Pharmaceuticals* **2022**, *15*, 602. [CrossRef] [PubMed]
13. Phan, T.T.V.; Phan, D.T.; Cao, X.T.; Huynh, T.C.; Oh, J. Roles of chitosan in green synthesis of metal nanoparticles for biomedical applications. *Nanomaterials* **2021**, *11*, 273. [CrossRef]
14. Fenton, O.S.; Olafson, K.N.; Pillai, P.S.; Mitchell, M.J.; Langer, R. Advances in biomaterials for drug delivery. *Adv. Mater.* **2018**, *30*, 1705328. [CrossRef] [PubMed]
15. Nair, A.; Haponiuk, J.T.; Thomas, S.; Gopi, S. Natural carbon-based quantum dots and their applications in drug delivery: A review. *Biomed. Pharmacother.* **2020**, *132*, 110834. [CrossRef]
16. Ayiloor Rajesh, G.; John, V.L.; Pookunnath Santhosh, A.; Krishnan Nair Ambika, A.; Thavarool Puthiyedath, V. Carbon dots from natural sources for biomedical applications. *Part. Part. Syst. Charact.* **2022**, *39*, 2200017. [CrossRef]
17. George, B.; Suchithra, T.V. Plant-derived bioadhesives for wound dressing and drug delivery system. *Fitoterapia* **2019**, *137*, 104241. [CrossRef]
18. Goksen, G.; Demir, D.; Dhama, K.; Kumar, M.; Shao, P.; Xie, F.; Echegaray, N.; Lorenzo, J.M. Mucilage polysaccharide as a plant secretion: Potential trends in food and biomedical applications. *Int. J. Biol. Macromol.* **2023**, *230*, 123146. [CrossRef]
19. Johnstone, R.M.; Adam, M.; Hammond, J.R.; Orr, L.; Turbide, C. Vesicle formation during reticulocyte maturation. Association of plasma membrane activities with released vesicles (exosomes). *J. Biol. Chem.* **1987**, *262*, 9412–9420. [CrossRef]
20. Zhang, Y.; Liu, Y.; Liu, H.; Tang, W.H. Exosomes: Biogenesis, biologic function and clinical potential. *Cell Biosci.* **2019**, *9*, 19.
21. Sen, S.; Xavier, J.; Kumar, N.; Ahmad, M.Z.; Ranjan, O.P. Exosomes as natural nanocarrier-based drug delivery system: Recent insights and future perspectives. *3 Biotech* **2023**, *13*, 101. [PubMed]
22. Tenchov, R.; Sasso, J.M.; Wang, X.; Liaw, W.S.; Chen, C.A.; Zhou, Q.A. Exosomes–Nature's Lipid Nanoparticles, a Rising Star in Drug Delivery and Diagnostics. *ACS Nano* **2022**, *16*, 17802–17846. [CrossRef] [PubMed]
23. Pirtarighat, S.; Ghannadnia, M.; Baghshahi, S. Biosynthesis of silver nanoparticles using Ocimum basilicum cultured under controlled conditions for bactericidal application. *Mater. Sci. Eng. C* **2019**, *98*, 250–255. [CrossRef] [PubMed]
24. Iravani, S.; Varma, R.S. Biofactories: Engineered nanoparticles via genetically engineered organisms. *Green Chem.* **2019**, *21*, 4583–4603. [CrossRef]

25. Nadagouda, M.N.; Varma, R.S. A greener synthesis of core (Fe, Cu)-shell (Au, Pt, Pd, and Ag) nanocrystals using aqueous vitamin C. *Cryst. Growth Des.* **2007**, *7*, 2582–2587. [CrossRef]
26. Lu, Y.; Ozcan, S. Green nanomaterials: On track for a sustainable future. *Nano Today* **2015**, *10*, 417–420. [CrossRef]
27. Küp, F.Ö.; Çoşkunçay, S.; Duman, F. Biosynthesis of silver nanoparticles using leaf extract of Aesculus hippocastanum (horse chestnut): Evaluation of their antibacterial, antioxidant and drug release system activities. *Mater. Sci. Eng. C* **2020**, *107*, 110207. [CrossRef]
28. Il Kim, M.; Park, C.Y.; Seo, J.M.; Kang, K.S.; Park, K.S.; Kang, J.; Hong, K.S.; Choi, Y.; Lee, S.Y.; Park, J.P.; et al. In situ biosynthesis of a metal nanoparticle encapsulated in alginate gel for imageable drug-delivery system. *ACS Appl. Mater. Interfaces* **2021**, *13*, 36697–36708. [CrossRef]
29. Fang, C.; Ma, Z.; Chen, L.; Li, H.; Jiang, C.; Zhang, W. Biosynthesis of gold nanoparticles, characterization and their loading with zonisamide as a novel drug delivery system for the treatment of acute spinal cord injury. *J. Photochem. Photobiol. B Biol.* **2019**, *190*, 72–75. [CrossRef]
30. Patra, J.K.; Ali, M.S.; Oh, I.G.; Baek, K.H. Proteasome inhibitory, antioxidant, and synergistic antibacterial and anticandidal activity of green biosynthesized magnetic Fe_3O_4 nanoparticles using the aqueous extract of corn (*Zea mays* L.) ear leaves. *Artif. Cells Nanomed. Biotechnol.* **2017**, *45*, 349–356. [CrossRef]
31. Wu, S.; Yang, X.; Luo, F.; Wu, T.; Xu, P.; Zou, M.; Yan, J. Biosynthesis of flower-shaped Au nanoclusters with EGCG and their application for drug delivery. *J. Nanobiotechnol.* **2018**, *16*, 90. [CrossRef]
32. Stephanie, R.; Kim, B.B.; Xu, P.; Choi, Y.; Park, C.Y.; Park, T.J. In vitro biosynthesis of iron selenide nanoparticles for imageable drug delivery platform. *Inorg. Chem. Commun.* **2022**, *145*, 109973. [CrossRef]
33. Gul, A.R.; Shaheen, F.; Rafique, R.; Bal, J.; Waseem, S.; Park, T.J. Grass-mediated biogenic synthesis of silver nanoparticles and their drug delivery evaluation: A biocompatible anti-cancer therapy. *Chem. Eng. J.* **2021**, *407*, 127202. [CrossRef]
34. Flieger, J.; Flieger, W.; Baj, J.; Maciejewski, R. Antioxidants: Classification, natural sources, activity/capacity measurements, and usefulness for the synthesis of nanoparticles. *Materials* **2021**, *14*, 4135. [CrossRef]
35. Gulia, K.; James, A.; Pandey, S.; Dev, K.; Kumar, D.; Sourirajan, A. Bio-inspired smart nanoparticles in enhanced cancer theranostics and targeted drug delivery. *J. Funct. Biomater.* **2022**, *13*, 207. [CrossRef]
36. Atanase, L.I. Micellar drug delivery systems based on natural biopolymers. *Polymers* **2021**, *13*, 477. [CrossRef] [PubMed]
37. Vijayakumar, S.; Saravanakumar, K.; Malaikozhundan, B.; Divya, M.; Vaseeharan, B.; Durán-Lara, E.F.; Wang, M.H. Biopolymer K-carrageenan wrapped ZnO nanoparticles as drug delivery vehicles for anti MRSA therapy. *Int. J. Biol. Macromol.* **2020**, *144*, 9–18. [CrossRef]
38. Shehabeldine, A.; Hasanin, M. Green synthesis of hydrolyzed starch–chitosan nano-composite as drug delivery system to gram negative bacteria. *J. Environ. Nanotechnol.* **2019**, *12*, 100252. [CrossRef]
39. Almeida, G.F.B.D.; Cardoso, M.R.; Zancanela, D.C.; Bernardes, L.L.; Norberto, A.M.Q.; Barros, N.R.; Paulino, C.G.; Chagas, A.L.D.; Herculano, R.D.; Mendonça, C.R. Controlled drug delivery system by fs-laser micromachined biocompatible rubber latex membranes. *Appl. Surf. Sci.* **2020**, *506*, 144762. [CrossRef]
40. Mokhtari, P.; Ghaedi, M. Water compatible molecularly imprinted polymer for controlled release of riboflavin as drug delivery system. *Eur. Polym. J.* **2019**, *118*, 614–618. [CrossRef]
41. Markam, R.; Bajpai, A.K. Functionalization of ginger derived nanoparticles with chitosan to design drug delivery system for controlled release of 5-amino salicylic acid (5-ASA) in treatment of inflammatory bowel diseases: An in vitro study. *React. Funct. Polym.* **2020**, *149*, 104520. [CrossRef]
42. Wang, M.; Yang, D.; Xu, Q.; Li, P.; Yi, C.; Qian, Y.; Qiu, X. Highly efficient evaporation method to prepare pH-responsive lignin-hollow-nanosphere with controllable size and its application in oral drug delivery. *Ind. Crop. Prod.* **2021**, *162*, 113230. [CrossRef]
43. Günter, E.A.; Popeyko, O.V. Delivery system for grape seed extract based on biodegradable Pectin-Zn-alginate gel particles. *Int. J. Biol. Macromol.* **2021**, *219*, 1021–1033. [CrossRef] [PubMed]
44. Limiti, E.; Mozetic, P.; Giannitelli, S.M.; Pinelli, F.; Han, X.; Del Rio, D.; Abbruzzese, F.; Basoli, F.; Rosanò, L.; Scialla, S.; et al. Hyaluronic acid–polyethyleneimine nanogels for controlled drug delivery in cancer treatment. *ACS Appl. Nano Mater.* **2022**, *5*, 5544–5557.
45. Zhu, L.; Yin, Y.; Wang, C.F.; Chen, S. Plant leaf-derived fluorescent carbon dots for sensing, patterning and coding. *J. Mater. Chem. C* **2013**, *1*, 4925–4932. [CrossRef]
46. Meng, W.; Bai, X.; Wang, B.; Liu, Z.; Lu, S.; Yang, B. Biomass-derived carbon dots and their applications. *Energy Environ. Mater.* **2019**, *2*, 172–192. [CrossRef]
47. Farooq, I.; Noor, S.; Sajjad, S.; Ashraf, S.; Sadaf, S. Functionalization of Biosynthesized CQDs Capped AgO/ZnO Ternary Composite Against Microbes and Targeted Drug Delivery to Tumor Cells. *J. Clust. Sci.* **2023**, *34*, 2681–2693. [CrossRef]
48. Vatanparast, M.; Shariatinia, Z. Revealing the role of different nitrogen functionalities in the drug delivery performance of graphene quantum dots: A combined density functional theory and molecular dynamics approach. *J. Mater. Chem. B* **2019**, *7*, 6156–6171. [CrossRef]
49. Mehta, V.N.; Chettiar, S.S.; Bhamore, J.R.; Kailasa, S.K.; Patel, R.M. Green synthetic approach for synthesis of fluorescent carbon dots for lisinopril drug delivery system and their confirmations in the cells. *J. Fluoresc.* **2017**, *27*, 111–124. [CrossRef]

50. Shao, Y.; Zhu, C.; Fu, Z.; Lin, K.; Wang, Y.; Chang, Y.; Han, L.; Yu, H.; Tian, F. Green synthesis of multifunctional fluorescent carbon dots from mulberry leaves (*Morus alba* L.) residues for simultaneous intracellular imaging and drug delivery. *J. Nanopart. Res.* **2020**, *22*, 229. [CrossRef]
51. Chung, H.K.; Wongso, V.; Sambudi, N.S.; Isnaeni. Biowaste-derived carbon dots/hydroxyapatite nanocomposite as drug delivery vehicle for acetaminophen. *J. Sol-Gel Sci. Technol.* **2020**, *93*, 214–223. [CrossRef]
52. Tejwan, N.; Kundu, M.; Ghosh, N.; Chatterjee, S.; Sharma, A.; Singh, T.A.; Das, J.; Sil, P.C. Synthesis of green carbon dots as bioimaging agent and drug delivery system for enhanced antioxidant and antibacterial efficacy. *J. Chem. Soc. D* **2022**, *139*, 109317. [CrossRef]
53. Amiri, M.S.; Mohammadzadeh, V.; Yazdi, M.E.T.; Barani, M.; Rahdar, A.; Kyzas, G.Z. Plant-based gums and mucilages applications in pharmacology and nanomedicine: A review. *Molecules* **2021**, *26*, 1770. [CrossRef]
54. Alur, H.H.; Pather, S.I.; Mitra, A.K.; Johnston, T.P. Evaluation of the gum from Hakea gibbosa as a sustained-release and mucoadhesive component in buccal tablets. *Pharm. Dev. Technol.* **1999**, *4*, 347–358. [CrossRef] [PubMed]
55. Vendruscolo, C.W.; Andreazza, I.F.; Ganter, J.L.M.S.; Ferrero, C.; Bresolin, T.M.B. Xanthan and galactomannan (from *M. scabrella*) matrix tablets for oral controlled delivery of theophylline. *Int. J. Pharm.* **2005**, *296*, 1–11. [CrossRef] [PubMed]
56. Venkataraju, M.P.; Gowda, D.V.; Rajesh, K.S.; Shivakumar, H.G. Xanthan and locust bean gum (from *Ceratonia siliqua*) matrix tablets for oral controlled delivery of metoprolol tartrate. *Curr. Drug Ther.* **2008**, *3*, 70–77. [CrossRef]
57. Alvarez-Manceñido, F.; Landin, M.; Lacik, I.; Martínez-Pacheco, R. Konjac glucomannan and konjac glucomannan/xanthan gum mixtures as excipients for controlled drug delivery systems. Diffusion of small drugs. *Int. J. Pharm.* **2008**, *349*, 11–18. [CrossRef]
58. Singh, K.; Kumar, A.; Langyan, N.; Ahuja, M. Evaluation of Mimosa pudica seed mucilage as sustained-release excipient. *AAPS PharmSciTech* **2009**, *10*, 1121–1127. [CrossRef]
59. Ganesh, G.N.K.; Sureshkumar, R.; Jawahar, N.; Senthil, V.; Venkatesh, D.N.; Srinivas, M.S. Preparation and evaluation of sustained release matrix tablet of diclofenac sodium using natural polymer. *J. Pharm. Sci. Res.* **2010**, *2*, 360.
60. Jian, H.; Zhu, L.; Zhang, W.; Sun, D.; Jiang, J. Galactomannan (from *Gleditsia sinensis* Lam.) and xanthan gum matrix tablets for controlled delivery of theophylline: In vitro drug release and swelling behavior. *Carbohydr. Polym.* **2012**, *87*, 2176–2182. [CrossRef]
61. Sharma, N.; Kulkarni, G.T.; Sharma, A.; Bhatnagar, A.; Kumar, N. Natural mucoadhesive microspheres of Abelmoschus esculentus polysaccharide as a new carrier for nasal drug delivery. *J. Microencapsul.* **2013**, *30*, 589–598. [CrossRef]
62. Nayak, A.K.; Pal, D.; Santra, K. Plantago ovata F. Mucilage-alginate mucoadhesive beads for controlled release of glibenclamide: Development, optimization, and in vitro-in vivo evaluation. *Int. J. Pharm.* **2013**, *2013*, 151035. [CrossRef] [PubMed]
63. Olayemi, O.J.; Allagh, S.T.; Oyi, A.R.; Isah, A.B.; Olayemi, A.G. Ibuprofen tablets compression-coated with Grewia mollis gum for colonic delivery. *Br. J. Pharm. Res.* **2015**, *6*, 107–120. [CrossRef]
64. Dhamija, K.; Arora, V.; Kulkarni, G.T. Formulation of Prunus Amygdalus (Family: Rosaceae) Gum Based Compression Coated Tablet for Colon Targeted Delivery of 5-Aminosalicylic Acid. *Nov. Approaches Drug Des. Dev.* **2017**, *2*, 67–70.
65. Balde, A.; Hasan, A.; Joshi, I.; Nazeer, R.A. Preparation and optimization of chitosan nanoparticles from discarded squilla (*Carinosquilla multicarinata*) shells for the delivery of anti-inflammatory drug: Diclofenac. *J. Air Waste Manag. Assoc.* **2020**, *70*, 1227–1235. [CrossRef]
66. Mahmood, A.; Erum, A.; Tulain, U.R.; Shafiq, S.; Malik, N.S.; Sidra; Khan, M.T.; Alqahtani, M.S. Aloe vera-Based Polymeric Network: A Promising Approach for Sustained Drug Delivery, Development, Characterization, and in Vitro Evaluation. *Gels* **2023**, *9*, 474. [CrossRef]
67. Rajalakshmi, M.; Sangeetha, S. Okra Mucilage-Method of Extraction and A Novel Strategy for Pharmaceutical Drug Delivery System. *J. Pharm. Negat. Results* **2023**, *14*, 2473–2481.
68. Narkar, N.; Singh, S.; Chatur, V.M.; Kaple, P.R.; Chauhan, L.; Lamjane, A. Formulation and Evaluation of Fast Disintegrating Tablet of Diclofenac Potassium Using plantago ovata Seed Mucilage Powder as a Natural Superdisintegrant. *Eur. Chem. Bull.* **2023**, *12*, 15380–15389.
69. Priya, P.S.; Sundari, I.B.T. Formulation and Evaluation of Oral Disintegrating Tablets Containing Loratadine Using Natural Super Disintegrants (Ispaghula Mucilage Powder). *Int. J. Pharm. Res. Appl.* **2023**, *8*, 1004–1017.
70. Patil, S.M.; Sawant, S.S.; Kunda, N.K. Exosomes as drug delivery systems: A brief overview and progress update. *Eur. J. Pharm. Biopharm.* **2020**, *154*, 259–269. [CrossRef]
71. Jyothi, V.G.S.; Bulusu, R.; Rao, B.V.K.; Pranothi, M.; Banda, S.; Bolla, P.K.; Kommineni, N. Stability characterization for pharmaceutical liposome product development with focus on regulatory considerations: An update. *Int. J. Pharm.* **2022**, *624*, 122022. [CrossRef]
72. Sundaram, K.; Miller, D.P.; Kumar, A.; Teng, Y.; Sayed, M.; Mu, J.; Lei, C.; Sriwastva, M.K.; Zhang, L.; Yan, J.; et al. Plant-derived exosomal nanoparticles inhibit pathogenicity of Porphyromonas gingival is. *Iscience* **2019**, *21*, 308–327. [CrossRef]
73. Cho, J.H.; Hong, Y.D.; Kim, D.; Park, S.J.; Kim, J.S.; Kim, H.M.; Yoon, E.J.; Cho, J.S. Confirmation of plant-derived exosomes as bioactive substances for skin application through comparative analysis of keratinocyte transcriptome. *Appl. Biol. Chem.* **2022**, *65*, 8. [CrossRef]
74. Fang, Z.; Liu, K. Plant-derived extracellular vesicles as oral drug delivery carriers. *J. Control. Release* **2022**, *350*, 389–400. [CrossRef] [PubMed]

75. Kim, J.; Li, S.; Zhang, S.; Wang, J. Plant-derived exosome-like nanoparticles and their therapeutic activities. *Asian J. Pharm.* **2022**, *17*, 53–69. [CrossRef] [PubMed]
76. Rutter, B.D.; Innes, R.W. Extracellular vesicles isolated from the leaf apoplast carry stress-response proteins. *Plant Physiol.* **2017**, *173*, 728–741. [CrossRef]
77. Cai, Q.; Qiao, L.; Wang, M.; He, B.; Lin, F.M.; Palmquist, J.; Huang, S.D.; Jin, H. Plants send small RNAs in extracellular vesicles to fungal pathogen to silence virulence genes. *Science* **2018**, *360*, 1126–1129. [CrossRef]
78. Stanly, C.; Alfieri, M.; Ambrosone, A.; Leone, A.; Fiume, I.; Pocsfalvi, G. Grapefruit-derived micro and nanovesicles show distinct metabolome profiles and anticancer activities in the A375 human melanoma cell line. *Cells* **2020**, *9*, 2722. [CrossRef]
79. Barry, C.S.; Llop-Tous, M.I.; Grierson, D. The regulation of 1-aminocyclopropane-1-carboxylic acid synthase gene expression during the transition from system-1 to system-2 ethylene synthesis in tomato. *Plant Physiol.* **2000**, *123*, 979–986. [CrossRef]
80. Chen, Q.; Li, Q.; Liang, Y.; Zu, M.; Chen, N.; Canup, B.S.; Luo, L.; Wang, C.; Zeng, L.; Xiao, B. Natural exosome-like nanovesicles from edible tea flowers suppress metastatic breast cancer via ROS generation and microbiota modulation. *Acta Pharm. Sin. B* **2022**, *12*, 907–923. [CrossRef]
81. Xu, X.H.; Yuan, T.J.; Dad, H.A.; Shi, M.Y.; Huang, Y.Y.; Jiang, Z.H.; Peng, L.H. Plant exosomes as novel nanoplatforms for microRNA transfer stimulate neural differentiation of stem cells in vitro and in vivo. *Nano Lett.* **2021**, *21*, 8151–8159. [CrossRef]
82. Mahdipour, E. Beta vulgaris juice contains biologically active exosome-like nanoparticles. *Tissue Cell* **2022**, *76*, 101800. [CrossRef]
83. Tabeshpour, J.; Hosseinzadeh, H.; Hashemzaei, M.; Karimi, G. A review of the hepatoprotective effects of hesperidin, a flavanon glycoside in citrus fruits, against natural and chemical toxicities. *DARU J. Pharm. Sci.* **2020**, *28*, 305–317. [CrossRef]
84. Hirata, T.; Fujii, M.; Akita, K.; Yanaka, N.; Ogawa, K.; Kuroyanagi, M.; Hongo, D. Identification and physiological evaluation of the components from Citrus fruits as potential drugs for anti-corpulence and anticancer. *Bioorg. Med. Chem.* **2009**, *17*, 25–28. [CrossRef] [PubMed]
85. Hung, W.L.; Suh, J.H.; Wang, Y. Chemistry and health effects of furanocoumarins in grapefruit. *J. Food Sci.* **2017**, *25*, 71–83. [CrossRef]
86. Homayoun, M.; Targhi, R.G.; Soleimani, M. Anti-proliferative and anti-apoptotic effects of grape seed extract on chemo-resistant OVCAR-3 ovarian cancer cells. *Res. Pharm. Sci.* **2020**, *15*, 390. [PubMed]
87. Vislocky, L.M.; Fernandez, M.L. Biomedical effects of grape products. *Nutr. Rev.* **2010**, *68*, 656–670. [CrossRef]
88. Nemati, M.; Singh, B.; Mir, R.A.; Nemati, M.; Babaei, A.; Ahmadi, M.; Rasmi, Y.; Golezani, A.G.; Rezaie, J. Plant-derived extracellular vesicles: A novel nanomedicine approach with advantages and challenges. *J. Cell Commun. Signal.* **2022**, *20*, 69. [CrossRef]
89. Mo, F.; Jiang, K.; Zhao, D.; Wang, Y.; Song, J.; Tan, W. DNA hydrogel-based gene editing and drug delivery systems. *Adv. Drug Deliv. Rev.* **2021**, *168*, 79–98. [CrossRef]
90. Sanwlani, R.; Fonseka, P.; Chitti, S.V.; Mathivanan, S. Milk-derived extracellular vesicles in inter-organism, cross-species communication and drug delivery. *Proteomes* **2020**, *8*, 11. [CrossRef] [PubMed]
91. Munagala, R.; Aqil, F.; Jeyabalan, J.; Agrawal, A.K.; Mudd, A.M.; Kyakulaga, A.H.; Singh, I.P.; Vadhanam, M.V.; Gupta, R.C. Exosomal formulation of anthocyanidins against multiple cancer types. *Cancer Lett.* **2017**, *393*, 94–102. [CrossRef]
92. Negi, J.S. Nanolipid materials for drug delivery systems: A comprehensive Review. *Charact. Biol. Nanomater. Drug Deliv.* **2019**, *69*, 137–163.
93. Pathan, R.A.; Bhandari, U. Preparation & characterization of embelin–phospholipid complex as effective drug delivery tool. *J. Incl. Phenom. Macrocycl. Chem.* **2011**, *69*, 139–147.
94. Zhang, M.; Wang, X.; Han, M.K.; Collins, J.F.; Merlin, D. Oral administration of ginger-derived nanolipids loaded with siRNA as a novel approach for efficient siRNA drug delivery to treat ulcerative colitis. *Nanomedicine* **2017**, *12*, 1927–1943. [CrossRef] [PubMed]
95. Zhang, M.; Xiao, B.; Wang, H.; Han, M.K.; Zhang, Z.; Viennois, E.; Xu, C.; Merlin, D. Edible ginger-derived nano-lipids loaded with doxorubicin as a novel drug-delivery approach for colon cancer therapy. *Mol. Ther.* **2016**, *24*, 1783–1796. [CrossRef] [PubMed]
96. Zhang, M.; Collins, J.F.; Merlin, D. Do ginger-derived nanoparticles represent an attractive treatment strategy for inflammatory bowel diseases? *Nanomedicine* **2016**, *12*, 3035–3037. [CrossRef] [PubMed]
97. Wang, X.; Zhang, M.; Woloshun, R.R.; Yu, Y.; Lee, J.K.; Flores, S.R.; Merlin, D.; Collins, J.F. Oral administration of ginger-derived lipid nanoparticles and Dmt1 siRNA potentiates the effect of dietary iron restriction and mitigates pre-existing iron overload in hamp KO mice. *Nutrients* **2021**, *13*, 1686. [CrossRef]
98. Comparetti, E.J.; Lins, P.M.; Quitiba, J.V.; Zucolotto, V. Cancer cell membrane-derived nanoparticles improve the activity of gemcitabine and paclitaxel on pancreatic cancer cells and coordinate immunoregulatory properties on professional antigen-presenting cells. *Mate. Adv.* **2020**, *1*, 1775–1787. [CrossRef]
99. Zhao, J.; Ruan, J.; Lv, G.; Shan, Q.; Fan, Z.; Wang, H.; Du, Y.; Ling, L. Cell membrane-based biomimetic nanosystems for advanced drug delivery in cancer therapy: A comprehensive review. *Colloids Surf. B* **2022**, *215*, 112503. [CrossRef]
100. Gu, C.; Yang, S.; Liu, X.; Jin, Y.; Yu, Y.; Lu, L. A biomimetic adipocyte mesenchymal stem cell membrane-encapsulated drug delivery system for the treatment of rheumatoid arthritis. *Nano Res.* **2023**, *16*, 11401–11410. [CrossRef]

101. Dogbey, D.M.; Torres, V.E.S.; Fajemisin, E.; Mpondo, L.; Ngwenya, T.; Akinrinmade, O.A.; Perriman, A.W.; Barth, S. Technological advances in the use of viral and non-viral vectors for delivering genetic and non-genetic cargos for cancer therapy. *Drug Deliv. Transl. Res.* **2023**, 1–20. [CrossRef] [PubMed]
102. Farheen, M.; Akhter, M.H.; Chitme, H.; Akhter, M.S.; Tabassum, F.; Jaremko, M.; Emwas, A.H. Harnessing Folate-Functionalized Nasal Delivery of Dox–Erlo-Loaded Biopolymeric Nanoparticles in Cancer Treatment: Development, Optimization, Characterization, and Biodistribution Analysis. *Pharmaceuticals* **2023**, *16*, 207. [CrossRef] [PubMed]

Journal of
Functional
Biomaterials

MDPI

Article

Development of Nanosuspension of *Artemisia absinthium* Extract as Novel Drug Delivery System to Enhance Its Bioavailability and Hepatoprotective Potential

Nazish Jahan [1,†], Fareeha Kousar [1], Khalil Ur Rahman [2], Syeeda Iram Touqeer [1] and Naseem Abbas [3,*,†]

1 Natural Products Lab, Department of Chemistry, University of Agriculture, Faisalabad 38000, Pakistan; nazishjahan@uaf.edu.pk (N.J.); fareehakousar87@gmail.com (F.K.); iram_touqeer@yahoo.com (S.I.T.)
2 Department of Biochemistry, Riphah International University, Faisalabad 38000, Pakistan; khaliluaf@yahoo.com
3 Department of Mechanical Engineering, Sejong University, Seoul 05006, Republic of Korea
* Correspondence: naseem.abbas@sejong.ac.kr
† These authors contributed equally to this work.

Abstract: A nanosuspension of *Artemisia absinthium* extract was formulated and characterized for the enhancement of bioavailability and better hepatoprotective efficacy. The nanosuspension of *A. absinthium* extract was formulated using an antisolvent precipitation technique, and various formulation parameters were optimized using response surface methodology (RSM). The optimized nanosuspension was characterized using AFM and FT–IR spectroscopy. The drug-release profile and oral bioavailability of the optimized nanosuspension were assessed with reference to coarse suspension. The DPPH radical scavenging method was used to measure the nanosuspension's antioxidant activity, and its in vivo hepatoprotective potential was assessed against CCl4-induced hepatic injury in rats. The developed optimized nanosuspension had suitable zeta potential of −11.9 mV, PDI of 0.285, and mean particle size of 253.8 nm. AFM study demonstrated a homogeneous population of nanoparticles with average size of 25 nm. The formulated nanosuspension of *A. absinthium* showed faster dissolution rate and 1.13-fold enhanced bioavailability as compared to the coarse suspension (plant extract). Furthermore, the nanoformulation had stronger antioxidant and hepatoprotective potential as compared to the unprocessed coarse extract. These results demonstrated that nanosuspension is a promising strategy for improving the oral bioavailability and bioactivities of *A. absinthium* extract.

Keywords: *Artemisia absinthium*; nanosuspension; response surface methodology; bioavailability

1. Introduction

Recently, the use of medicinal plants has increased all over the world due to their promising health benefits and safety [1,2]. The World Health Organization (WHO) is giving prime importance to the evaluation of secondary metabolites derived from natural products for the treatment of diseases due to broad spectrum management [3]. About 80% of the population in developing countries uses natural products for their primary health needs [4]. Wormwood, also known as *Artemisia absinthium* L., is a significant perennial shrubby medicinal plant that is indigenous to Asia, the Middle East, Europe, and North Africa [5]. *A. absinthium* exhibits several pharmacological activities including antimalarial [6], antimicrobial, antioxidant, anti-inflammatory [7], and nephroprotective activities, as well as an excellent hepatoprotective potential [8]. Aerial parts are used in gastric herbal preparations, in dietary supplements, and in alcoholic beverages [9]. Various phytochemicals such as essential oil, absinthin, anabsinthin, anabsin, lactones, and organic acids have been reported in *A. absinthium* extract. It also possesses flavonoids such as quercetin, myrecetin, hesperidin, rutin [10], and artemisnin and phenolic acids such as salicylic, coumaric, syringic, vanillic, and chlorogenic acids, which are probably involved in the mechanism of free-radical scavenging activity [11]. Many medicinal activities of *Artemisia* are reported, but the formulation of nanosuspension and pharmacokinetic studies of *A. absinthium* extract are reported for the first time in this study.

It is evident that most of the bioactive constituents of herbal extracts are unable to cross the lipid membrane due to their large molecular diameter and low water solubility that further results in poor systemic absorption and low bioavailability [12,13]. Nanotechnology has recently emerged as a novel technique to address the difficulties of solubility and bioavailability of poorly water-soluble pharmaceuticals. The herbal extracts processed through nanotechnology may enhance the efficacy of bioactive phytopharmaceuticals by increasing their water solubility and bioavailability as well as by reducing the treatment dose and side effects [14]. Various novel drug delivery systems like polymeric nanoparticles, liposomes, nano emulsions, and phytosomes for plant extracts and their bioactive compounds have been reported [15]. Formulation of nanosuspension is an engrossing strategy for increasing the dissolution velocity and bioavailability of synthetic drugs and phytochemicals due to the increased surface area of nanoparticles. [16]. The medication delivery method known as nanosuspension uses nanosized drug particles that are stabilized by polymers or surfactants [17,18]. Pharmaceutical nanosuspension of herbal medicines is a bewildering and fascinating strategy because it increases saturation solubility, and it poses fewer side effects with high drug loading. Moreover, various administration routes of oral, parenteral, intravenous, and pulmonary delivery systems can be applied to nanosuspensions. A variety of formulation techniques, such as micronization, solid dispersion, inclusion complexes, lipid carriers and liposomes, and emulsions and micro-emulsions are extensively used to overcome the solubility problem of poorly soluble drugs. However, the main difficulty associated with these approaches is their lack of universal applicability to all kinds of drugs. Nanosuspension technology has revealed greater potential to resolve the problem because of simplicity and the advantages it bestows over other techniques. Pharmaceutical nanosuspensions are extremely fine, dispersed solid drug particles in an aqueous phase stabilized by surfactants, polymers, or a mixture of both. The size of nanoformulated drug particles is usually smaller than 1 micrometer with an average size ranging from 200 nm to 600 nm. This formulation has low processing cost, high dug loading, and diminutive side effects for excipients. Owing to the improved surface-to-volume ratio of nanosuspensions, drug particles exhibit greater saturation solubility and faster dissolution rates, which ultimately improve bioavailability [18]. Therefore, the goal of the current research was to formulate an *A. absinthium* extract nanosuspension with increased oral bioavailability and dissolution.

2. Materials and Methods

2.1. Plant Extract Preparation

The aerial portions of *Artemisia absinthium* were purchased from a local market in Faisalabad and identified from a plant taxonomist from the Department of Botany, University of Agriculture, Faisalabad. N-hexane was used to remove the fat of the plant material. Plant ethanol extract was prepared using the Soxhlet device. Briefly, 30 g of defatted plant material was introduced to the Soxhlet extractor's thimble, and 300mL of ethanol (99.9%, MERCK Germany, Darmstadt, Germany) was taken in flask and heated for 8 h. The resulting ethanolic extract was filtered and concentrated on Rotary evaporators (Buchi, CH-9230 Flawil 1, Flawil, Switzerland) at low temperature (40 °C) and pressure (50 torr). The concentrated ethanolic extract was kept in the refrigerator (2–8 °C) for additional examination.

2.2. Formulation and Optimization of Nanosuspension

A. absinthium extract was made into a nanosuspension utilizing the antisolvent precipitation method reported by Thadkala et al., 2014, with some modification. Plant extract (0.25 g) was thoroughly diluted in 10mL ethanol (*w*/*v*) (99.9%, MERCK, Germany); then this organic solution was slowly injected (1 mL/min) with the help of a syringe connected to a thin Teflon tube into aqueous phase containing hydroxypropyl methylcellulose (HPMC) (K4M, Sigma-Aldrich Germany, Taufkirchen, Germany) with continuous mechanical stirring at 6000 rpm for 6 h at room temperature [19]. RSM was used to optimize various nanosuspension parameters. Average particle size, poly dispersity index (PDI), and zeta potential were the study's response variables, whereas stabilizer-to-plant extract ratio, antisolvent/solvent ratio, and stirring time were its input components. Stabilizer-to-plant extract ratio (*w*/*w*) varied from 0.20:1 to 1:1, antisolvent/solvent ratio (*v*/*v*) from 5:1 to 15:1, and stirring time was varied from and 2 to 6 h. The design of the experiment was used to optimize the selected parameters. Based on the number of factors and their levels, central composite design (CCD) was used to investigate the effects of various parameters on physical properties of prepared nanosuspensions. The design consists of a total of 20 experiments and data obtained via these experiments were analyzed using Design Expert software (Minneapolis, MN, USA). Optimized nanosuspensions were lyophilized at −60 °C for 72 h. Freeze-dried samples were ground to fine powder and used for solid-state characterization.

2.3. Stability of Nanosuspension

At two different temperatures, the physical stability of the optimized nanosuspension was assessed. For this use, the prepared nanosuspension was kept at 4 °C in the refrigerator for three months and at room temperature between 25 and 30 °C. Aliquots of samples were taken after three months, and their particle size, PDI, and zeta potential were all examined.

2.4. Characterization of Nanosuspension

Freshly prepared nanosuspension particle size, PDI, and zeta potential were measured using the DLS (Dynamic Light Scattering) technique and the Zetasizer (Nano ZS, Malvern Instruments, Malvern, UK). The optimized nanosuspension surface morphology and topography were assessed using a scanning electron microscope (JEOL, JSM-6400, Tokyo, Japan) at various magnifications. An atomic force microscope (AFM Shimadzu WET-SPM 9600, Tokyo, Japan) was used to obtain three-dimensional (3D) pictures of the optimized nanosuspension. On an FT–IR spectrometer (Perkin Elmer Spectrum, Version 10.4.3, USA), the molecular interactions of stabilizer-optimized nanosuspensions were captured. For this, FT–IR analysis was performed on HPMC (stabilizer), designed nanosuspension, and coarse plant extract. The spectra were collected from the KBr disc. A small amount of material was applied to the lens, and scans were made with a 4000–450 cm^{-1} scanning range.

2.5. Dissolution Investigation

The optimized nanosuspension dissolution profile with reference to coarse extract were determined in phosphate buffer using USP dissolution Type-II (pharma test de, ISO 9001, Germany). Equivalent amounts of lyophilized powder of optimized nanosuspension and coarse plant extract were poured into empty gelatin capsules. The dissolution medium was phosphate buffer (pH 7.4, 900 mL) at 37 °C, and the rotation speed was 100 rpm. An amount of 10 mL of the dissolution liquid were removed at predetermined intervals (10, 20, 30, 50, 60, 90, and 120 min), and the amount of medication dissolved was determined spectrophotometrically at 237 nm using quercetin (≥95%, HPLC grade, Merck Germany) as the standard compound. The percentage drug release of nanosuspension was compared with coarse suspension. Results of the dissolution test, which was carried out in triplicate, are expressed as Mean ± SD (n = 3) [20].

2.6. Pharmacokinetic Study

Healthy Sprague Dawley rats weighing 250–300 g were used as experimental rats to perform pharmacokinetic studies of nanosuspensions. Before doing the experiments, the animals were fed a regular diet for one week. The rats fasted for twelve hours before the experiment but with free access to water. The coarse extract and nanosuspension at doses of 50 mg kg^{-1} were orally administered to rats. Blood samples of about 0.5 mL were collected using cardiac puncture under mild anesthesia into heparinized tubes at 0.5 h, 1 h, 2 h, 4 h, 6 h, and 24 h time intervals. For separation of plasma, the collected blood samples were centrifuged at 4000 rpm for ten minutes. All plasma samples were stored at −20 °C for further analysis [21].

HPLC Analysis

For extraction of quercetin, plasma (200 µL) was mixed with 400 µL methanol (99.9%, HPLC grade, Merck, Germany) and HCl (200 µL, 25%, analytical grade, Merck, Germany). The resulting mixture was vortexed in a vortex shaker for 90 s and incubated at 50 °C for fifteen minutes [22]. Then, this mixture was centrifuged at 10,000 rpm for ten minutes. The supernatant (20 µL) was injected into the column for determination of quercetin in plasma. The mixture of Na_2HPO_4 (≥99%, HPLC grade, Merck, Germany) (30 mM), acetonitrile (99.9%, HPLC grade, Merck, Germany), and methanol (65:29:6, $v/v/v$) was used as a mobile phase at the flow rate of 1 mL min^{-1}. The column effluent was analyzed at 370 nm using a UV–Visible detector. The standard plots of quercetin were constructed, and pharmacokinetic parameters were determined using MS Excel, 2010. Maximum peak concentration in plasma (C_{max}), the time required for maximum concentration (T_{max}), was determined from concentration time curves. Area under curve (AUC) was determined using the trapezoidal method. Results were expressed as Mean ± SD (n = 3).

2.7. *In Vitro Antioxidant Activity*

In vitro antioxidant activity of the coarse extract (ethanolic extract suspended in water) and nanosuspension were evaluated via 2, 2-Diphenyl-1-picrylhydazyl (DPPH) radical scavenging method [23,24]. Five concentrations of nanosuspension and coarse extract ranging from 0.02 to 0.1 mg/mL were made. Then, 1 mL of freshly prepared DPPH (99% Merck, Germany) solution (0.1 mM in methanol) was added to 3 mL of each sample solution, and the reaction mixture was incubated in the dark for half an hour. The absorbance of the reaction mixture was measured at 517 nm after incubation. Ascorbic acid was utilized as the standard, and DPPH solution as the blank. The decrease in absorbance indicated that plant extracts inhibited the DPPH radical to a larger extent. All experiments were carried out in three replicates, and the average results were provided. Percent inhibition of DPPH free radical was calculated using formula given below:

$$\text{Inhibition of DPPH free radical (\%)} = A_c - A_s/A_c \times 100$$

where A_c represents absorbance of control, and A_s represents absorbance of samples.

2.8. *In Vivo Hepatoprotective Potential*

The in vivo hepatoprotective potential study was carried out in accordance with international ethical guidelines and was overseen by a veterinarian at the Clinical Medicine and Surgery Department, UAF. The proposal was approved by the synopsis scrutiny committee of the Department of Chemistry, University of Agriculture, Faisalabad and endorsed by the graduate research board through letter No. DGS-20525-28. In this investigation, healthy Sprague Dawley rats of either sex weighing 200–250 g were employed. Animals were housed in the Clinical Medicine and Surgery department of the University of Agriculture in Faisalabad. Rats were acclimatized for seven days before starting the experiment.

For evaluation of hepatoprotective potential of nanosuspensions and plant extract, hepatotoxicity in rats was induced via oral administration of CCl_4 (1 mL/kg body weight) for two consecutive days. After inducing hepatotoxicity, various curative treatments were given to these CCl_4-intoxicated rats. The curative hepatoprotective potential of plant extracts were compared with nanosuspension.

Experimental Design

Rats were randomly divided into different treatment groups with four rats in each group. The detailed treatment protocol was as follows:

Group I: (normal control) received a normal diet during all the experiment.
Group II: (positive control) rats were orally administrated with CCl_4 at the dose 1 mL/kg body weight mixed with olive oil (1:1).
Group III (CCl4 + AA NS): Rats were orally administered CCl_4 to induce liver toxicity. Then these rats received nanosuspension at dose of 100 mg/kg for four consecutive days. Blood samples were collected daily after twenty-four hours of each treatment.
Group IV (CCl4 + AA CE): These rats were orally administered carbon tetrachloride (1 mL/kg body weight) for two consecutive days to induce liver toxicity. After that, plant extract (150 mg/kg body weight) was given to these CCl_4-intoxicated rats for four days. Blood samples were collected after twenty-four hours of each curative treatment.

After collection, blood samples were centrifuged at 3000 rpm, and serum was analyzed for different biochemical parameters such as aspartate aminotransferase (AST), alanine aminotransferase (ALT), alkaline phosphatase (ALP), albumin (Alb), total protein (TP), and total bilirubin (TB) using a chemistry analyzer (Semar-S1000 elite, Prato, Italy). On the last day of experiment, all the animals were slaughtered, and liver tissues were removed and washed with buffered saline. Liver homogenate was prepared by homogenizing the liver tissues in ice-cold phosphate buffer (pH 7.4). Superoxide dismutase (SOD), catalase (CAT), and glutathione peroxidase (GPX) were among the antioxidant enzymes measured in the homogenate mixture after centrifugation at 10,000 rpm

2.9. Statistical Analysis

CCD was used to improve the parameters of the nanosuspensions, and Design Ex-pert (version 7.1, Stat-Ease, Inc., Minneapolis, MN, USA) was utilized to examine the data. The statistical difference in means was analyzed using ANOVA, followed by Tukey's test, and $p < 0.05$ was considered statistically significant. All data were reported as Mean ± SD.

3. Results and Discussion

3.1. Optimization of Nanosuspension

In the present study, CCD (central composite design) was used to study the effect of various formulation variables on particle size, PDI (polydispersity index), and zeta potential. The experimental data of all experimental runs with response variables are given in Table 1. The ranges of three responses Y_1, Y_2, and Y_3 were found to be 224.3 nm to 605 nm, 0.295 to 0.590, and −2.00 mV to −24.50 mV, respectively. The responses obtained via experiments were treated with linear, cubic, and quadratic model functions to select the best fitting models for optimization study. The quadratic model was chosen in the end to establish the mathematical connection between the input variables and the results. Analysis of variance (ANOVA) was used to determine the importance of the selected model. The coefficient of determination (R^2) is an important statistical parameter used to check the fitness of a model. A high value of R^2 indicates a significant correlation between observed and predicted values of response [25]. The values of R^2 for particle size, PDI, and zeta potential are all 0.9963, 0.9416, and 0.8896, respectively, demonstrating strong correlations between experimental and predicted values. The polynomial regression equations in terms of coded factors describing the relationship between the input variables and response variables were also generated. The positive sign with a factor indicates increase in the response variable with the factor and vice versa.

$$\text{Particle size (nm)} = +349.09 - 86.71A - 48.21B - 69.16C + 51.09AB + 0.16AC - 12.69BC + 26.18A^2 + 4.37B^2 + 37.39C^2 \quad (1)$$

$$\text{PDI} = +0.47 - 0.081A - 0.053B - 0.064C + 0.055AB + 0.064AC - 0.022BC + 3.574E - 003A^2 + 0.023B^2 + 0.040C^2 \quad (2)$$

$$\text{Zeta potential (mV)} = +10.73 - 1.42A + 0.48B - 0.013C - 0.013AB + 0.71AC + 0.74BC + 1.30A^2 + 0.16B^2 - 0.19C^2 \quad (3)$$

Table 1. The effect of formulation factors on nanosuspension particle size, PDI, and zeta potential.

Formulation Code	Stabilizer-to-Plant Extract Ratio (*w*/*w*)	AS/S Ratio (*v*/*v*)	Stirring Time (Hours)	Particle Size (nm)	PDI	Zeta Potential (−mV)
A1	0.40	15.00	2.00	481.60	0.453	14.60
A2	0.70	18.41	4.00	277.00	0.295	11.40
A3	0.40	5.00	6.00	540.00	0.671	11.80
A4	0.70	10.00	0.64	578.00	0.682	9.70
A5	0.70	10.00	7.36	337.80	0.451	10.10
A6	1.00	15.00	6.00	250.00	0.285	13.10
A7	0.70	10.00	4.00	348.70	0.493	9.60
A8	0.20	10.00	4.00	572.20	0.536	16.50
A9	1.00	5.00	2.00	374.30	0.526	10.60
A10	1.00	15.00	2.00	417.60	0.503	9.70
A11	0.40	15.00	6.00	328.20	0.513	13.90
A12	0.70	10.00	4.00	352.00	0.481	12.50
A13	0.70	1.59	4.00	452.00	0.483	10.40
A14	0.40	5.00	2.00	656.20	0.718	14.20
A15	0.70	10.00	4.00	332.50	0.424	9.80
A16	0.70	10.00	4.00	358.00	0.416	10.30
A17	1.20	10.00	4.00	280.20	0.352	11.70
A18	0.70	10.00	4.00	342.00	0.468	11.40
A19	0.70	10.00	4.00	360.30	0.523	10.90
A20	1.00	5.00	6.00	271.00	0.242	9.80

As = antisolvent, S = solvent.

Effect of Formulation Variables

Three-dimensional (3D) response surface plots were generated to study the main and interaction effects of formulation variables on response variables. Figure 1a illustrates the interaction effect of stabilizer-to-extract ratio and AS/S ratio at a fixed level of factor C. The graph shows that the particle size was significantly decreased by increasing the stabilizer-to-extract ratio and AS/S ratio. During nanonization, the reduction in particle size resulted in tremendous increase in the surface area. The process of coverage of new surfaces with stabilizer competes with agglomeration of nanoparticles. At a higher stabilizer-to-drug ratio, more molecules of stabilizer would be able to shield the newly forming nanoparticles, which prevents agglomeration [26]. In this study, nanosuspension prepared with HPMC showed the best stability and suitable particle size. HPMC is a nonionic polymer provided with a hydrodynamic boundary layer around the nanoparticles, which prevents the nanoparticles from agglomeration [27]. The hydroxypropyl and methoxy groups of HPMC can form hydrogen bonds with polyphenols and flavonoids molecules present in *A. absinthium* extract, and the strong adsorption of HPMC on the surface of the nanoparticles inhibits the particle crystal growth and aggregation [23]. At a constant AS/S ratio, increasing the stirring time and stabilizer/extract ratio considerably reduced particle size (Figure 1b). The reduction in particle size of nanosuspensions caused by increasing stirring time revealed that longer stirring times were superior in preventing crystal formation and aggregation.

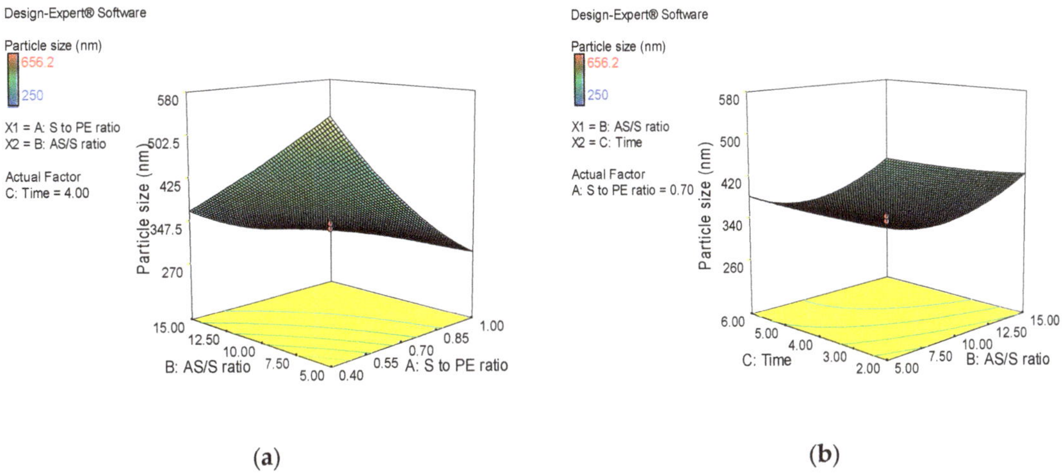

Figure 1. 3D plots showing the combined effect of formulation variables on particle sizes of *A. absinthium* nanosuspensions. (**a**) the interaction effect of stabilizer-to-extract ratio and AS/S ratio (**b**) the interaction effect stirring time and stabilizer-to-extract ratio.

The influence of selected parameters on PDI of *A. absinthium* nanosuspensions are displayed in Figure 2. At fixed level of factor C, the interaction effect of stabilizer-to-extract ratio and AS/S ratio was found to be significant in the formulation of homogeneous particle size distribution as a sharp decreasing trend in PDI was observed by increasing the stabilizer-to-extract ratio and AS/S ratio (Figure 2a). The decreasing trend in PDI was also observed by increasing stirring time and stabilizer-to-extract ratio at a fixed AS/S ratio (Figure 2b). The observed reduction in PDI indicates that a greater amount of stabilizer with longer stirring favored the production of more uniform particle size distribution. Zeta potential is the magnitude of surface charge. It is an index of stability of a nanosuspension system [28]. High values of zeta potential are required for providing repulsion between nanoparticles with a similar charge to prevent them from aggregation [29]. The zeta potential values were significantly decreased with increasing factor A, which indicated that the adsorption layer of steric stabilizer on the surface of nanosized particles increases the distance to the plane of shear at which the zeta potential was measured (Figure 3a).

For optimization of *A. absinthium* nanosuspensions, constraints were applied on independent response variables. In the current study, optimization was based upon minimum particle size, lower PDI, and maximization of zeta potential. The optimum values of input variables obtained via software were 1:1 of A (stabilizer-to-extract ratio), 15:1 of B (AS/S ratio), and 6 of C (stirring time) to attain the required values of response Y_1 (251.18 nm), Y_2 (0.294), and Y_3 (−12.5) in the optimized formulation of *A. absinthium* extract. The fresh formulation was prepared and evaluated. The optimized formulation has a PDI of 0.258, a zeta potential of −11.9, and an average particle size of 253.8 nm (Figure 4). The observed values of the responses (dependent variables) were discovered to be in strong agreement with the values projected by the model. These findings supported the chosen model's accuracy in predicting how input variables would affect response variables.

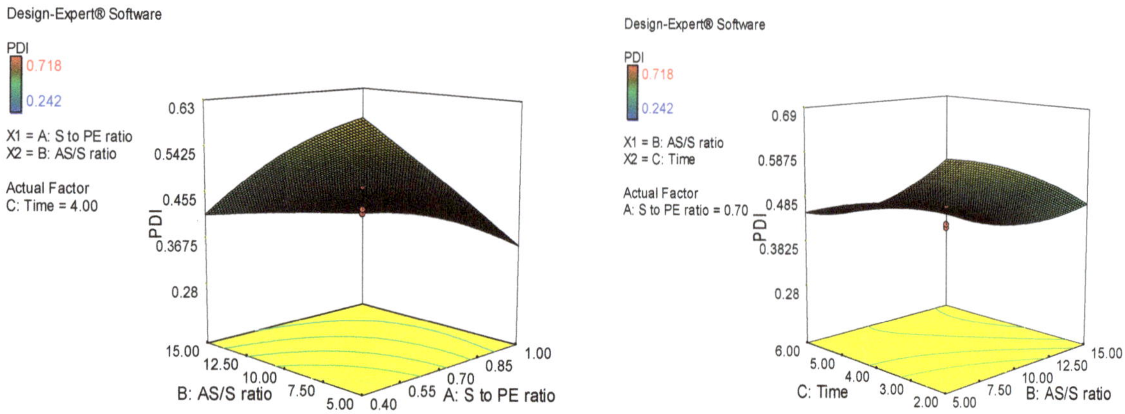

(**a**) (**b**)

Figure 2. 3D plots showing the combined effect of formulation variables on PDI of *A. absinthium* nanosuspensions. (**a**) the interaction effect of stabilizer-to-extract ratio and AS/S ratio (**b**) the interaction effect stirring time and stabilizer-to-extract ratio.

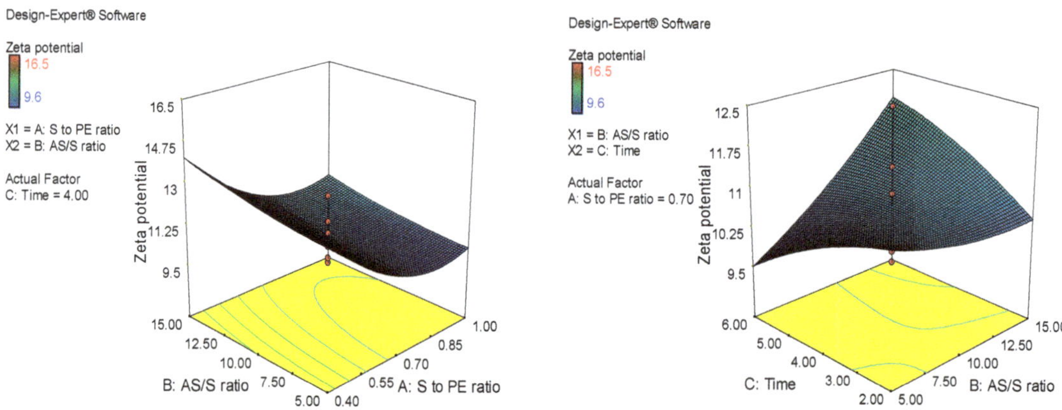

(**a**) (**b**)

Figure 3. 3D plots showing the combined effect of formulation variables on zeta potential of *A. absinthium* nanosuspensions. (**a**)the interaction effect of stabilizer-to-extract ratio and AS/S ratio (**b**) the interaction effect stirring time and stabilizer-to-extract ratio.

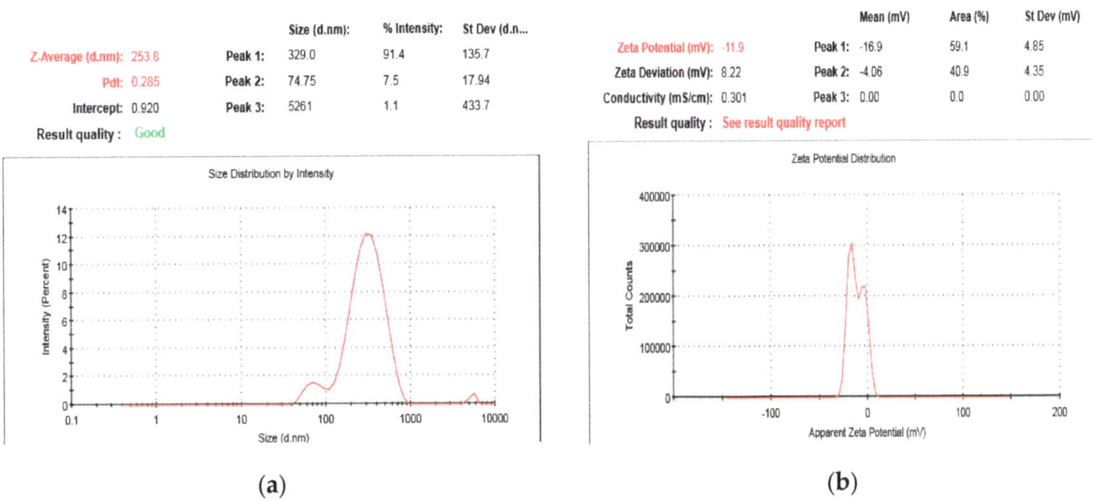

Figure 4. Particle size, PDI (**a**), and zeta potential (**b**) of *A. absinthium* optimized nanosuspensions.

3.2. Stability Studies

After storage at 25 °C and 4 °C (for 3 months), the stability of the A. absinthium extract formulation was assessed. Over the course of three months at two temperatures, no visible deposition of particles was seen. A slight increase in average particle size and PDI values were observed at both temperatures after the storage period (Table 2). The results showed that the optimized nanosuspension of *A. absinthium* extract was physically stable due to presence of HPMC, which acts as particle growth inhibitor by providing steric repulsion.

Table 2. Stability of *A. absinthium* nanosuspension at two different temperatures.

Storage Temperatures	Particle Size (nm)	PDI	Zeta Potential (mV)
25 °C	271.0 ± 0.02	0.706 ± 0.001	−10.6 ± 0.03
4 °C	286.6 ± 0.01	0.434±0.003	−9.22 ± 0.04

Every value is shown as the Mean ± SD (n = 3).

3.3. Characterization of Nanosuspension

3.3.1. Atomic Force Microscopy

An AFM analysis of *A. absinthium* nanosuspension revealed that particles were uniform with an approximate size of 25 nm. The AFM 3D topography image clearly indicated a well-defined homogeneous population of nanoparticles with good surface characteristics (Figure 5). The particle size measured using AFM is smaller than that with Zeta sizer (DLS). Particle size variations may be observed when using different methodologies to measure the size of nanoparticles. The difference between the diameters evaluated using the two approaches is clear since AFM examines the physical diameter of the nanoparticles, and DLS evaluates hydrodynamic diameter. Before the measurement of particle size using AFM and DSL, the lyophilized nanosuspension was suspended in distilled water and sonicated to obtain a homogenous suspension. During this process, nanoparticles may dissolve. The size measurement using DLS involved a solvation shell, so the size measurement using DLS should be a little bit greater than AFM. Solvation of nanoparticles is the reason for the greater particle size measured using DLS [30]. When lyophilized nanosuspension is suspended in distilled water and sonicated to create a homogeneous suspension prior to the determination of particle size, nanoparticles may aggregate. The inclusion of water during the lyophilization process may have caused aggregate flaws by promoting Ostwald ripening. Atomic force microscopy (AFM) demonstrated the successful preparation of plant nanosuspensions with nanoscale particle size and acceptable shape. To characterize the formulated nanosuspensions and identify their precise particle size and morphology, atomic force microscopy (AFM) is preferred [31].

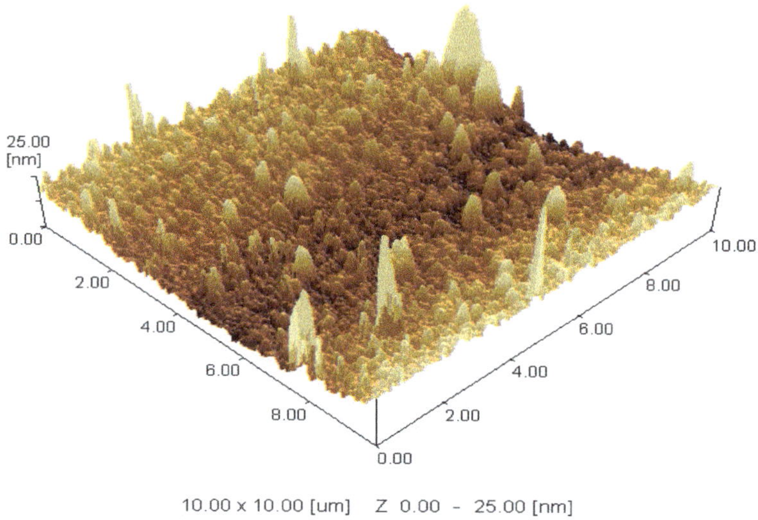

Figure 5. AFM image of *A. absinthium* nanosuspension.

3.3.2. FT–IR Spectra

The FT–IR spectra of *A. absinthium* extract, *A. absinthium* nanosuspension, and HPMC (stabilizer) are compared in Figure 6a–c. The spectrum of *A. absinthium* coarse extract presenting a strong and broad band at 3213 cm^{-1} was assigned to the stretching vibrations of the –OH group of flavonoids. This peak shifted to 3381 cm^{-1} and became less broad in the nanosuspension, which revealed inter-molecular hydrogen bonding between the phenolic -OH group and HPMC. The peaks observed at 1598 cm^{-1} (C=C aromatic stretching) and 1404 cm^{-1} (–C-H bending of aromatic hydrocarbon) in *A. absinthium* extract shifted to 1577 cm^{-1} and 1408 cm^{-1}, respectively, in the nanosuspension spectrum. Other peaks in the *A. absinthium* extract were observed at 2962 cm^{-1}, 1054 cm^{-1}, and 620 cm^{-1}. However, these peaks were not found in the spectrum of *A. absinthium* nanosuspension. These results indicated that during formulation of nanosuspension some sort of interaction developed between plant phytoconstituents and the stabilizer.

3.4. Dissolution Study

The dissolution rate of the nanosuspension of *A. absinthium* was compared with the coarse extract by measuring the concentration of quercetin, and results are depicted in Figure 7. The dissolution medium was phosphate buffer (pH 7.4, 900 mL) at 37 °C. The release profile of the *A. absinthium* extract showed slow dissolution with 21.45% release within the first ten minutes. On the other hand, the *A. absinthium* nanosuspension indicated faster dissolution as 35.96% quercetin was released within the first ten minutes. After complete dissolution (within 120 min), the amount of quercetin released from the *A. absinthium* nanosuspension (89.71%) was still greater than the *A. absinthium* coarse extract (55.50%). The dissolving velocity of the nanosuspension was dramatically accelerated by the smaller particle size and increased surface area of nanoparticles [32,33]. Due to the presence of surface stabilizers, poorly soluble flavonoids in plant extract have higher solubility and wettability in the dissolving medium, which could also account for the increased dissolution rate of nanosuspensions [34].

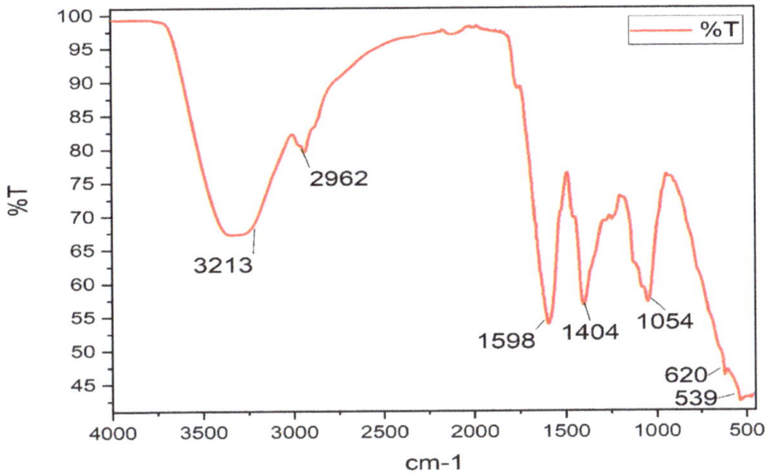

(a)

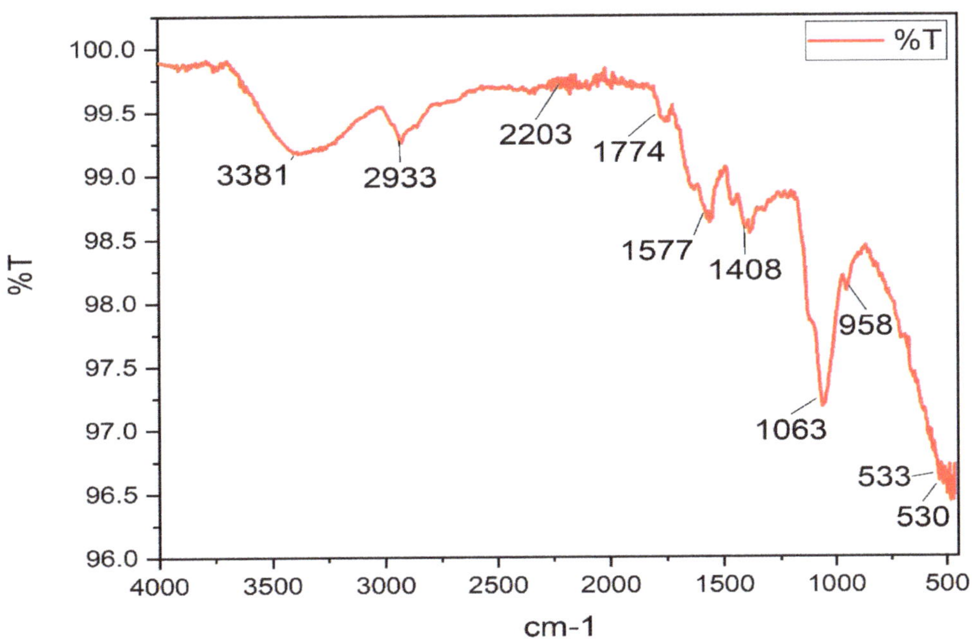

(b)

Figure 6. *Cont.*

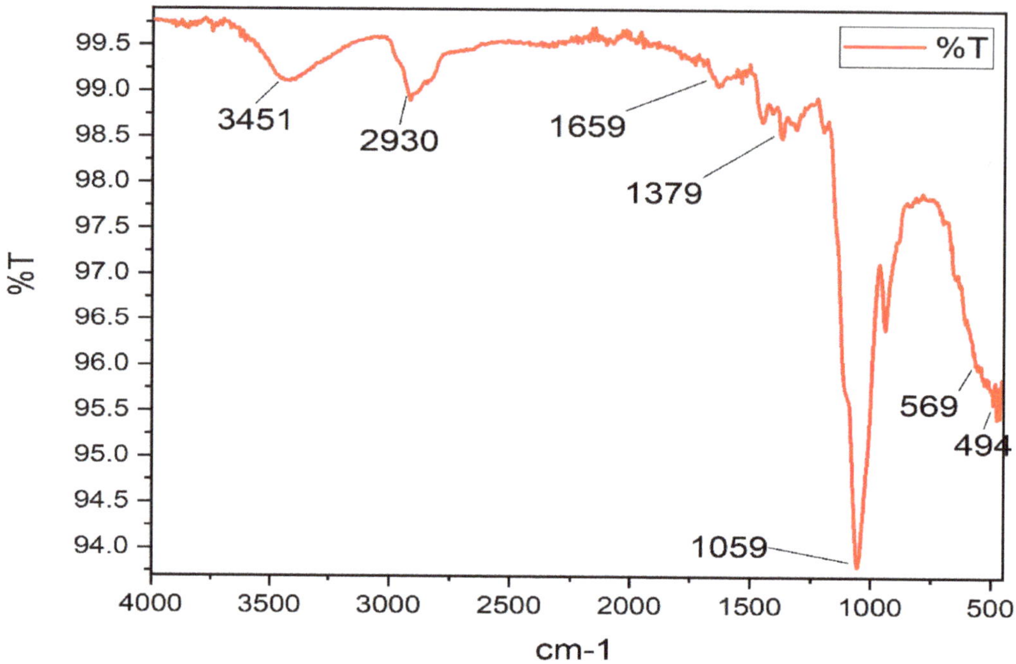

(c)

Figure 6. (**a**) FT–IR spectrum of *A. absinthium* extract. (**b**) FT–IR spectrum of *A. absinthium* nanosuspension. (**c**) FT–IR spectrum of HPMC.

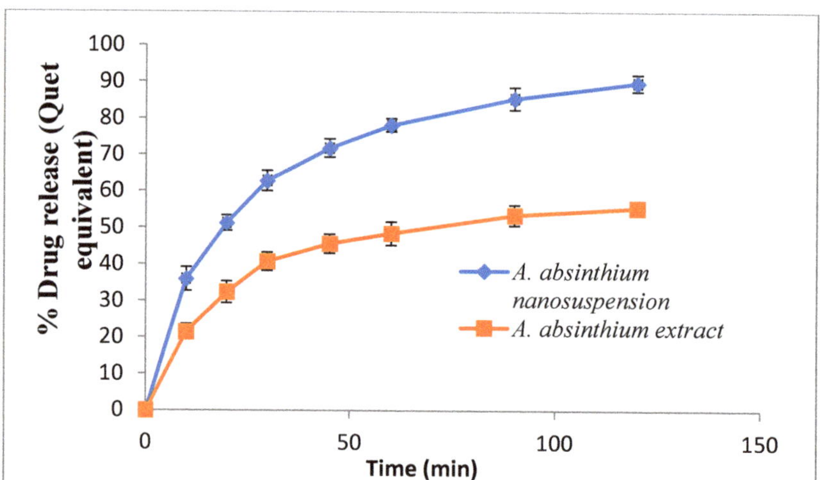

Figure 7. *A. absinthium* nanosuspension and coarse extract dissolution profiles. The results are presented as Mean ± SD (n = 3).

3.5. Pharmacokinetic Study

Figure 8 displays the mean plasma concentration versus time curves following oral administration of *A. absinthium* nanosuspension and coarse extract at doses of 50 mg/kg (with reference to quercetin). Plants contain many bioactive phytoconstituents, and it is immensely difficult to evaluate the concentration of all these constituents, so in the ongoing research only one key bioactive component was used as the standard compound to compare results. For this purpose, quercetin, which is the major constituent of Artemisia extract, was used as the standard compound to evaluate the dissolution profile as well as for pharmacokinetic studies of nanosuspensions. The dissolution profile of the *Artemisia* extract and nanosuspension was expressed as "quercetin equivalent". After 1 h of oral administration, the value of C_{max} of *A. absinthium* nanosuspension (521.2 µg/mL) was significantly ($p < 0.05$) higher than coarse extract (324.93 µg/mL). The value of $AUC_{0–24h}$ of nanoformulation was 1.13-fold greater than coarse extract. In the present investigation, the larger C_{max} and AUC values indicated improved absorption of the nanosuspension. Nanosuspension technology significantly increased the saturation solubility and dissolution rate due to smaller particle size and greater surface area results in enhanced bioavailability [35,36]. In addition, nanoparticles exhibited increased bio adhesion to intestinal villi that might prolong the retention time of nanosuspensions in the gut and enhance the passive absorption [37].

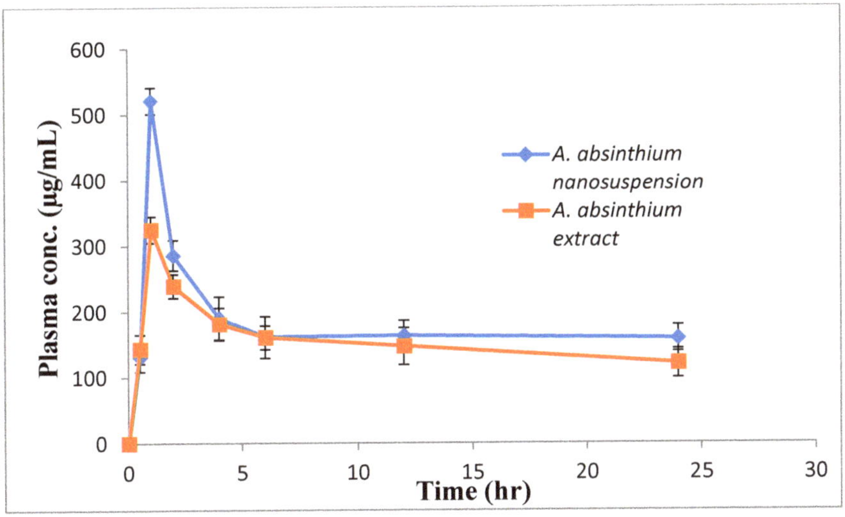

Figure 8. Plasma concentration–time curves after oral administration of *A. Absinthium* nanosuspension and coarse extract (quercetin equivalent) to rats. Results are expressed as Mean ± SD (n = 3).

3.6. In Vitro Antioxidant Activity

Antioxidant potentials of nanosuspensions and coarse extract were determined using the DPPH radical scavenging method. The DPPH test based on the ability of DPPH to decolorize via antioxidants is a reliable and easy method for determining radical scavenging potential of pure compounds and plant extracts [32]. The results of antioxidant potential were represented in terms of IC50 value (Table 3). Ascorbic acid, a natural antioxidant, was utilized as a control molecule and demonstrated the highest antioxidant activity with an IC50 value of 125.94 g/mL. The nanosuspension of *A. absinthium* revealed a stronger DPPH radical scavenging potential as indicated by its lower IC50 value (196.93 µg/mL) compared to the coarse extract (248.32 µg/mL).

Table 3. Antioxidant activity of *A. absinthium* nanosuspension.

Treatments	IC50 Value (μg/mL)
A. absinthium nanosuspension	196.93 ± 0.13
A. absinthium extract	248.32 ± 0.21
Ascorbic acid	125.94 ± 021

Every value is shown as the Mean ± SD (n = 3).

3.7. In Vivo Hepatoprotective Activity

Rats given CCl4 revealed a large ($p < 0.05$) increase in AST, alanine transaminase (ALT), ALP, and total bilirubin levels, as well as a significant ($p < 0.05$) decrease in albumin and total protein levels, confirming the presence of hepatic injury. Significant liver damage was induced by CCl4 administration, as shown by rising levels of marker enzymes in the serum. After cellular I jury, these enzymes are typically present in the cytoplasm and released into the blood. The raised levels of serums AST and ALT are highly sensitive and specific clinical biomarkers of hepatotoxicity and represent damage to the hepatocytes. Another crucial indicator of liver health is ALP, which is also widely used to assess the integrity of plasma membranes. Pathological alterations in biliary flow were detected via an elevated level of ALP in the serum. Additionally, mice treated with CCl4 had considerably lower levels of total protein and albumin. Low levels of total proteins suggested hepatic disease, as protein synthesis is a function of a healthy liver. Low albumin levels are a sign of hepatotoxicity.

Treatment with *A. absinthium* nanosuspension at 100 mg/kg significantly reduced the activities of AST (56.24 ± 0.46 IU/L), ALT (29.27 ± 0.21 IU/L), and ALP (242.39 ± 8.25 IU/L) as well as the level of total bilirubin (0.52 ± 0.25 mg/dL) as compared to the positive control group after four days of treatment. The decreased levels of AST, ALT, ALP, and total bilirubin suggest a hepatoprotective potential of *A. absinthium* nanosuspension. Moreover, average levels of albumin (3.85 ± 0.26 g/dL) and total protein (8.78 ± 0.38 g/dL) were significantly improved in rats treated with 100mg/kg of *A. absinthium* nanosuspension. It was observed that the ameliorative effect of *A. absinthium* nanosuspension at 100 mg/kg was comparable to 150 mg/kg of *A. absinthium* coarse extract (Table 4).

Table 4. Effects of *A. absinthium* nanosuspension on hepatic biomarkers.

Hepatic Biomarkers	Normal Control G-I	Positive Control (CCl4) G-II	CCl4 + AA NS (100 mg/Kg)	CCl4 + AA CE (150 mg/Kg)
AST (IU/L)	56.00 ± 0.27	108.17 ± 0.67 #	56.31 ± 0.46 *	56.45 ± 0.20 *
ALT (IU/L)	29.43 ± 0.18	98.23 ± 0.45 #	29.27 ± 0.21 *	29.18 ± 0.44 *
ALP (IU/L)	164.47 ± 8.98	387.23 ± 5.32 #	242.39 ± 8.25 *	240.00 ± 7.25 *
Bilirubin (mg/dL)	0.54 ± 0.16	0.83 ± 0.12 #	0.52 ± 0.25 *	0.52 ± 0.27 *
Albumin (g/dL)	3.90 ± 0.28	2.61 ± 0.43 #	3.85 ± 0.26 *	3.85 ± 0.47 *
Total protein (g/dL)	9.15 ± 0.18	5.52 ± 0.33 #	8.78 ± 0.38 *	8.76 ± 0.20 *

Every value is shown as the Mean SEM (n = 4). AANS: # Significant difference ($p < 0.05$) from normal control group, * significant difference ($p < 0.05$) from positive control group. AA: *Artemisia absinthium*, NS: nanosuspension, CE: coarse extract.

The hepatoprotective activity of *A. absinthium* extract and nanosuspension could be explained due to presence of polyphenols and flavonoids, which exert strong antioxidant activity and are involved in hampering the formation of toxic metabolites of CCl_4. Quercetin has been reported as a promising hepatoprotective compound due to its antioxidative, anti-inflammatory, and anti-apoptotic activities against various liver disorders [33]. The findings are consistent with earlier research that found quercetin, the primary bioactive component of hydroalcoholic extract flavonoid C. spinosa, to be hepatoprotective against tertiary butyl hydroperoxide (t-BHP)-induced liver damage [34]. These results indicated that *A. absinthium* nanosuspension at 100 mg/kg showed equivalent hepatoprotective activity as 150 mg/kg of *A. absinthium* coarse extract. The enhanced hepatoprotective activity of *A. absinthium* nanosuspension was due to improved bioavailability, which is in line with the results of dissolution and pharmacokinetic studies.

Antioxidant Enzymes

A remarkable ($p < 0.05$) reduction in activities of GPx, CAT, and SOD were observed in CCl_4-treated rats as compared to normal healthy rats. Treatment with *A. absinthium* nanosuspension at 100 mg/kg restored the levels of GPx, CAT, and SOD, which was comparable to 150 mg/kg of *A. absinthium* coarse extract (Table 5). The in vivo antioxidant potential of *A. absinthium* nanosuspension directly linked to the flavonoids like quercetin, rutin, apigenin, and myricetin. These flavonoids have potent antioxidant activity that prevents the harmful effects caused by reactive oxygen species by neutralizing the free radicals and elevating the activities of antioxidant enzymes [38].

Table 5. Effect of *A. absinthium* nanosuspensions on antioxidant enzymes.

Groups	GPx (IU/mg Protein)	CAT (IU/mg Protein)	SOD (IU/mg Protein)
Normal control	4.70 ± 0.18	42.21 ± 0.34	22.23 ± 0.25
Positive control	2.92 ± 0.32 #	20.49 ± 0.17 #	15.61 ± 0.20 #
AA CE (150 mg/kg)	4.39 ± 0.20 *	41.68 ± 0.34 *	20.49 ± 0.46 *
AA NS (100 mg/Kg)	4.01 ± 0.25 *	40.86 ± 0.22 *	20.78 ± 0.25 *

Results are shown as Mean SEM (n = 4) with significant differences ($p < 0.05$) between the normal control group and the positive control group. AA: *Artemisia absinthium*, NS: nanosuspension, CE: coarse extract, GPx: glutathione peroxidase, CAT: catalase, SOD: superoxide dismutase. # Significant difference ($p < 0.05$) from normal control group, * significant difference ($p < 0.05$) from positive control group. AA: *Artemisia absinthium*, NS: nanosuspension, CE: coarse extract.

A. absinthium extract has been reported to possess antioxidant and antiparasitic activities, and its aqueous methanolic extract provides hepatoprotection against CCl_4 and acetaminophen-induced liver injury [39]. *A. absinthium* was used to treat epilepsy, urinary disorders, and gastric problems and for wound healing. However, most of the phytochemicals such as quercetin and myrecetin suffered poor water solubility and low bioavailability [40–42]. In the present work, a nanosuspension of *A. absinthium* extract was developed to enhance bioavailability and bioactivity. No other research is available on the formulation of nanosuspensions of *A. absinthium* extract. In recent years, nanosuspensions have proven a promising strategy for the delivery of poorly water-soluble drugs and phytoconstituents as it increases solubility and dissolution of drug molecules. The reduced particle size offers high surface area, which dramatically increases the saturation solubility and dissolution velocity and ultimately translates into improved bioavailability of therapeutic candidates [43].

The comparison between *A. absinthium* CS- and NS-treatment groups indicated that NS at 100 mg/kg showed comparable hepatoprotective activity as 150 mg/kg of *A. absinthium* CS. The nanosuspension showed hepatoprotective potential at a smaller dose, which ultimately reduces side effects. The enhanced hepatoprotective activity of *A. absinthium* NS was due to improved bioavailability. The results agree with the study of Mishra et al. (2015), which demonstrated that nanosuspension formulation of *Phyllanthus amarus* (PA) extract showed better hepatoprotective potential than coarse extract. Nanoparticles of PA at a dose of 50 mg/kg were more effective than 125 mg/kg of PA coarse extract in providing hepatoprotection against paracetamol-induced hepatic injury. Devara et al. (2015) also reported that curcumin in the form of intravenous nanosuspension showed better liver protection as compared to the coarse suspension of the drug. Many other reports are also available on the formulation of nanosuspensions from medicinal plants such as *Azadirachta indica*, *Chrysanthemum coronarium* [44], and *Rauvolfia serpentina* [45], and the results reveal that nanoformulation has enhanced the bioavailability and potential of medicinal plants.

4. Conclusions

A nanosuspension of *Artemisia absinthium* extract with suitable particle size was successfully prepared. *Artemisia absinthium* nanosuspension is an appropriate pharmaceutical formulation with faster dissolution rate, enhanced bioavailability, and hepatoprotective ability. The study suggested that the prepared *Artemisia absinthium* nanosuspension is a potent hepatoprotective formulation having potential for commercialization in the pharmaceutical industry.

Author Contributions: Writing—original draft preparation, conceptualization, N.J.; Writing—original draft preparation, investigation, methodology, F.K.; Formal analysis, project administration, K.U.R.; Formal analysis, data curation, S.I.T.; Writing—review and editing, data curation, N.A. All authors have read and agreed to the published version of the manuscript.

Funding: Financial support was received from the Higher Education Commission of Pakistan through research project grant No. 66441.

Institutional Review Board Statement: The current study was a part of research project No. 66441 funded by the Higher Education Commission of Pakistan, and its protocol for the research synopsis was approved by the departmental technical committee followed by the Directorate of Graduate Studies, University of Agriculture Faisalabad.

Data Availability Statement: Not applicable.

Conflicts of Interest: The authors declare no conflict of interest.

References

1. Ananth, D.A.; Tietela, Z.; Aseervatham, G.S.B.; Garlapatic, D.; Sivasudhad, T. Phytochemical and pharmacological status of indigenous medicinal plant *Pedalium murex* L.—A review. *Biomed. Pharmacother.* **2018**, *103*, 1456–1463.
2. Tlili, N.; Tir, M.; Feriani, A.; Yahia, Y.; Allagui, M.S.; Saadaoui, E.; Cafsi, M.E.; Nasri, N. Potential health advantages of *Periploca laevigata*: Preliminary phytochemical analysis and evaluation of in vitro antioxidant capacity and assessment of hepatoprotective, anti-inflammatory and analgesic effects. *J. Funct. Foods* **2018**, *48*, 234–242. [CrossRef]
3. Junejo, J.A.; Gogoi, G.; Islam, J.; Rudrapal, M.; Mondal, P.; Hazarika, H.; Zaman, K. Exploration of antioxidant, antidiabetic and hepatoprotective activity of *Diplazium esculentum*—A wild edible plant from North Eastern India. *Future J. Pharm. Sci.* **2018**, *4*, 93–101. [CrossRef]
4. Shazhni, J.R.A.; Renu, A.; Vijayaraghavan, P. Insights of antidiabetic, anti-inflammatory and hepatoprotective properties of antimicrobial secondary metabolites of corm extract from *Caladium x hortulanum*. *Saudi J. Biol. Sci.* **2018**, *25*, 1755–1761. [CrossRef]
5. Moaca, E.; Pavel, I.Z.; Danciu, C.; Crainiceanu, Z.; Minda, D.; Ardelean, F.; Antal, D.S.; Ghiulai, R.; Cioca, A.; Derban, M.; et al. Romanian Wormwood (*Artemisia absinthium* L.): Physicochemical and nutraceutical screening. *Molecules* **2019**, *24*, 3087. [CrossRef]
6. Msaada, K.; Salem, N.; Bachrouch, O.; Bousselmi, S.; Tammar, S.; Alfaify, A.; Sane, K.A.; Ammar, W.B.; Azeiz, S.; Brahim, A.H.; et al. Chemical composition and antioxidant and antimicrobial activities of wormwood (*Artemisia absinthium* L.) essential oils and phenolics. *J. Chem.* **2015**, *2015*, 804658. [CrossRef]
7. Amat, N.; Upur, H.; Blazekovic, B. In vivo hepatoprotective activity of the aqueous extract of *Artemisia absinthium* L. against chemically and immunologically induced liver injuries in mice. *J. Ethnopharmacol.* **2010**, *131*, 478–484. [CrossRef] [PubMed]
8. Antonio, S.W.; Carmen, S.; Victor, V.T.; Jose, C.; Abhel, C.; Cinthya, A.; Cesar, G.; Segundo, R.; Juana, C. Hepatoprotective and nephroprotective activity of *Artemisia absinthium* L. on diclofenac-induced toxicity in rats. *Pharmacogn J.* **2020**, *12*, 1032–1041. [CrossRef]
9. Aberham, A.; Cicek, S.S.; Schneider, P.; Stuppner, H. Analysis of sesquiterpene lactones, lignans, and flavonoids in wormwood (*Artemisia absinthium* L.) using High-Performance Liquid Chromatography (HPLC)-Mass Spectrometry, Reversed Phase HPLC, and HPLC-Solid Phase Extraction-Nuclear Magnetic Resonance. *J. Agric. Food Chem.* **2010**, *58*, 10817–10823. [CrossRef]
10. Sahin, S.; Aybastier, O.; Isik, E. Optimization of ultrasonic-assisted extraction of antioxidant compounds from *Artemisia absinthium* using response surface methodology. *Food Chem.* **2013**, *141*, 1361–1368. [CrossRef]
11. Batiha, G.E.; Olatunde, A.; El-Mleeh, A.; Hetta, H.F.; Al-Rejaie, S.; Alghamdi, S.; Zahoor, M.; Beshbishy, A.M.; Murata, T.; Zaragoza-Bastida, A.; et al. Bioactive compounds, pharmacological actions, and pharmacokinetics of wormwood (*Artemisia absinthium*). *Antibiotics* **2020**, *9*, 353. [CrossRef] [PubMed]
12. Raj, N.; Krishnakumar, K.; Dineshkumar, B. Green herbs nanosuspensions: A review. *Pharm. Biol.* **2016**, *6*, 82–85.
13. Yin, T.; Zhang, Y.; Liu, Y.; Chen, Q.; Fu, Y.; Liang, J.; Zhou, J.; Tang, X.; Liu, J.; Huo, M. The efficiency and mechanism of N-octyl-O, N-carboxymethyl chitosan-based micelles to enhance the oral absorption of silybin. *Int. J. Pharm.* **2018**, *536*, 231–240. [CrossRef] [PubMed]
14. Bajaj, H.; Bisht, S.; Yadav, M.; Singh, V. Bioavailability enhancement: A review. *Int. J. Pharma Bio Sci.* **2011**, *2*, 202–216.

15. Ajazuddin; Saraf, S. Applications of novel drug delivery system for herbal formulations. *Fitoterapia* **2010**, *81*, 680–689. [CrossRef]
16. Koradia, K.D.; Sheth, N.R.; Koradia, H.D.; Dabhi, M.R. Ziprasidone nanocrystals by wet media milling followed by spray drying and lyophilization: Formulation and process parameter optimization. *J. Drug Deliv. Sci. Technol.* **2018**, *43*, 73–84. [CrossRef]
17. Zong, L.; Li, X.; Wang, H.; Cao, Y.; Yin, L.; Li, M.; Wei, Z.; Chen, D.; Pu, X.; Han, J. Formulation and characterization of biocompatible and stable I.V. itraconazole nanosuspensions stabilized by a new stabilizer polyethylene glycol-poly(β-Benzyl-L-aspartate) (PEG-PBLA). *Int. J. Pharm.* **2017**, *531*, 108–117. [CrossRef]
18. Lai, F.; Pireddu, R.; Corrias, F.; Fadda, A.M.; Valenti, D.; Pini, E.; Sinico, C. Nanosuspension improves tretinoin photostability and delivery to the skin. *Int. J. Pharm.* **2013**, *458*, 104–109. [CrossRef]
19. Thadkala, K.; Prema, K.N.; Bathini, R.; Chinta, S.; Jithan, A. Preparation and characterization of amorphous ezetimibe nanosuspensions intended for enhancement of oral bioavailability. *Int. J. Pharm. Investig.* **2014**, *4*, 131–137.
20. Mishra, S.; Pandey, H.; Pandey, A.C. Nanosuspension of *Phyllanthus amarus* extract for improving oral bioavailability and prevention of paracetamol induced hepatotoxicity in Sprague–Dawley rats. *Adv. Nat. Sci: Nanosci.* **2013**, *4*, 035007. [CrossRef]
21. Yu, P.; Lu, S.; Zhang, S.; Zhang, S.; Li, Y.; Liu, J. Enhanced oral bioavailability and diminished food effect of lurasidone hydrochloride nanosuspensions prepared by facile nanoprecipitation based on dilution. *Powder Technol.* **2017**, *312*, 11–20. [CrossRef]
22. Zu, Y.; Wu, W.; Zhao, X.; Li, Y.; Wang, W.; Zhong, C.; Zhang, Y.; Zhao, X. Enhancement of solubility, antioxidant ability and bioavailability of taxifolin nanoparticles by liquid antisolvent precipitation technique. *Int. J. Pharm.* **2014**, *471*, 366–376. [CrossRef] [PubMed]
23. Sun, M.; Gao, Y.; Pei, Y.; Guo, C.; Li, H.; Cao, F.; Yu, A.; Zhai, G. Development of nanosuspension formulation for oral delivery of quercetin. *J. Biomed. Nanotechnol.* **2010**, *6*, 325–332. [CrossRef] [PubMed]
24. Jahan, N.; Rahman, K.U.; Ali, S.; Bhatti, I. Antioxidant activity of gemmo therapeutically treated indigenous medicinal plants. *Asian J. Chem.* **2011**, *23*, 3461–3470.
25. Abdous, B.; Sajjadi, S.M.; Mamani, L. β-Cyclodextrin modified mesoporous silica nanoparticles as a nano-carrier: Response surface methodology to investigate and optimize loading and release processes for curcumin delivery. *J. Appl. Biomed.* **2017**, *15*, 210–218. [CrossRef]
26. Mishra, B.; Sahoob, J.; Dixit, P.K. Formulation and process optimization of naproxen nanosuspensions stabilized by hydroxy propyl methyl cellulose. *Carbohydr. Polym.* **2015**, *127*, 300–308. [CrossRef]
27. Mishra, B.; Sahoo, J.; Dixit, P.K. Enhanced bioavailability of cinnarizine nanosuspensions by particle size engineering: Optimization and physicochemical investigations. *Mater. Sci. Eng.* **2016**, *63*, 62–69. [CrossRef]
28. Steffi, P.F.; Srinivasan, M. Preparation, characterization, and stabilization of curcumin nanosuspension. *Int. J. Pharm. Tech. Res.* **2014**, *6*, 842–849.
29. Santos, A.M.; Carvalho, F.C.; Teixeira, D.A.; Azevedo, D.L.; Barros, W.M.; Gremiao, M.P.D. Computational and experimental approaches for development of methotrexate nanosuspensions by bottom-up nanoprecipitation. *Int. J. Pharm.* **2017**, *524*, 330–338. [CrossRef]
30. Humera, I.; Nazish, J.; Khalil-ur-Rahman; Saba, J. Formulation and characterization of *Azadirachta indica* nano biopesticides for ecofriendly control of wheat pest *Tribolium castaneum* and *Rhyzopertha dominica*. *J. Microencapsul.* **2022**, *39*, 638–653.
31. Fritzen-Garcia, M.B.; Zanetti-Ramos, B.G.; Oliveira, C.S.D.; Soldi, V.; Pasa, A.A.; Creczynski-Pasa, T.B. Atomic force microscopy imaging of polyurethane nanoparticles onto different solid substrates. *Mater. Sci. Eng.* **2009**, *29*, 405–409. [CrossRef]
32. Han, M.; Xiaoli, L.; Guo, Y.; Wang, Y.; Wang, X. Preparation, characterization, biodistribution and antitumor efficacy of hydroxycamptothecin nanosuspensions. *Int. J. Pharm.* **2013**, *455*, 85–92. [CrossRef] [PubMed]
33. Li, Y.; Zhao, X.; Zu, Y.; Zhang, Y. Preparation and characterization of paclitaxel nanosuspension using novel emulsification method by combining high speed homogenizer and high pressure homogenization. *Int. J. Pharm.* **2015**, *490*, 324–333. [CrossRef] [PubMed]
34. Salem, H.F.; Kharshoum, R.M. Nanoprecipitation technique for preparation of sterically stabilized risperidone nanosuspension: *In vitro* and *in vivo* study. *Int. J. Pharm. Pharm.* **2016**, *8*, 136–142.
35. Zhang, J.; Huang, Y.; Liu, D.; Gao, Y.; Qian, S. Preparation of apigenin nanocrystals using supercritical antisolvent process for dissolution and bioavailability enhancement. *Eur. J. Pharm. Sci.* **2013**, *48*, 740–747. [CrossRef]
36. Singh, M.K.; Pooja, D.; Ravuri, H.G.; Gunukula, A.; Kulhari, H.; Sistla, R. Fabrication of surfactant-stabilized nanosuspension of naringenin to surpass its poor physicochemical properties and low oral bioavailability. *Phytomedicine* **2018**, *40*, 48–54. [CrossRef]
37. Yang, H.; Teng, F.; Wang, P.; Tian, B.; Lin, X.; Hu, X.; Zhang, L.; Zhang, K.; Zhang, Y.; Tang, X. Investigation of a nanosuspension stabilized by Soluplus to improve bioavailability. *Int. J. Pharm.* **2014**, *477*, 88–95. [CrossRef]
38. Miltonprabu, S.; Tmczyk, M.; Wozniak, K.S.; Rastrelli, L.; Daglia, M.; Nabavi, S.F.; Alavian, S.M.; Nabbavi, S.M. Hepatoprotective effect of quercetin: From chemistry to medicine. *Food Chem. Toxicol.* **2016**, *108*, 365–374. [CrossRef]
39. Kalantari, H.; Foruozandeh, H.; Khodayar, M.J.; Sianpoosh, A.; Saki, N.; Kheradamand, P. Antioxidant and hepatoprotective effects of *Capparis spinosa* L. fractions and quercetin on tert-butyl hydroperoxide-induced acute liver damage in mice. *J. Tradit. Complement. Med.* **2018**, *8*, 120–127. [CrossRef]
40. Peralta, M.A.; Ortega, M.G.; Cabrera, J.L.; Paraje, M.G. The antioxidant activity of a prenyl flavonoid alters its antifungal toxicity on Candida albicans biofilms. *Food Chem. Toxicol.* **2018**, *114*, 285–291. [CrossRef]

41. Tang, X.; Olatunji, O.J.; Zhou, Y.; Hou, X. *Allium tuberosum*: Antidiabetic and hepatoprotective activities. *Food Res. Int.* **2017**, *102*, 681–689. [CrossRef] [PubMed]
42. Vahid, Z.; Jalal, M.; Mostafa, M.; Mohammad, M.; Ali, V. Antioxidant and hepatoprotective effects of *Artemisia dracunculus* against CCl_4-induced hepatotoxicity in rats. *Avicenna J. Phytomed.* **2018**, *8*, 51–62.
43. Hao, J.; Gao, Y.; Zhao, J.; Zhang, J.; Li, Q.; Zhao, Z.; Liu, J. Preparation and optimization of resveratrol nanosuspensions by antisolvent precipitation using boxbehnken design. *AAPS Pharm. Sci. Tech.* **2015**, *16*, 118–128. [CrossRef] [PubMed]
44. Hazafa, A.; Nazish, J.; Anjum, Z.; Rahman, K.-U.; Muhammad, S.; Naeem, M. Evaluation and optimization of nanosuspensions of *Chrysanthemum coronarium* and *Azadirachta indica* using Response Surface Methodology for pest management. *Chemosphere* **2022**, *292*, 133411. [CrossRef] [PubMed]
45. Irum, T.S.; Nazish, J.; Nadeem, A.; Ali, A. Formulation and Process Optimization of *Rauvolfia serpentina* Nanosuspension by HPMC and In Vitro Evaluation of A CE Inhibitory Potential. *J. Funct. Biomater.* **2022**, *13*, 268.

Journal of
Functional Biomaterials

MDPI

Article

Natural Biomolecule Ovomucin–Chitosan Oligosaccharide Self-Assembly Nanogel for Lutein Application Enhancement: Characterization, Environmental Stability and Bioavailability

Qi Xu [1,2,*,†], Haoye Teng [1,2,†], Xuanchen Li [2], Zhenqing Zhang [2], Yumeng Han [2] and Haixin Sun [1,*]

1 College of Life Science, Qingdao University, Qingdao 266000, China; hy12122021@163.com
2 Institute of Advanced Cross-Field Science, Qingdao University, Qingdao 266000, China; lxc1559360735@163.com (X.L.); zhangzhenqing0330@163.com (Z.Z.); hanym0105@163.com (Y.H.)
* Correspondence: xq@qdu.edu.cn (Q.X.); sunhaixin@qdu.edu.cn (H.S.)
† These authors contribute equally to this work.

Abstract: As an essential nutrient, lutein (LUT) has the ability to aid in the prevention of eye diseases, cardiovascular diseases, and cancer. However, the application of LUT is largely restricted by its poor solubility and susceptibility to oxidative degradation. Thus, in this study, LUT-loaded nanogel (OVM-COS-LUT) was prepared by a self-assembly of ovomucin (OVM) and chitosan oligosaccharide (COS) to enhance the effective protection and bioavailability of LUT. The nanogel had excellent dispersion (PDI = 0.25) and an 89.96% LUT encapsulation rate. XRD crystal structure analysis confirmed that the encapsulated LUT maintained an amorphous morphology. In addition, the nanogel showed satisfactory stability with pH levels ranging from 2 to 9 and high ionic strengths (>100 mM). Even under long-term storage, the nanogel maintained an optimistic stabilization and protection capacity; its effective retention rates could reach 96.54%. In vitro, digestion simulation showed that the bioaccessibility and sustained release of OVM-COS-LUT nanogel was superior to that of free LUT. The nanogel provided significant antioxidant activity, and no significant harmful effects were detected in cytotoxicity analyses at higher concentrations. In summary, OVM-COS-LUT can be utilized as a potential safe oral and functional carrier for encapsulating LUT.

Keywords: nanogel; lutein; stability; bioavailability; oral delivery

1. Introduction

Carotenoids are one of the essential nutrients for physiological health [1]. As a member of the carotenoid family, LUT has shown benefits in preventing diseases and easing symptoms, such as reducing the risk of cataracts or age-related macular degeneration [2,3], cancer prevention [4], and immunomodulation [5].

However, natural carotenoids are found only in plants or microorganisms. For humans, uptake through daily ingestion rather than synthesis is the only way to obtain LUT [6]. Although foods like corn are an abundant source of LUT, its poor water solubility limits its bioavailability via oral administration [7]. In addition, its unique chemical structure makes LUT sensitive to light, heat, and oxygen. Therefore, the oral application of LUT in medicine and nutritional supplements faces severe challenges [8].

One of the current strategies to solve this problem is to encapsulate bioactive substances into nano-delivery systems [9]. There is great potential to utilize nanomaterials' large surface area-to-volume ratio to improve bioavailability, controlled release, and sensory improvement of active ingredients [10]. There are two main methods for generating nanoparticle systems; one is a "top-down" approach where larger-sized materials are dispersed and milled [11]. This method is prone to raw material waste and requires higher energy support. The other is the "bottom-up" approach, where small molecules are chemically synthesized or self-assembled into nanostructures [11]. Among them, self-assembly from natural biomolecules, especially proteins or polysaccharides, possesses advantages for the design or manufacture of nanocarriers [12]. Those nanocarriers become catabolized and absorbed as nutrients after entering the digestive tract; therefore, they have low immunogenicity and high biocompatibility [13]. In addition, without using other chemical cross-linking agents, natural protein–polysaccharide nano-systems can self-assemble through electrostatic interactions and hydrogen bonding, which is also more eco-friendly and safer. Ma et al. prepared nanoemulsion loaded with β-carotene using soy protein isolate (SPI) and citrus pectin (CP), and the ultrasound-treated group showed excellent storage stability [14]. Li et al. encapsulated lutein using zein-soluble soybean polysaccharide composite nanoparticles, and the bioaccessibility of encapsulated lutein was significantly higher than that of the free group [15].

OVM, an anionic protein isolated from eggs, consists of low-carbohydrate α1- subunits, α2-subunits, and high-carbohydrate β-subunits polymerized by disulfide bonds [16]. OVM has a variety of functional activities, such as antiviral [17], anti-tumor [18], and anti-inflammatory [19] effects. The application of OVM as a novel functional component in nano-delivery systems is yet to be explored. Due to its unique molecular structure, OVM has excellent gelling properties, which makes it a potential material for constructing nanogel [20]. The natural amphiphilicity of OVM also provides sufficient hydrophobic space for the payload of hydrophobic substances. In addition, to enhance the stability of the protein delivery body after encapsulating the cargo, a low molecular weight in COS was utilized to induce the construction further. COS, a cationic polysaccharide derived from chitin/chitosan, has good biocompatibility, water solubility, and adhesion [21], and can be self-assembled by electrostatic force binding to OVM.

Given the factors above, OVM and COS were used to prepare lutein-coated oral-delivery-based nanogel. A structure analysis showed that all the components bonded to each other through self-assembly during the formation of nanogel. The nanogel exhibited a wide pH range, ionic strength, and long-term storage stability. Meanwhile, LUT's antioxidant ability and bioavailability were raised through binding with nanogel. The biocompatibility of nanogel was also verified by a cytotoxicity assay. In summary, this study provides new insights into the nano-delivery applications of OVM-COS, offering a potential strategy for effectively utilizing hydrophobic LUT.

2. Materials and Methods

2.1. Materials

Lutein (purity > 90%), chitosan oligosaccharide (molecular weight < 2000), ethyl acetate, 1,1-diphenyl-2-pyridine-hydrazyl radical (DPPH), methanol, and acetonitrile for HPLC were purchased from Macklin Biochemical Co., Ltd. (Shanghai, China). All other chemicals were of analytical grade.

Ovomucin (purity > 90%) was extracted from fresh eggs by a two-step salt ion precipitation method [22]. The extracted ovomucin was ultrasound-treated (Scientz, Ningbo, China), and after centrifugation (15,000 rpm, 4 °C, 30 min), the supernatant was separated to obtain the ovomucin solution.

2.2. Preparation of OVM-COS and OVM-COS-LUT Nanogel

Under stirring at 200 rpm, 500 μL of an LUT solution (2 mg/mL, DMSO) was slowly added to a 10 mL OVM solution (1.25 mg/mL), and the mixture was ultrasound-treated (100 W, On/Off 5 s) in an ice bath for 5 min. Then, 500 μL of COS solution (1 mg/mL) was slowly added to the above mixture, and stirring was continued at 200 rpm for 60 min. The solution was slightly centrifuged (5000× *g*, 10 min) to remove insoluble matter and then transferred to a dialysis bag for 12 h to remove DMSO. The prepared nanogel was stored at 4 °C for further research. Meanwhile, OVM-COS nanogel without the addition of LUT was prepared.

2.3. Determination of Average Particle Size, Zeta Potential, and PDI

Determination was performed using Zetasizer Nano (Malvern Instruments Corp., Malvern, UK). Before measurement, the nanogel samples were diluted with deionized water to a protein concentration of 0.5 mg/mL and equilibrated at 25 °C for 2 min.

2.4. Encapsulation Efficiency (EE) and Loading Capacity (LC) of Lutein

The EE and LC of LUT by OVM-COS-LUT nanogel were determined by ethyl acetate extraction [23]. Utilizing the insolubility of ethyl acetate with the aqueous phase, the free lutein in the aqueous phase nanogel was effectively extracted. Briefly, 1 mL of LUT-loaded nanogel was mixed with 3 mL of ethyl acetate. The mixture was vortexed vigorously for 30 s and centrifuged at 5000 rpm for 5 min. The supernatant phase of the mixture was separated, and the absorbance of free lutein dissolved in ethyl acetate was measured at 448 nm using a UV–visible spectrophotometer (UV-2600, Shimadzu, Kyoto, Japan). A standard curve was established for the standard lutein solution in 0–20 µg/mL ($y = 0.065x - 0.0049$, $R^2 = 0.9999$). The encapsulation efficiency (EE) and loading capacity (LC) of lutein was calculated according to the following equation:

$$\mathrm{EE}(\%) = \frac{\text{Total lutein content} - \text{Free lutein}}{\text{Total lutein content}} \times 100\% \tag{1}$$

$$\mathrm{LC}(\%) = \frac{\text{Total lutein content} - \text{Free lutein}}{\text{Total nanogel content}} \times 100\% \tag{2}$$

2.5. Morphology Analysis

The morphology of OVM-COS-LUT nanogel was observed using a transmission electron microscope (HT7700, Hitachi Ltd., Tokyo, Japan). A total of 20 µL of the newly prepared sample was dropped on a 200-mesh carbon-coated copper grid. After 5 min, excess samples were removed from the copper grid with filter paper and dried naturally at room temperature. Samples were observed under 80 kV accelerated voltage.

2.6. Ultraviolet–Visible (UV–Vis) Spectroscopy

The UV–visible spectra of OVM-COS and OVM-COS-LUT nanogel dispersion were measured using a UV–visible spectrophotometer. Wavelength scans were observed in a range of 300–700 nm.

2.7. Fluorescence Spectroscopy

Protein endogenous fluorescence spectra of OVM, OVM-COS, and OVM-COS-LUT were measured using a fluorescence spectrophotometer (Spectrofluorometer FS5, Edinburgh Instruments, Livingston, UK). The sample protein concentration was diluted to 0.5 mg/mL; the excitation wavelength was 274 nm. The wavelength scan range was 280–500 nm; the excitation and emission slit widths were set to 2 nm.

2.8. Circular Dichroism (CD) Spectroscopy

Circular dichroism spectra of OVM, OVM-COS, and OVM-COS-LUT were measured using a circular dichroism spectrometer (J-810, JASCO, Tokyo, Japan). Sample protein concentrations were diluted to 0.3 mg/mL, temperature to 25 °C, quartz cell optical path length to 0.1 cm, wavelength scan range to 190–240 nm, speed to 10 nm/s, and resolution to 0.1 nm.

2.9. Fourier-Transform Infrared (FTIR) Spectroscopy

The infrared spectra of LUT, COS, OVM, OVM-COS, and OVM-COS-LUT powders were determined using a Fourier-Transform Infrared (FTIR) spectrophotometer (Nicolet iS50, Thermo Fisher Scientific Inc., Madison, WI, USA). The powder samples were pressed into flakes at room temperature. Then, 32 scans were repeated, and spectra were recorded in the range of 4000–500 cm^{-1}.

2.10. X-ray diffraction (XRD)

X-ray diffraction spectra of LUT, OVM, COS, OVM-COS, and OVM-COS-LUT powders were determined using an X-ray diffractometer (XRD) (Smart Lab 3KW, Rigaku Inc., Tokyo, Japan) with a test voltage of 40 kV, a current of 40 mA, a 2θ range of 10–30°, and a speed of 5°/min.

2.11. Stability Analysis

2.11.1. pH Stability

Freshly prepared OVM-COS-LUT nanogel was mixed with twice the volume of deionized water. The samples were then adjusted to the desired pH (2–9) with 0.1 mol/L NaOH or HCl. After 6 h of standing, the average particle size, PDI, and zeta potential of the OVM-COS-LUT nanogel were measured at different pH environments. Before measurement, the sample was equilibrated at 25 °C for 2 min.

2.11.2. Ionic Strength Stability

The pH environment of the newly prepared OVM-COS-LUT nanogel was adjusted to 6 with 0.1 mol/L HCL and then mixed with equal volumes of different concentrations of NaCl solutions (pH = 6), with the final NaCl concentrations being 0, 50, 100, 200, 300, 400, and 500 mM. After 6 h of standing, the average particle size and PDI of the OVM-COS-LUT nanogel were measured at different ionic strengths. Before measurement, the sample was equilibrated at 25 °C for 2 min.

2.11.3. Storage Stability

Freshly prepared OVM-COS-LUT nanogel was stored at 4 °C for 30 days. Every 5 days, equal amounts of nanogel were aspirated, and the average particle size and PDI of the OVM-COS-LUT nanogel were measured. Before measurement, the sample was equilibrated at 25 °C for 2 min. The UV absorption intensity of the nanogel was measured by a UV–Vis spectrophotometer. Changes in the nanogel were observed by optical photo documentation.

2.12. Antioxidant Activity

The antioxidant capacity of free LUT, OVM-COS, and OVM-COS-LUT nanogel was determined using the DPPH radical scavenging ability [24]. First, 1 mL of different sample concentrations was homogenously mixed with 2.0 mL of DPPH (0.02 mM), and the reaction was carried out at 25 °C for 30 min under light-proof conditions. The absorbance of the samples was measured at 517 nm. Ethanol was used in place of the DPPH solution for blanks, and deionized water was used in place of the sample solution for controls. The DPPH radical scavenging rate was calculated according to the following equation:

$$\text{DPPH radical scavenging capacity}(\%) = 1 - \frac{(A_1 - A_2)}{A_0} \times 100\% \quad (3)$$

A_1 represents the absorbance of the sample group; A_2 and A_0 represent the absorbance of the blank and control groups, respectively.

2.13. In Vitro Digestion Behavior

2.13.1. Bioaccessibility

An in vitro digestion method suitable for food standardization to evaluate the bioaccessibility of LUT was referenced [25].

Simulated gastric fluid (SGF): 10 mL fresh OVM-COS-LUT nanogel was mixed with 10 mL of simulated gastric fluid (SGF, 1 mg/mL pepsin). The 20 mL mixture was adjusted to pH 2.0 with 0.5 mol/L HCl and incubated in a shaker at 100 rpm at 37 °C for 2 h.

Small intestinal fluid (SIF): The above gastric mock mixture was adjusted to pH 7.0 with 0.5 mol/L NaOH to inactivate the pepsin. Trypsin was added to the 20 mL mixture to simulate the small intestinal fluid (SIF, 2 mg/mL trypsin). The mixture was then incubated in a shaker at 100 rpm at 37 °C for 3 h.

At the end of gastric and intestinal digestion, 1 mL of each reaction mixture was centrifuged at 10,000× *g* for 30 min. After centrifugation, the supernatant was filtered through a 0.45 μm filter to obtain soluble LUT. The filtrate was diluted in ethanol absolute and passed through a 0.22 μm filter membrane, and LUT release was determined by high-performance liquid chromatography (HPLC) [26]. For free LUT, it was treated using the same digestion simulation described above. The in vitro bioaccessibility of LUT was calculated according to the following equation:

$$\text{Bioaccessibility}(\%) = \frac{A_0}{A_1} \times 100\% \quad (4)$$

where A_0 represents the weight of LUT in the supernatant after simulated gastric or intestinal digestion, and A_1 represents the initial weight of LUT before simulated digestion.

HPLC analysis was performed on an Agilent 1260 liquid chromatography system (1260 Infinity II, Agilent Technologies Inc., Santa Clara, CA, USA) equipped with an SB-C18 HPLC column (4.6 mm, 250 mm, 5 μm). The mobile phase was 90% acetonitrile + 10% methanol at a flow rate of 1 mL/min, with an injection volume of 20 μL, detection at 470 nm, and a column temperature of 25 °C. The standard curve was made with 2–10 μg/mL of ethanolic solution of LUT (y = 62.391x + 7.1939, R^2 = 0.9973).

The average particle size of the nanogel was determined by Zetasizer Nano during the simulation of gastrointestinal digestion.

2.13.2. In Vitro Release

To create conditions for hydrophobic LUT release, the release medium consisted of a 50% gastrointestinal simulating solution mixed with 50% anhydrous ethanol [27]. A total of 5 mL of OVM-COS-LUT nanogel or LUT was placed into a dialysis bag, after which the airtight dialysis bag was placed into a release medium containing 100 mL of SGF (pH = 2, 0.5 mg/mL pepsin) and then incubated for 2 h in a shaker at 100 rpm, 37 °C. The dialysis bag was then transferred to another one containing 100 mL of an SIF (pH = 7, 1 mg/mL trypsin) release medium, and the incubation was continued for 3 h. The amount of lutein released was determined using a UV–visible spectrophotometer by aspirating 5 mL of the release medium every 30 min, and an equal volume of the release medium was replenished. The release rate of lutein was calculated according to the following equation:

$$\text{Release rate}(\%) = \frac{C_0}{C_1} \times 100\% \quad (5)$$

C_0 is the concentration of LUT in the release medium after a certain time interval, and C_1 is the initial concentration of LUT in the dialysis bag.

2.14. Cytotoxicity Analysis

The effect of OVM-COS-LUT nanogel on the activity of L929 cells (Shanghai Jining Industrial Co., Ltd., Shanghai, China) was determined using the MTT (3-(4,5-dimethylthiazol-2)-2,5-diphenyltetrazolium bromide salt) method [28]. Cells were cultured in DMEM containing 10% fetal bovine serum, 100 μg/mL penicillin, and 100 μg/mL streptomycin at 37 °C in a 5% CO_2 humidified environment. L929 cells were inoculated in 96-well plates at 8 × 10^3 cells/well cell density. The cell suspension was 80 μL/well and incubated at 37 °C for 24 h. Then, 20 μL of OVM-COS-LUT nanogel at different concentrations was added to the 96-well plates. The final concentration of nanogel in the cell culture mixture was 0, 25, 50, 75, 100, 150, and 200 μg/mL, and the final volume of cell suspension was 100 μL/well. After 24 h of incubation, 40 μL of an MTT solution was added to each well, and incubation continued for 4 h. After incubation, the medium was removed, 150 μL of dimethyl sulfoxide (DMSO) was added to each well, and the absorbance was measured at 492 nm after incubation for 30 min in the dark.

2.15. Data Analysis

Analysis of variance (ANOVA) was performed using IBM SPSS Statistical version 26.0 software. Data were processed with Origin 2018 software. Results were expressed as mean ± SD value of three replicates.

3. Results and Discussion

3.1. Characterization of Nanogel

Table 1 shows the characteristics of OVM, COS, OVM-COS, and OVM-COS-LUT, including size, PDI, zeta potential, EE, and LC. OVM carried a plentiful negative charge due to the presence of groups such as sialic acid or glycan sulfate. As a cationic polysaccharide, COS had the property of carrying positively charged groups. Compared with OVM, the ζ-potential of OVM-COS was altered, demonstrating the existence of electrostatic interactions between COS and OVM. In addition, COS did not have the characteristics of a colloidal particle with a PDI of 1. However, COS could act as a small molecular weight inducer, which induced a more homogeneous system (PDI 0.44–0.29) of OVM-COS with only a slight increase in average particle size. Generally, it can be considered a homogeneous system when PDI is below 0.3 [29].

Table 1. Particle size, PDI, zeta potential, EE, and LC of OVM, COS, OVM-COS, and OVM-COS-LUT.

Sample	Size (nm)	PDI	Zeta Potential (mV)	EE (%)	LC (%)
OVM	117.26 ± 2.54	0.44	−26.32 ± 0.38	—	—
COS	3036 ± 614.49	1	+1.95 ± 0.22	—	—
OVM-COS	127.33 ± 2.01	0.29	−20.05 ± 0.31	—	—
OVM-COS-LUT	209.16 ± 1.71	0.25	−20.71 ± 0.68	89.96 ± 0.32	6.47 ± 0.02

The electrostatic repulsion force was an important element in the stability of nano-systems. The surface charge of colloidal particles affects the strength of the intermolecular electrostatic repulsion, and too low an electrostatic repulsion can cause aggregation between colloidal particles [30]. The interaction of COS with OVM reduced the surface charge of the nanogel, but it still exhibited the highly negative charge characteristic of OVM, indicating that low molecular weight COS may have been interspersed between OVM during the nanogel formation, thus facilitating the cross-linking between the components. The large charges gathered by OVM on the nanogel surface could still stabilize the nanogel through the formation of electrostatic repulsion between the particles. In addition, as a similar phenomenon described in a previous study [15], the particle size increased significantly (127.33 ± 2.01 to 209.16 ± 1.71 nm) after LUT loading. The interaction of LUT with OVM-COS had no influence on the homogeneity of OVM-COS-LUT (PDI = 0.25). Moreover, the high encapsulation efficiency (89.96 ± 0.32%) proved that the nanogel provided a strong loading capacity for LUT.

As shown in Figure 1, The macro and micro forms of OVM-COS-LUT were investigated. OVM-COS-LUT presented itself as a brownish-yellow solution with low scattering (Figure 1a). Due to the low water solubility of LUT, the LUT solution showed aggregation. The result showed that LUT was stably dispersed in the solution by nanogel encapsulation. Compared to OVM-COS, OVM-COS-LUT showed a strong absorption peak in UV–Vis spectra around 390 nm (Figure 1b). The TEM morphology of the OVM-COS-LUT nanogel is shown in Figure 1c. Colloidal particles in the image were approximately spherical with a size of about 200 nm, consistent with DLS measurement. Furthermore, the shadow in the center and the surrounding light halo indicated that the colloidal particles had a characteristic core–shell structure.

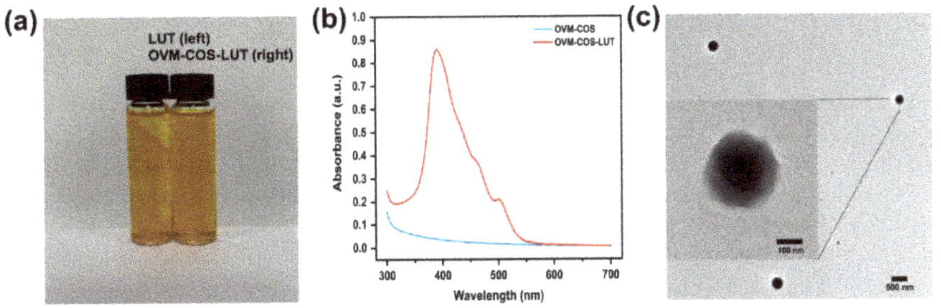

Figure 1. Optical pictures of LUT and OVM-COS-LUT (**a**). UV–Vis spectrum of OVM-COS and OVM-COS-LUT, ranging 300–700 nm (**b**). TEM image (scale bar = 100/500 nm) of OVM-COS-LUT (**c**).

3.2. Structure Analysis

Circular dichroism is a rapid and accurate method to determine the changes in secondary structure [31]. The CD spectra of OVM, OVM-COS, and OVM-COS-LUT nanogel are shown in Figure 2a, and the percentage of secondary structure is listed in Table 2. For each sample, the negative bands near 210 nm and 218 nm were ascribed to the α-helix, and the positive bands at 196 nm and 198 nm were ascribed to the β-sheet [31]. As shown in Table 2, COS hardly changed the α-helix, but the content of the β-sheet increased. The main reason causing this phenomenon was attributed to the electrostatic attraction between OVM and COS [32,33]. An increase in the β-sheet usually appeared with protein aggregation [34]. Those results corresponded with the scene in which COS gathered OVM molecules through electrostatic interaction. For LUT-loaded nanogel, the upward shift in spectrum near 210 nm signified a decrease in the α-helix, amounting to 4.56%. Nevertheless, the content of the β-sheet was further expanded to 43.53%, induced by LUT. The transformation could be attributed to the changes in hydrogen bonds and the hydrophobic interaction of OVM, eventually leading to recombination in the secondary structure.

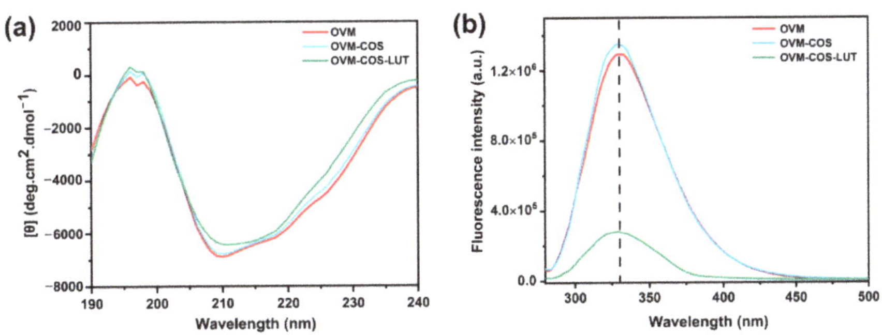

Figure 2. Circular dichroism (CD) spectra (**a**) and fluorescence spectra (**b**) of OVM, OVM-COS, and OVM-COS-LUT.

Table 2. The secondary structure percentage of OVM, OVM-COS, and OVM-COS-LUT.

Sample	α-Helix	β-Sheet	β-Turn	Random Coil
OVM	16.53 ± 0.45^{a}	30.80 ± 1.80^{a}	20.23 ± 0.89^{a}	32.37 ± 0.76^{a}
OVM-COS	15.83 ± 0.62^{a}	34.67 ± 0.74^{b}	18.33 ± 0.49^{b}	31.13 ± 0.62^{ab}
OVM-COS-LUT	11.97 ± 0.49^{b}	43.53 ± 0.84^{c}	14.36 ± 0.71^{c}	30.06 ± 0.55^{b}

Different letters marked on the same column indicate significant differences ($p < 0.05$).

The formation of nanogel is also coupled with changes in tertiary structure. Figure 2b shows the fluorescence tendency of OVM, OVM-COS, and OVM-COS-LUT using tyrosine as a probe. An increase or decline in fluorescence generally accompanies structure transformation in protein. The conformation and folding state of OVM were changed in OVM-COS formation, resulting in changes in intrinsic fluorescence intensity. The fluorescence peak shift was considered the signal representing microenvironment changes to the amino acid. As shown in Figure 2b, no band shift was exhibited in the spectrum before LUT addition, but a blue shift was exhibited in OVM-COS-LUT (329 to 323 nm). Some regions within OVM, especially hydrophobic ones, could curl inward in LUT binding. Hence, the tyrosine residues entered a hydrophobic environment, leading to a peak shift in nanogel [35]. In addition, with the addition of LUT, the fluorescence intensity of OVM decreased sharply. The quenching effect further indicated that the conformation of OVM was altered by the interaction between components.

3.3. FT-IR and XRD Analysis

FT-IR spectroscopy is a classical method in interaction studies. The FT-IR bands of all samples are shown in Figure 3a. Free LUT showed several characteristic peaks in a wide range, including the stretch vibration peak of -C-H (2918.25 cm^{-1} and 2851.72 cm^{-1}), the peak of the dimethyl splitting group (1362.46 cm^{-1}) or trans-conjugated alkene -CH=CH- (961.34 cm^{-1}), and some others [36,37]. Remarkably, compared with OVM-COS, the presence of LUT characteristic peaks in LUT-OVM-COS indicated successful LUT encapsulation. The wide band between 3600 and 3200 cm^{-1} could be assigned to the stretch vibration peak of -OH [38]. The peak shifted from 3277.43 cm^{-1} to 3274.54 cm^{-1} after OVM-COS-LUT formation, indicating a hydrogen bond linking LUT to OVM. Indeed, the amide bands shift was evidence of the electrostatic interaction between protein and polysaccharide [39]. After the addition of COS, the amide I and amide II bands in OVM were shifted from 1632.45 to 1632.93 cm^{-1} and 1528.79 to 1532.17 cm^{-1}. Therefore, electrostatic interaction was likely the main driving force for the colloidal particle formation between OVM and COS. All these results supported these inferences; nanogel was formed by electrostatic force, and LUT was anchored in the system by hydrogen bonding.

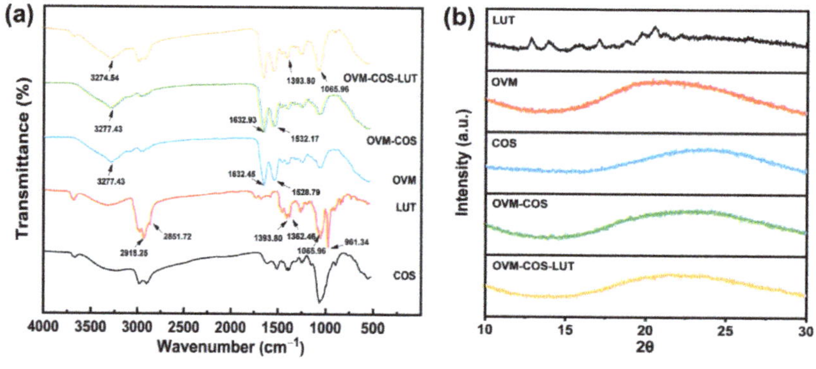

Figure 3. FT-IR spectra (**a**) and XRD spectra (**b**) of COS, LUT, OVM, OVM-COS, and OVM-COS-LUT.

The form of function molecules determines their biological activity to some extent. The crystal structure is an essential factor in this aspect. As shown in Figure 3b, the crystal form of all samples was measured by XRD. For the band of LUT, several strong diffraction peaks were found in the range over 10–25°, indicating a high degree of crystallinity. On the contrary, COS and OVM only exhibited an amorphous broadband. Meanwhile, the effect of COS on OVM was just peak shifting. Those phenomena indicated that polysaccharide derivatives, proteins, or their complexes were amorphous structures. However, no crystal diffraction peaks of LUTs were found in OVM-COS-LUT. The interaction between LUT and the nanocarrier might be the primary cause of crystalline state transformation [40].

In addition, amorphous nutrients were considered as holding better bioavailability [41]. Therefore, lutein-loaded nanogel may lead to better absorption or acceptability in oral administration.

3.4. pH Stability Analysis

When ingested by the body, nanogel faces a complex digestive environment, especially floating pH. Thus, investigating the stability of nanogel at different pH levels is essential. Figure 4a shows the particle size and PDI of nanogel at pH 2–9. In the beginning, the size of the nanogel increased with pH 2 to 5. When the pH was 6–9, the particle size was maintained at around 200 nm. Under acidic conditions (pH $\leq$ 3), OVM and COS maintain the same surface charge, which may cause repulsion between the two components, manifested as a slight swelling of the colloidal particles. Furthermore, particle aggregation at pH = 4 or 5 (near the OVM isoelectric point) resulted in a larger average size. However, this aggregation might result in a decrease in smaller particles, exhibiting lower PDI.

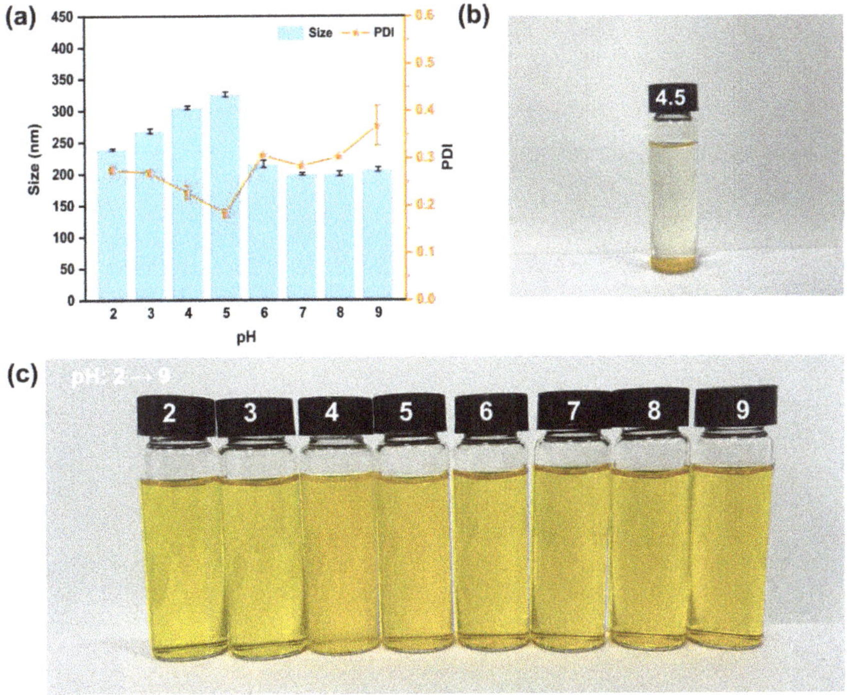

Figure 4. Particle size, PDI of OVM-COS-LUT at pH 2–9 (**a**). Optical image of OVM-COS-LUT at pH = 4.5 (**b**). Optical images of OVM-COS-LUT at different pH 2–9 (**c**).

As analyzed by the nanogel construction, the external characteristics of OVM-COS-LUT with a core–shell structure was closer to the OVM shell. Thus, the nanogel was altered to sediment only when the pH was the isoelectric point of OVM (about 4.5, Figure 4b). The strength of the surface charge of the particles can reflect the magnitude of the inter-particle electrostatic repulsion, and a smaller electrostatic repulsion may not be able to maintain the inter-particle stability. As shown in Table 3, at pH 4.5, the electrostatic charge of the particles only wrapped −3.1 mv, resulting in a decline of electrostatic repulsion, which made it hard to prevent the particles from approaching each other. Finally, the particles gradually aggregated to form precipitation. In an environment that gradually deviates from the OVM isoelectric point, the surface charge of the particles gradually increases, maintaining the stability of the system. As humans' dominant digestion and absorption area, the small intestine was responsible for most LUT absorption. This specific scenario should be considered here. Although the size fluctuated, the nanogel maintained its stability under acidic pH. In addition, a related study has confirmed that OVM can resist protease to a certain extent [16]. It is reasonable to believe that OVM-COS-LUT can resist the interference of the gastric environment and stabilize in the intestinal tract. The high stability of OVM-COS-LUT in the alkaline environment also ensured the controlled release and utilization of LUT in the intestine.

Table 3. Zeta potential of OVM-COS-LUT at pH 2–9.

pH	Zeta Potential (mV)
2	26.30 ± 0.47
3	24.33 ± 0.07
4	7.63 ± 0.03
4.5	-3.11 ± 0.44
5	-15.11 ± 0.35
6	-22.66 ± 0.67
7	-28.18 ± 0.55
8	-31.62 ± 0.59
9	-32.65 ± 0.58

3.5. Ionic Strength Stability Analysis

System stability under various situations, such as ionic strength, is of great importance for cargo-delivery vehicles. When the NaCl concentration was 50 mM, aggregate deposition was observed in the nanogel (Figure 5a,c). The phenomenon above might be attributed to the sharp decrease in the electrostatic repulsion between colloidal particles caused by the electrostatic shielding effect of ions (e.g., Na^+ and Cl^-) [42]. With the increase in NaCl addition, the agglomeration tendency gradually degraded. At the concentration of 100 mM, the colloidal particles returned to a steady state of homogeneous dispersion and the particle size exhibited a slight expansion (about 344.53 nm). After the concentration exceeded 200 mM, the average particle size stabilized at about 200 nm and returned to the initial level, which did not change with a further increase in NaCl concentration. In actual gastrointestinal digestion, gastric fluid ionic strength was around 100 mM in the fasting state [43]. After energy intake, a change in ionic concentration >100 mM was often accompanied due to additional external ionic intake. The stabilization of the nanogel at >50 mM ionic concentration contributes to the protection and utilization of the delivered cargo.

In order to further understand the physical properties of OVM and its constructed nanogels, the OVM at different NaCl concentrations was analyzed (Figure 5b). The OVM and OVM-COS-LUT behaved similarly in terms of variation, which was consistent with the structure of the OVM shell of the nanogel. When NaCl concentration approached about 50 mM, the particle size of the OVM increased rapidly, forming larger agglomerates. On the contrary, when the salt concentration covered the threshold, these aggregates were more likely to disintegrate and eventually maintain a stable state. This tendency was also reflected in apparent turbidity. With the increase in NaCl concentration, the OVM presented a clear–turbid–clear change.

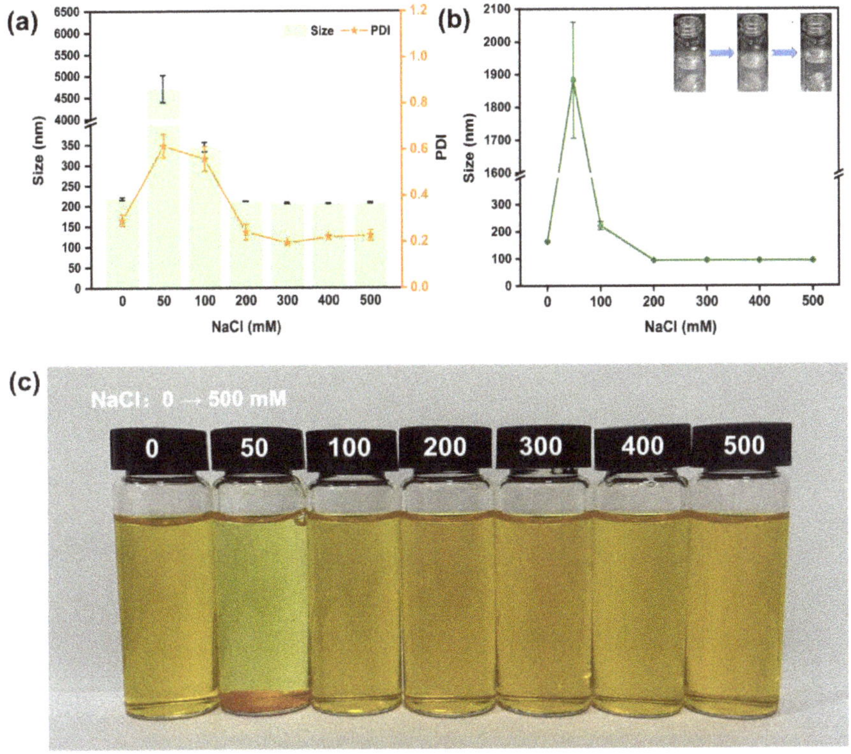

Figure 5. Particle size and PDI of OVM-COS-LUT (**a**). Particle size and solution state changes in OVM (**b**). Optical images of OVM-COS-LUT under different NaCl concentrations (0–500 mM) (**c**).

3.6. Storage Stability Analysis

A principal concern when designing carriers is the protection of functional components within the system. Therefore, the retention of LUT could be a reliable and important index for evaluating the storage stability of OVM-COS-LUT [8]. Due to its unique molecular structure, absorbance measurement could be a reliable way to judge LUT retention. Free LUT is susceptible to oxidative degradation in processing and storage, which is one of the main challenges in achieving effective LUT utilization [44]. As shown in Figure 6a, the absorbance values remained essentially constant during the early stages of the storage period. From 25 days onward, the absorbance began to decrease slightly. After 30 days of storage, the effective retention of LUT by the nanogel was able to reach 96.54%, indicating that the nanogel had long-term LUT protection ability. Meanwhile, in the particle size determination of the nanogel, as shown in Figure 6b, the particle size of OVM-COS-LUT were almost unchanged with the storage time, and the PDI were all kept around 0.25. The results showed that the nanogel had satisfactory storage stability. In addition, the change in macroscopic morphology could reflect the stability of the delivery system, which was usually associated with the interactions between particles. No signs of nanogel deposition were found in the optical photographs (Figure 6c). This indicates that after long-time storage, the colloidal particles could still retain strong interactions to maintain the stability of the system. In summary, OVM-COS-LUT has effective long-term cargo protection and strong storage stability.

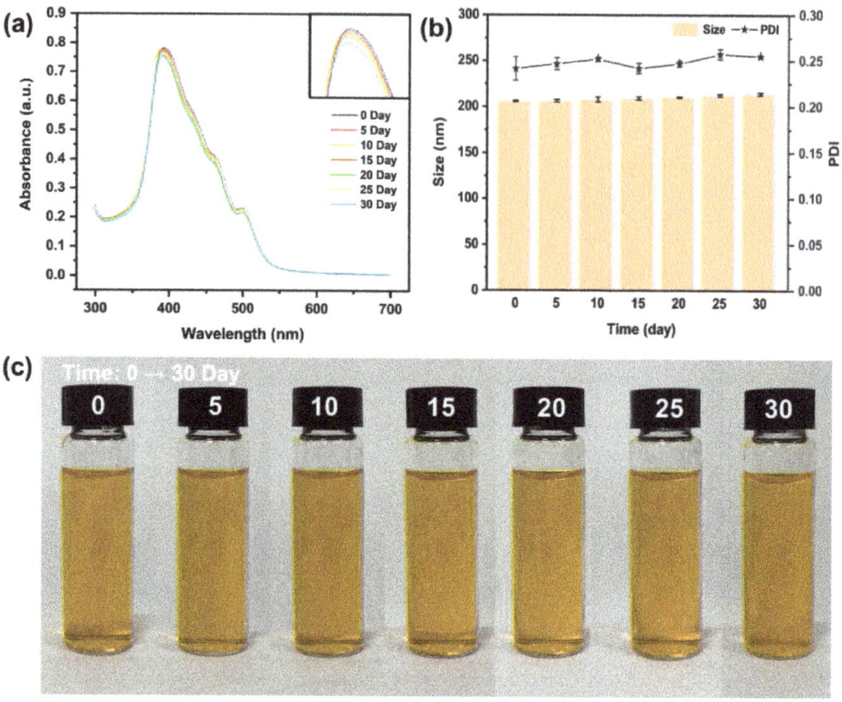

Figure 6. UV–Vis spectrum (**a**); particle size and PDI (**b**); optical images (**c**) of OVM-COS-LUT during 30-day storage.

3.7. *Antioxidant and Bioavailability of Lutein*

3.7.1. Antioxidant Activity

Antioxidant capacity is considered to be one main bioactivity of LUT. DPPH, a free radical, is widely used to evaluate antioxidant activity in several fields. As shown in Figure 7a, the antioxidant capacity of all samples in different concentrations was analyzed. By contrast, OVM-COS exhibited weaker antioxidant capacity than the two others. It was suggested that the dominant antioxidant capacity from OVM-COS-LUT was not derived from body materials but from the cargo. In addition, under the same LUT level, a significant scavenging differential could be found between OVM-COS-LUT and free LUT ($p < 0.001$). Similar results have been described in a study that prepared a glycosylated zein protein–lutein nanoparticle [45]. The enhancement of scavenging capacity might be explained by the equable LUT dispersibility [46], which was attributed to the binding between LUT and carriers.

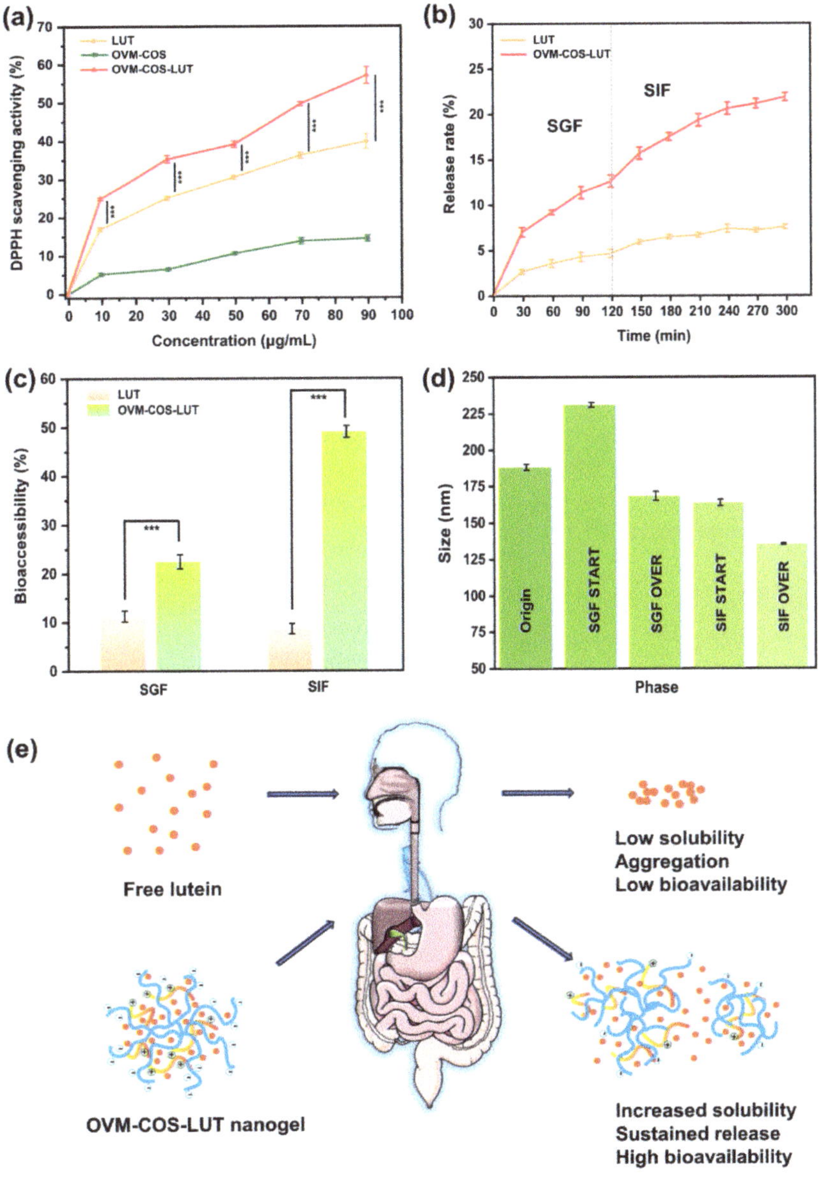

Figure 7. DPPH scavenging activity of LUT, OVM-COS, and OVM-COS-LUT at different lutein concentrations (***: $p < 0.001$) (**a**). Release behavior of LUT and OVM-COS-LUT nanogel in a simulated medium (**b**). Bioaccessibility of LUT and OVM-COS-LUT in simulated gastrointestinal digestion (***: $p < 0.001$) (**c**). Size changes in OVM-COS-LUT in successive gastrointestinal digestion (**d**). Schematic diagram of the simulated release of free lutein and OVM-COS-LUT nanogel (In the schematic structure of OVM-COS-LUT nanogel, the blue line represents OVM, and the gradient red line represents COS.) (**e**). Parts of Figure 7e were drawn using pictures from Server Medical Art. Servier Medical Art by Servier is licensed under Creative Commons Attribution 4.0. https://creativecommons.org/licenses/by/4.0/ (accessed on 15 November 2023).

3.7.2. Release Behavior

The biodegradation, diffusion, and dissolution of nanoparticles guide the release process, and most drugs have stronger solubility and sustained release ability through nanocarrier encapsulation. As shown in Figure 7b, the release behavior of LUT and OVM-COS-LUT nanogel in a simulated medium was investigated. Free LUT maintained a low release rate throughout the simulated release process, which may be related to its own hydrophobicity. During the release process, free LUT exhibits aggregated deposition, which prevents it from effectively crossing the dialysis bag barrier. By contrast, the release rate of OVM-COS-LUT nanogel for lutein was apparently higher than that of free LUT. The nanogel maintained stable dispersion during the release process, and the enhanced water solubility of LUT allowed for efficient and sustainable release into external media.

3.7.3. Digestion Behavior

In order to understand the behavior of OVM-COS-LUT in complex digestion processing, the effects of the nanogel against degradation in a simulated GI fluid was analyzed through particle size variation. When the nanogel was in SGF incubation, the particle size increased due to component rejection caused by low pH (Section 3.4). The loose structure might have allowed for pepsin cleavage and some LUT to escape, which leads to size reduction (Figure 7d). At the beginning of intestinal digestion, particle swelling was weakened, as the repulsive force was lost due to changes in pH. Perhaps benefiting from the compaction of colloidal particles, the particle size cut dominated by trypsin (163.67 $\pm$ 2.23 to 135.40 $\pm$ 0.49, about 17%) was weaker than pepsin (231.07 $\pm$ 1.59 to 168.33 $\pm$ 3.04, about 27%). Meanwhile, compact particles were conducive to the stabilization of LUT, which was ultimately reflected in higher bioaccessibility (26.6% higher than SGF, Figure 7c). Ma et al. found that in in vitro digestion simulations using zein/tea saponin composite nanoparticles to deliver lutein, the nanoparticles had similar results for the improvement of lutein bioaccessibility [33].

According to previous studies, possible physicochemical factors affecting the bioaccessibility of hydrophobic compounds pointed more to their solubility in the gastrointestinal tract [47]. Based on the results, no indication of aggregation and precipitation in nanogel was detected during successive gastrointestinal digestion simulations, which marked the finding that LUT could be stabilized in a dissolved state by wrapping it in nanogel. Related studies have confirmed that precipitation triggered by low water solubility is the main cause of hydrophobic compounds' low bioaccessibility [47]. From this perspective, the stable dissolution of OVM-COS-LUT throughout the simulated digestion might give it a bioaccessibility far superior to free LUT. Overall, all the phenomena suggested that encapsulation within nanogel could be a practical tool to improve the bioaccessibility of LUT.

3.8. Cytotoxicity Analysis

Safety is an essential index for evaluating an oral delivery system. The effects of OVM-COS-LUT nanogel on cell viability was measured through the MTT method. In Figure 8, compared to the control group, no statistical difference in absorbance could be found in a wide concentration range. It was suggested that incubation with OVM-COS-LUT was hardly harmful to cell viability. Similar to expectation, the design project formed by natural biomolecules conferred a high safety level on nanogel. Hence, OVM-COS-LUT could be considered a reliable strategy for LUT supplements.

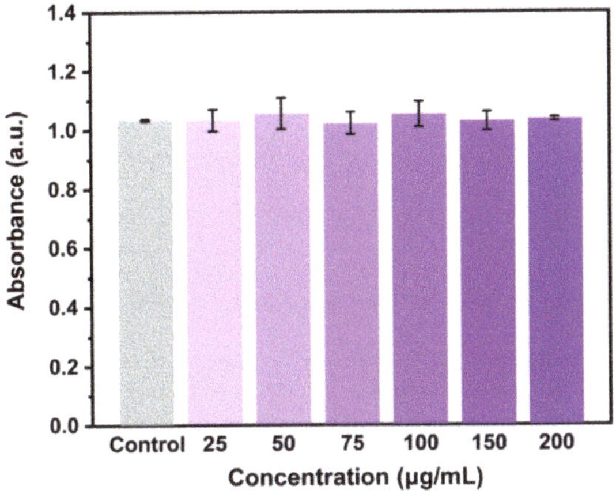

Figure 8. Effect of different concentrations of OVM-COS-LUT nanogel on cell viability (control: no nanogel was added).

4. Conclusions

In this study, nanogel was prepared with OVM and COS to encapsulate LUT in order to improve its bioavailability. The results showed that OVM-COS-LUT appeared to be approximately spherical with a smaller size and narrow particle size distribution. Hydrogen bonding, hydrophobic effects, or other interactions made LUT well encapsulated in a nanogel with an amorphous form, and this enhanced LUT solubility and dispersion, thus exhibiting better antioxidant capacity and bioavailability. In addition, this carrier–cargo interaction helped the nanogel maintain stability in a gastrointestinal environment, enabling the controlled release of LUT. Meanwhile, OVM-COS-LUT also showed good stability in different situations (such as under various pH or ionic strength conditions). Compared with lutein carriers such as liposomes or chemical polymer nanoparticles, OVM-COS-LUT was prepared entirely from natural edible molecules, which gives it a high degree of biocompatibility. Furthermore, its self-assembly method could effectively control the use of organic solvents, reduce the residue of harmful components, and ensure the safety of nanogel. In summary, OVM-COS-LUT could be used as an effective lutein carrier to deliver and improve its stability and bioavailability. This present work presents a simple, efficient, and safe construction strategy for OVM-COS nanocarriers, and it can serve as a reference for applying hydrophobic LUT in the pharmaceutical field.

Author Contributions: Conceptualization, Q.X.; methodology, Z.Z.; software, Y.H.; validation, H.T.; formal analysis, X.L.; investigation, H.T. and Z.Z.; resources, X.L.; data curation, Q.X.; writing—original draft preparation, H.T.; writing—review and editing, Q.X. and H.S.; visualization, Y.H.; supervision, H.S.; project administration, H.S.; funding acquisition, Q.X. All authors have read and agreed to the published version of the manuscript.

Funding: This work was supported by the Natural Science Foundation of Shandong Province (No. ZR2020ME063, No. ZR2020QC009 and No. ZR2023QC037).

Data Availability Statement: The original contributions presented in the study are included in the article, and further inquiries can be directed to the corresponding authors.

Conflicts of Interest: The authors declare no conflicts of interest.

References

1. Krinsky, N.I.; Johnson, E.J. Carotenoid actions and their relation to health and disease. *Mol. Asp. Med.* **2005**, *26*, 459–516. [CrossRef]
2. Carpentier, S.; Knaus, M.; Suh, M. Associations between lutein, zeaxanthin, and age-related macular degeneration: An overview. *Crit. Rev. Food Sci. Nutr.* **2009**, *49*, 313–326. [CrossRef]

3. Arnal, E.; Miranda, M.; Almansa, I.; Muriach, M.; Barcia, J.M.; Romero, F.J.; Diaz-Llopis, M.; Bosch-Morell, F. Lutein prevents cataract development and progression in diabetic rats. *Graefes Arch. Clin. Exp. Ophthalmol.* **2009**, *247*, 115–120. [CrossRef]
4. Freudenheim, J.L.; Marshall, J.R.; Vena, J.E.; Laughlin, R.; Brasure, J.R.; Swanson, M.K.; Nemoto, T.; Graham, S. Premenopausal breast cancer risk and intake of vegetables, fruits, and related nutrients. *J. Natl. Cancer Inst.* **1996**, *88*, 340–348. [CrossRef]
5. Lo, H.M.; Chen, C.L.; Yang, C.M.; Wu, P.H.; Tsou, C.J.; Chiang, K.W.; Wu, W.B. The carotenoid lutein enhances matrix metalloproteinase-9 production and phagocytosis through intracellular ROS generation and ERK1/2, p38 MAPK, and RARbeta activation in murine macrophages. *J. Leukoc. Biol.* **2013**, *93*, 723–735. [CrossRef]
6. Eggersdorfer, M.; Wyss, A. Carotenoids in human nutrition and health. *Arch. Biochem. Biophys.* **2018**, *652*, 18–26. [CrossRef]
7. Uzun, S.; Kim, H.; Leal, C.; Padua, G.W. Ethanol-induced whey protein gels as carriers for lutein droplets. *Food Hydrocoll.* **2016**, *61*, 426–432. [CrossRef]
8. Boon, C.S.; McClements, D.J.; Weiss, J.; Decker, E.A. Factors influencing the chemical stability of carotenoids in foods. *Crit. Rev. Food Sci. Nutr.* **2010**, *50*, 515–532. [CrossRef]
9. Soukoulis, C.; Bohn, T. A comprehensive overview on the micro- and nano-technological encapsulation advances for enhancing the chemical stability and bioavailability of carotenoids. *Crit. Rev. Food Sci. Nutr.* **2018**, *58*, 1–36. [CrossRef]
10. Zahin, N.; Anwar, R.; Tewari, D.; Kabir, M.T.; Sajid, A.; Mathew, B.; Uddin, M.S.; Aleya, L.; Abdel-Daim, M.M. Nanoparticles and its biomedical applications in health and diseases: Special focus on drug delivery. *Environ. Sci. Pollut. Res.* **2020**, *27*, 19151–19168. [CrossRef]
11. Pareek, V.; Bhargava, A.; Gupta, R.; Jain, N.; Panwar, J. Synthesis and applications of noble metal nanoparticles: A review. *Adv. Sci. Eng. Med.* **2017**, *9*, 527–544. [CrossRef]
12. Cho, Y.H.; Jones, O.G. Assembled protein nanoparticles in food or nutrition applications. *Adv. Food Nutr. Res.* **2019**, *88*, 47–84. [CrossRef]
13. Kianfar, E. Protein nanoparticles in drug delivery: Animal protein, plant proteins and protein cages, albumin nanoparticles. *J. Nanobiotechnol.* **2021**, *19*, 159. [CrossRef]
14. Ma, X.; Yan, T.; Miao, S.; Mao, L.; Liu, D. In vitro digestion and storage stability of β-carotene-loaded nanoemulsion stabilized by soy protein isolate (SPI)-citrus pectin (CP) complex/conjugate prepared with ultrasound. *Foods* **2022**, *11*, 2410. [CrossRef]
15. Li, H.; Yuan, Y.; Zhu, J.; Wang, T.; Wang, D.; Xu, Y. Zein/soluble soybean polysaccharide composite nanoparticles for encapsulation and oral delivery of lutein. *Food Hydrocoll.* **2020**, *103*, 105715. [CrossRef]
16. Tu, A.; Zhao, X.; Shan, Y.; Lu, X. Potential role of ovomucin and its peptides in modulation of intestinal health: A review. *Int. J. Biol. Macromol.* **2020**, *162*, 385–393. [CrossRef]
17. Xu, Q.; Shan, Y.; Wang, N.; Liu, Y.; Zhang, M.; Ma, M. Sialic acid involves in the interaction between ovomucin and hemagglutinin and influences the antiviral activity of ovomucin. *Int. J. Biol. Macromol.* **2018**, *119*, 533–539. [CrossRef]
18. Watanabe, K.; Tsuge, Y.; Shimoyamada, M.; Ogama, N.; Ebina, T. Antitumor effects of pronase-treated fragments, glycopeptides, from ovomucin in hen egg white in a double grafted tumor system. *J. Agric. Food Chem.* **1998**, *46*, 3033–3038. [CrossRef]
19. Tu, A.; Wang, X.C.; Chen, H.; Jia, X.; Wang, T.; Yi, Y.; Liu, B.; Xin, W.; Lü, X.; Shan, Y. Ovomucin Ameliorates Intestinal Barrier and Intestinal Bacteria to Attenuate DSS-Induced Colitis in Mice. *J. Agric. Food Chem.* **2021**, *69*, 5887–5896. [CrossRef]
20. Li, X.; Yin, C.; Liu, B.; Zou, L.; Xu, Q.; Li, C.M. Glycerol-compressed self-assembly nanogel based on ovomucin and chito-oligosaccharide: A novel green strategy for curcumin delivery. *Food Hydrocoll.* **2023**, *134*, 107996. [CrossRef]
21. Naveed, M.; Phil, L.; Sohail, M.; Hasnat, M.; Baig, M.M.F.A.; Ihsan, A.U.; Shumzaid, M.; Kakar, M.U.; Khan, T.M.; Akabar, M. Chitosan oligosaccharide (COS): An overview. *Int. J. Biol. Macromol.* **2019**, *129*, 827–843. [CrossRef]
22. Omana, D.A.; Wu, J. A new method of separating ovomucin from egg white. *J. Agric. Food Chem.* **2009**, *57*, 3596–3603. [CrossRef]
23. Xu, Y.; Ma, X.Y.; Gong, W.; Li, X.; Huang, H.B.; Zhu, X.M. Nanoparticles based on carboxymethylcellulose-modified rice protein for efficient delivery of lutein. *Food Funct.* **2020**, *11*, 2380–2394. [CrossRef]
24. Cai, X.; Huang, Q.; Wang, S. Isolation of a novel lutein-protein complex from *Chlorella vulgaris* and its functional properties. *Food Funct.* **2015**, *6*, 1893–1899. [CrossRef]
25. Minekus, M.; Alminger, M.; Alvito, P.; Ballance, S.; Bohn, T.; Bourlieu, C.; Carriere, F.; Boutrou, R.; Corredig, M.; Dupont, D.; et al. A standardised static in vitro digestion method suitable for food—An international consensus. *Food Funct.* **2014**, *5*, 1113–1124. [CrossRef]
26. Liu, H.; Zhang, Y.; Li, Q.; Zou, Y.; Shao, J.; Lan, S. Quantification of Lutein and Zeaxanthin in Marigold (*Tagetes erecta* L.) and Poultry Feed by Ultra-Performance Liquid Chromatography and High Performance Liquid Chromatography. *J. Liq. Chromatogr. Relat.* **2011**, *34*, 2653–2663. [CrossRef]
27. Chang, C.; Wang, T.; Hu, Q.; Luo, Y. Caseinate-zein-polysaccharide complex nanoparticles as potential oral delivery vehicles for curcumin: Effect of polysaccharide type and chemical cross-linking. *Food Hydrocoll.* **2017**, *72*, 254–262. [CrossRef]
28. Mosmann, T. Rapid colorimetric assay for cellular growth and survival: Application to proliferation and cytotoxicity assays. *J. Immunol. Methods* **1983**, *65*, 55–63. [CrossRef]
29. Abd-Elhakeem, E.; Teaima, M.H.M.; Abdelbary, G.A.; El Mahrouk, G.M. Bioavailability enhanced clopidogrel -loaded solid SNEDDS: Development and in-vitro/in-vivo characterization. *J. Drug Deliv. Sci. Technol.* **2019**, *49*, 603–614. [CrossRef]
30. Xu, R. Progress in nanoparticles characterization: Sizing and zeta potential measurement. *Particuology* **2008**, *6*, 112–115. [CrossRef]
31. Kelly, S.M.; Price, N.C. The use of circular dichroism in the investigation of protein structure and function. *Curr. Protein Pept. Sci.* **2000**, *1*, 349–384. [CrossRef] [PubMed]

32. Yuan, Y.; Li, H.; Liu, C.; Zhang, S.; Xu, Y.; Wang, D. Fabrication and Characterization of Lutein-Loaded Nanoparticles Based on Zein and Sophorolipid: Enhancement of Water Solubility, Stability, and Bioaccessibility. *J. Agric. Food Chem.* **2019**, *67*, 11977–11985. [CrossRef] [PubMed]
33. Ma, M.; Yuan, Y.; Yang, S.; Wang, Y.; Lv, Z. Fabrication and characterization of zein/tea saponin composite nanoparticles as delivery vehicles of lutein. *Lwt* **2020**, *125*, 109270. [CrossRef]
34. Chen, S.; Han, Y.; Wang, Y.; Yang, X.; Sun, C.; Mao, L.; Gao, Y. Zein-hyaluronic acid binary complex as a delivery vehicle of quercetagetin: Fabrication, structural characterization, physicochemical stability and in vitro release property. *Food Chem.* **2019**, *276*, 322–332. [CrossRef] [PubMed]
35. Fu, X.; Belwal, T.; He, Y.; Xu, Y.; Li, L.; Luo, Z. Interaction and binding mechanism of cyanidin-3-O-glucoside to ovalbumin in varying pH conditions: A spectroscopic and molecular docking study. *Food Chem.* **2020**, *320*, 126616. [CrossRef] [PubMed]
36. He, Y.; He, Y.; Zhao, Y.; Zhang, C.; Sun, C.; Li, X.; Zhao, Y.; Zhang, C.; Sun, C.; Li, X. Determination of ß-Carotene and Lutein in Green Tea Using Fourier Transform Infrared Spectroscopy. *Trans. ASABE* **2019**, *62*, 75–81. [CrossRef]
37. Nalawade, P.; Gajjar, A. Preparation and characterization of spray dried complexes of lutein with cyclodextrins. *J. Incl. Phenom. Macrocycl. Chem.* **2015**, *83*, 77–87. [CrossRef]
38. Liu, J.; Chen, J.; Dong, N.; Ming, J.; Zhao, G. Determination of degree of substitution of carboxymethyl starch by Fourier transform mid-infrared spectroscopy coupled with partial least squares. *Food Chem.* **2012**, *132*, 2224–2230. [CrossRef]
39. Derkach, S.R.; Kuchina, Y.A.; Kolotova, D.S.; Voron'ko, N.G. Polyelectrolyte Polysaccharide-Gelatin Complexes: Rheology and Structure. *Polymers* **2020**, *12*, 12020266. [CrossRef]
40. Toragall, V.; Jayapala, N.; Vallikannan, B. Chitosan-oleic acid-sodium alginate a hybrid nanocarrier as an efficient delivery system for enhancement of lutein stability and bioavailability. *Int. J. Biol. Macromol.* **2020**, *150*, 578–594. [CrossRef]
41. Recharla, N.; Riaz, M.; Ko, S.; Park, S. Novel technologies to enhance solubility of food-derived bioactive compounds: A review. *J. Funct. Foods.* **2017**, *39*, 63–73. [CrossRef]
42. Wu, W.; Kong, X.; Zhang, C.; Hua, Y.; Chen, Y. Improving the stability of wheat gliadin nanoparticles—Effect of gum arabic addition. *Food Hydrocoll.* **2018**, *80*, 78–87. [CrossRef]
43. Acevedo-Fani, A.; Singh, H. Biopolymer interactions during gastric digestion: Implications for nutrient delivery. *Food Hydrocoll.* **2021**, *116*, 106644. [CrossRef]
44. Gombac, Z.; Crnivec, I.G.O.; Skrt, M.; Istenic, K.; Knafelj, A.K.; Pravst, I.; Ulrih, N.P. Stabilisation of Lutein and Lutein Esters with Polyoxyethylene Sorbitan Monooleate, Medium-Chain Triglyceride Oil and Lecithin. *Foods* **2021**, *10*, 10030500. [CrossRef] [PubMed]
45. Chang, Y.; Jiao, Y.; Li, D.J.; Liu, X.L.; Han, H. Glycosylated zein as a novel nanodelivery vehicle for lutein. *Food Chem.* **2021**, *376*, 131927. [CrossRef]
46. Yi, J.; Fan, Y.; Zhang, Y.; Wen, Z.; Zhao, L.; Lu, Y. Glycosylated α-lactalbumin-based nanocomplex for curcumin: Physicochemical stability and DPPH-scavenging activity. *Food Hydrocoll.* **2016**, *61*, 369–377. [CrossRef]
47. Sorasitthiyanukarn, F.N.; Muangnoi, C.; Rojsitthisak, P.; Rojsitthisak, P. Chitosan oligosaccharide/alginate nanoparticles as an effective carrier for astaxanthin with improving stability, in vitro oral bioaccessibility, and bioavailability. *Food Hydrocoll.* **2022**, *124*, 107246. [CrossRef]

Journal of
Functional
Biomaterials

MDPI

Article

Tailoring Microemulsification Techniques for the Encapsulation of Diverse Cargo: A Systematic Analysis of Poly (Urea-Formaldehyde) Microcapsules

Sivashankari P. Rajasekaran, Bao Huynh and Ana Paula P. Fugolin *

Division of Biomaterials & Biomedical Sciences, Department of Oral Rehabilitation and Biosciences, School of Dentistry, Oregon Health & Science University, 2730 S Moody Ave., Portland, OR 97201, USA; purushot@ohsu.edu (S.P.R.); huynhb@ohsu.edu (B.H.)
* Correspondence: fugolin@ohsu.edu

Abstract: Cargo encapsulation through emulsion-based methods has been pondered over the years. Although several microemulsification techniques have been employed for the microcapsule's synthesis, there are still no clear guidelines regarding the suitability of one technique over the others or the impacts on the morphological and physicochemical stability of the final particles. Therefore, in this systematic study, we investigated the influence of synthesis parameters on the fabrication of emulsion-based microcapsules concerning morphological and physicochemical properties. Using poly(urea-formaldehyde) (PUF) microcapsules as a model system, and after determining the optimal core/shell ratio, we tested three different microemulsification techniques (magnetic stirring, ultrasonication, and mechanical stirring) and two different cargo types (100% TEGDMA (Triethylene glycol dimethacrylate) and 80% TEGDMA + 20% DMAM (N,N-Dimethylacrylamide)). The resulting microcapsules were characterized via optical and scanning electron microscopies, followed by size distribution analysis. The encapsulation efficiency was obtained through the extraction method, and the percentage reaction yield was calculated. Physicochemical properties were assessed by incubating the microcapsules under different osmotic pressures for 1 day and 1, 2, or 4 weeks. The data were analyzed statistically with one-way ANOVA and Tukey's tests ($\alpha = 0.05$). Overall, the mechanical stirring resulted in the most homogeneous and stable microcapsules, with an increased reaction yield from 100% to 50% in comparison with ultrasonication and magnetic methods, respectively. The average microcapsule diameter ranged from 5 to 450 μm, with the smallest ones in the ultrasonication and the largest ones in the magnetic stirring groups. The water affinities of the encapsulated cargo influenced the microcapsule formation and stability, with the incorporation of DMAM leading to more homogeneous and stable microcapsules. Environmental osmotic pressure led to cargo loss or the selective swelling of the shells. In summary, this systematic investigation provides insights and highlights commonly overlooked factors that can influence microcapsule fabrication and guide the choice based on a diligent analysis of therapeutic niche requirements.

Keywords: microemulsification; microcapsules; poly (urea-formaldehyde); magnetic stirring; mechanical stirring; ultrasonication; Triethylene glycol dimethacrylate; N; N-dimethylacrylamide; physicochemical properties

1. Introduction

The sequestering of cargo in microcapsules is a well-established strategy aimed at maximizing its stability and shelf life, overcoming biological and chemical compatibility challenges, ensuring the possibility of its controlled and pre-programmed delivery, and facilitating its handling [1]. This strategy has proven useful in various fields, including pharmaceuticals, food, paint coatings, medicine, electronics, textiles, waste treatment, agriculture, energy storage, the household, and personal care, among others [2].

Numerous encapsulation techniques can be used for cargo sequestering, with the emulsion-based route standing out as a widely adopted approach due to its relative simplicity, cost-effectiveness, and versatility [3]. In this method, two immiscible liquids—one containing the cargo and the other with the shell precursors—are vigorously mixed to create a stable and homogeneous emulsion [4]. During this process, the dispersed phase, composed of the cargo, undergoes fragmentation into small droplets dispersed within the other liquid, which acts as the continuous phase. The incorporation of surfactants reduces the surface tension energy between the liquids, ensuring emulsion stability. As the chemical reaction progresses, the thermopolymerization of the shell precursors takes place, leading to the microcapsules' formation [4]. Various techniques can be employed to facilitate the breakdown of the dispersed phase and produce microemulsification, including magnetic stirring, ultrasonication, and mechanical propeller agitation. Magnetic stirring involves the rotation of a magnetic stir bar within a liquid using an external magnetic field [5]. Ultrasonication is based on high-frequency sound waves to generate cavitation bubbles that promote intense local agitation as they collapse [6]. Mechanical propeller agitation employs upper rotating blades to create turbulence and shear forces in the liquid [7]. Although various synthetic protocols exist for each microemulsification technique, their distinct impacts on the morphological characteristics and physicochemical properties of the resulting microcapsules remain unexplored, and there are no clear recommendations for when one technique should be chosen over the others. Similar microcapsule systems have been synthesized and reported in the literature utilizing various microemulsification techniques [8–10]. However, the selection of a particular technique in these studies has often been based on personal preferences or the replication of previously described protocols, rather than a clearly defined rationale.

To assess the impact of the microemulsification techniques on the properties of microcapsules, an oil-in-water system based on poly(urea-formaldehyde) (PUF) shells was chosen for this study. PUF microcapsules have found extensive use in various applications, spanning from the construction industry to self-healing biomedical materials [11,12]. While this versatility highlights the feasibility of employing different methods for the synthesis of PUF microcapsules, explicit recommendations regarding potential distinctions in microemulsification production methods have yet to be established. The PUF system was selected for this comprehensive and systematic analysis for two main reasons: (1) this system is utilized in numerous applications, including pharmaceuticals, food, paint coatings, medicine, electronics, textiles, waste treatment, agriculture, energy storage, the household, and personal care; and (2) the different microemulsification techniques tested in this study have been employed for the synthesis of PUF capsules in various studies without a specific rationale for choosing one over the other. Furthermore, two systems with distinct water affinities were chosen as cargo to examine their influence on emulsion stability and the selection of the microemulsification technique. Triethylene glycol dimethacrylate (TEGDMA) and a mixture of TEGDMA and N,N-dimethylacrylamide (DMAM) were selected as the cargo due to their differences in water affinity, mimicking hydrophobic and hydrophilic cores, respectively. In the present study, "cargo" refers to the compounds loaded into the microcapsules, constituting their core. Lastly, the physicochemical stability of the microcapsules was assessed by exposing them to diverse incubation conditions, mimicking varied application scenarios, and their respective responses were systematically monitored and analyzed over time.

Therefore, this study proposes a comprehensive and systematic analysis aimed at understanding the effects of different microemulsification techniques, namely magnetic, ultrasonication, and mechanical stirring, on the properties of PUF microcapsules that sequester cargo with different water affinities. The ultimate goal is to contribute to the development of a microemulsification technique toolkit that can assist in strategically tailoring the encapsulation of a diverse array of cargo forms designed for specific applications. The tested hypotheses are: (1) distinct microemulsification methods will yield capsules with varying physical characteristics, chemical stability, and mechanical properties; and

(2) the water affinity of the cargo will likely impact emulsion stability, thereby influencing encapsulation performance. To the best of the authors' knowledge, this is the first study to systematically compare the most common microemulsification techniques used for microencapsulation, investigating their impact on the final properties of the microcapsules. Understanding how each technique affects the morphological characteristics and stability of microcapsules can significantly aid the decision-making involved in developing tailored microcapsules for specific applications.

2. Materials and Methods

Triethylene glycol dimethacrylate (TEGDMA), poly (ethylene maleic anhydride) (pEMA; M.W: 100,000 to 500,000) (pEMA), Resorcinol (ACS Reagent $\geq$ 99%), and 4-(Dicyanomethylene)-2-methyl-6-(4-dimethylaminostyryl)-4H-pyran (DCM dye) were procured from Sigma Aldrich (Saint Louis, MO, USA). N, N-Dimethylacrylamide (DMAM; 99% purity) was obtained from Acros Organics (Geel, Antwerpen, Belgium), urea (Ultrapure™ Urea) from Invitrogen (Waltham, MA, USA), and ammonium chloride and formaldehyde (37%) from Fisher Scientific (Hampton, NH, USA). All chemicals were used without further purification.

To achieve the goal of this study, the research plan was divided into three phases. Firstly, the core/shell ratio was optimized. Secondly, the three most common microemulsification techniques were tested using cargo with different water affinities. Finally, in the last phase, the stability of the synthesized microcapsules was assessed by storing them under different conditions. Figure 1 outlines the main parameters studied in this research.

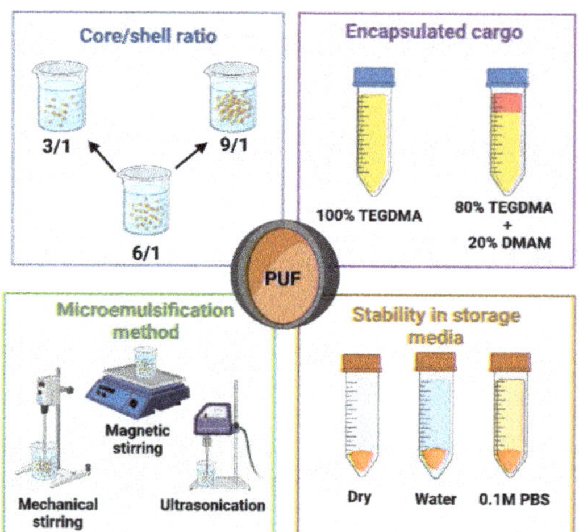

Figure 1. Schematic illustrating the key factors examined in this systematic study.

2.1. Phase 1—Synthesis and Characterization of Poly (Urea-Formaldehyde) (PUF) Microcapsules with Different Core/Shell Ratios

In the first phase of the project, PUF microcapsules with core/shell ratios of 3/1, 4.5/1, 6/1, 7.5/1, and 9/1 were synthesized utilizing the oil-in-water double emulsion technique, as previously described [13] (Figure 1). Briefly, 50 mL of distilled water was mixed with 13 mL of a 2.5% (wt./vol.) aqueous solution of the surfactant pEMA in a 250 mL 3-neck round-bottom flask. The temperature was set at 50 °C, and the stirring speed was adjusted to 300 rpm (stirring bar = 50 mm $\times$ 20 mm). Following these procedures, 0.125 g of ammonium chloride, 0.125 g of resorcinol, and 1.25 g of urea were added to the solution. The pH of the system was increased from 2.7 to 3.5 using a 1 M solution of NaOH. Subsequently, the speed stirring was increased to 400 rpm, and the cargo composed of TEGDMA tagged with DCM dye at 2 wt./wt.% was added dropwise to the solution to form the microdroplets. The amount of cargo added ranged from 15 g to 45 g to reflect the different tested core/shell ratios. After 10 min of emulsion stabilization, the temperature was raised to 55 °C, and 3.15 mL of 37% formaldehyde was added dropwise into the reaction mixture. The mixture was left to thermopolymerize for 4 h (Figure 2). At the end of this period, the reaction was cooled to room temperature, and the microcapsules were transferred to a beaker containing 500 mL of distilled water. They were allowed to settle for approximately 0.5 h and then, the supernatant, containing unreacted byproducts, was discarded. The microcapsules were collected, rinsed with distilled water, vacuum filtered, and washed with 200 mL of hexanes to remove any unencapsulated or adhered cargo. The resulting purified microcapsules were dried at room temperature for 24 h. Immediately following these procedures, the final mass of the microcapsules was measured to calculate the reaction percent yield, using the following equation:

$$Percent\ Yield(\%) = \frac{Actual\ Yield\ (g)}{Theoretical\ Yield\ (g)} \times 100\% \tag{1}$$

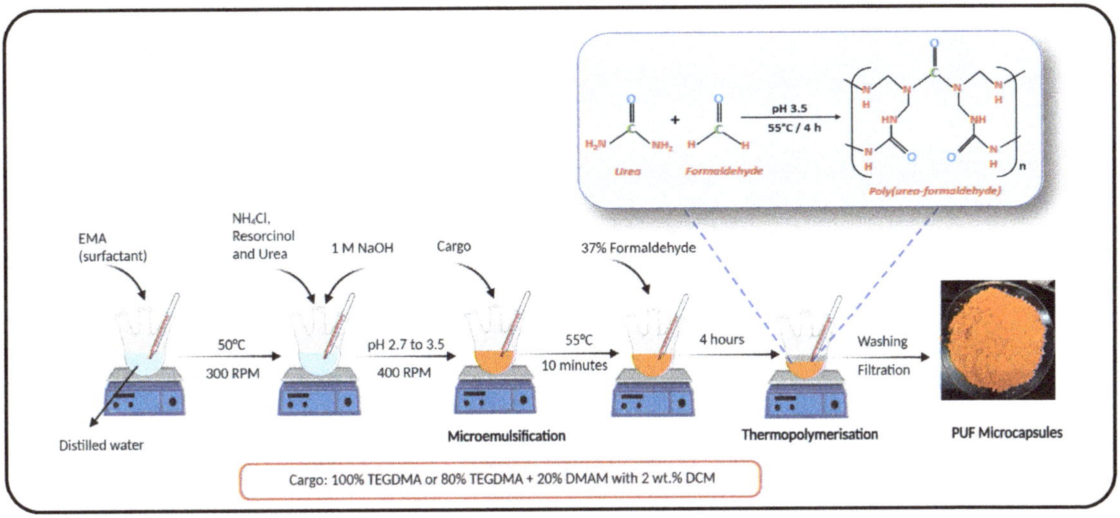

Figure 2. Representative depiction of the synthetic steps of PUF microcapsules based on oil-in-water double emulsion. The reaction encompasses 5 different phases: reaction medium preparation, the addition of the shell polymer precursors, emulsification via the dropwise incorporation of the cargo (oil phase), the addition of the crosslinking agent after emulsion stabilization for 10 min, thermopolymerization, and final product recovery after washing and filtration.

The morphology of the microcapsules was analyzed using optical microscopy. For the measurement of the microcapsules' diameter, the flasks were agitated to ensure a homogeneous distribution of the capsules. Subsequently, 10 mg of the sample was collected and dispersed in 20 μL of distilled water in an Eppendorf tube. Using a 5 mL transfer pipette with the tip cut to prevent high shear stress on the microcapsules, the mixture was transferred to a glass slide and covered with a cover slip. The samples were then imaged at 4× and 10× magnifications using an AmScope Trinocular Compound Microscope (Model BS1153-EPL, AmScope, Irvine, CA, USA). The images captured at 10× magnification were uploaded into ImageJ software (Version 1.53t, National Institutes of Health, Bethesda, MD, USA), and the diameters of 50 microcapsules were measured and averaged.

The core/shell ratio with the highest percent yield was selected to be used in the next phase of this study.

2.2. Phase 2—Synthesis and Characterization of Poly (Urea-Formaldehyde) (PUF) Microcapsules Using Different Emulsification Techniques

In this second phase, in addition to the commonly used magnetic stirring technique described above, two other microemulsification techniques based on ultrasonication with a homogenizer and mechanical stirring with a propeller were tested and compared. For the ultrasonication, the distilled water and surfactant solution were mixed in a 200 mL beaker. The cargo was added under magnetic stirring (400 RPM), followed by emulsification using a probe sonicator (Benchmark Pulse 150 Ultrasonic homogenizer, 6 mm tip sonication horn, and 150 W frequency, Benchmark Scientific, Sayreville, NJ, USA) for 4 min at 40% intensity (pulse on: 2 s; pulse off: 2 s), following a methodology previously described [14]. This procedure was followed by thermopolymerization under magnetic stirring (400 RPM) at 55 °C. For the mechanical stirring method, all the components were added to a 250 mL beaker, and a stainless-steel impeller with a blade diameter of 4.5 cm at 400 RPM was used for the emulsification, followed by thermopolymerization at 55 °C. The magnetic stirring synthesis and washing/filtration/drying procedures for all the synthesized microcapsules followed the methods outlined in Section 2.1. The only modification necessary was an additional washing step with 100 mL of chloroform for the DMAM-containing groups, which will be discussed later.

To gain insight into the robustness of the techniques, two different cargo systems were tested: one based solely on TEGDMA (logP = 1.6) and a second one composed of 80 wt.% TEGDMA and 20 wt.% DMAM (logP = 1.041—considering the mol concentrations of each component). In both cases, the cargo was tagged in orange with DCM dye to aid in microcapsule characterization and the monitoring of the volume of encapsulated cargo. Table 1 provides a concise overview of the experimental groups. Each synthesis was replicated three times, resulting in three batches for each experimental group.

Table 1. Overview of the six experimental groups, categorized by cargo systems and microemulsification techniques.

Experimental Group Name	Cargo System	Microemulsification Technique
100T-MA	100 wt.% TEGDMA	Magnetic Stirring
100T-U	100 wt.% TEGDMA	Ultrasonication
100T-ME	100 wt.% TEGDMA	Mechanical Stirring
80T/20D-MA	80 wt.% TEGDMA + 20 wt.% DMAM	Magnetic Stirring
80T/20D-U	80 wt.% TEGDMA + 20 wt.% DMAM	Ultrasonication
80T/20D-ME	80 wt.% TEGDMA + 20 wt.% DMAM	Mechanical Stirring

After the drying process, the determination of the reaction's percent yield and the morphological analysis of each batch of microcapsules, including diameter measurements, were conducted following the procedures described in Section 2.1. Additionally, complementary morphological analysis using scanning electron microscopy (SEM) was performed. The procedure involved dispersing the PUF microcapsules in distilled water, drop-casting them onto a silicon wafer secured with carbon tape, and allowing for water evaporation. Subsequently, the samples underwent gold sputter coating (Denton Vacuum Desk II sputter coater, Denton Vacuum, Moorestown. NJ, USA) and were examined with SEM (FEI Quanta 200, FEI, Hillsboro, OR, USA) in low-vacuum mode at 10 kV.

The encapsulation efficiency of each batch of PUF microcapsules, indicating the amount of cargo encapsulated within them, was also evaluated. In brief, approximately 100 mg of PUF microcapsules (W1) were placed in 2 mL microcentrifuge tubes and incubated with 1.5 mL of acetone. The microcapsules were then sonicated in a bath sonicator

(Fisher Scientific Ultrasonic Bath, Fisher Scientific, Pittsburgh, PA, USA) for 10 min to break them and extract the cargo (n = 3). Subsequently, the samples were centrifuged at 12,000 RPM for 10 min to pelletize the empty shells. The supernatant was removed, and the pelletized shells were dried in an oven at 37 °C until a stable weight was achieved (*W*2). The encapsulation efficiency of the microcapsules was calculated using the following equation:

$$Encapsulation\ Efficiency(\%) = \frac{(W1 - W2) \times 100}{W1} \quad (2)$$

2.3. Phase 3—Assessment of Physicochemical Stability of PUF Microcapsules under Different Osmotic Pressure Conditions and Times

The experimental microcapsules synthesized in phase 2 had their physicochemical stability assessed under different osmotic pressure and time conditions. Briefly, 100 mg of each batch of microcapsules was placed in 2 mL tubes containing 1.5 mL of distilled water (pH = 7, Osmolality = 0) or 0.1 M of phosphate-buffered saline buffer solution (pH = 7.4, Osmolality = 265–310 mOsm/kg). Microcapsules incubated in dry conditions served as control groups. The tested samples were stored at 4 °C for 24 h, 1 week, 2 weeks, or 4 weeks (n = 3). At the end of each time point, morphological changes in the microcapsules were examined using optical microscopy, following the method previously described. The percentage of the remaining cargo was determined by measuring the encapsulation efficiency (%) after the samples were removed from the storage solution and rinsed with either 2 mL of hexanes (100T groups) or 2 mL of hexanes followed by 1 mL of chloroform (80T/20D groups). The rinsing step was included to remove any potential cargo leaked during storage and adhered to the shell's surface, which could affect the accuracy of the measurements.

2.4. Statistical Analysis

The data from each study phase were assessed for normality and homoscedasticity using the Anderson–Darling and Levene tests, respectively. Subsequently, one-way ANOVA followed by Tukey's test for multiple comparisons was conducted. The significance level was set at 95%. It is important to note that the results presented in this analysis for phases 2 and 3 represent the average of different microcapsule batches.

3. Results

3.1. Phase 1—Influence of Core/Shell Ratio on Microcapsule Morphology and Reaction Percent Yield

The optimal core-to-shell ratio for the emulsification and encapsulation of TEGDMA in PUF shells was investigated and the results are shown in Figure 2. The percentage yield of the reactions ranged from 44.9% to 9.1%, with the highest results observed for the core/shell ratio of 6/1 and the lowest at 9/1 (Figure 3A). The performance of the microencapsulation reaction based on an oil-in-water emulsion is highly dependent on several factors, including the equilibrium between the inner oily and outer water phases. This equilibrium hinges on differences in hydrophilicity/hydrophobicity between the phases, emulsification stability, viscosity, the solubility of the shell precursor compounds in water, and reaction kinetics [15, 16]. In summary, under the influence of high shear stresses produced by the agitation, the formation of microdroplets during emulsification relies on the dispersion of TEGDMA into the water phase, resulting in droplets stabilized by the presence of the surfactant pEMA. These emulsion droplets undergo spherical-to-ellipsoidal shape deformation and subsequent breakup into smaller drops. This process is highly dependent on the media's viscosity, shear rate, and interfacial tension [17]. An intricate interplay exists between the media's viscosity and the concentration of surfactant. An increase in the volume of TEGDMA in the core/shell ratios of 7.5/1 to 9/1 may have significantly increased the viscosity of the emulsion. This increased viscosity may render the oily phase more resistant to the shear stress transmitted by the water phase due to agitation. In simpler terms, since the agitation rate was held constant for all the groups, emulsions with a higher viscosity experienced a lower magnitude of stress transmitted by the water phase, leading to reduced droplet formation. Moreover, the droplet coalescence and collision in these systems are favored due to the reduced distance between them caused by the increased concentration of cargo in the oil phase [15]. Additionally, surfactants are added to microemulsions to lower interfacial tension and, consequently, the internal pressure of microdroplets [18]. This reduction in tension is essential for microdroplet formation and preventing their coalescence. In these groups, the lower overall concentration of surfactant, due to the increased volume of TEGDMA, may not have been sufficient to migrate toward the interface within the interfacial film, lower the stress, facilitate microdroplet formation, and prevent coalescence. As a result, there was a significantly decreased reaction yield and an agglomeration of the shell polymer precursors in the water phase, forming sheet-like networks (Figure 3B) [18]. Lastly, limited shell polymer precursors may also impose a limitation to completely cover the healing microdroplets and often result in the formulation of thin and fragile shells that are susceptible to the shear forces during the synthesis.

A

Core/ shell ratio	Reaction Percent Yield (%) – Final Mass of Dried Microcapsules (g)	Microcapsules Diameter (μm)
3/1	10.53% – 2.11g	104.5 ± 63.5
4.5/1	19.21% – 5.28g	131.2 ± 97.3
6/1	44.9% – 15.68g	85.8 ± 64.5
7.5/1	13.46% – 5.72g	62.3 ± 30.7
9/1	9.1% – 4.53g	79.4 ± 61.4

B

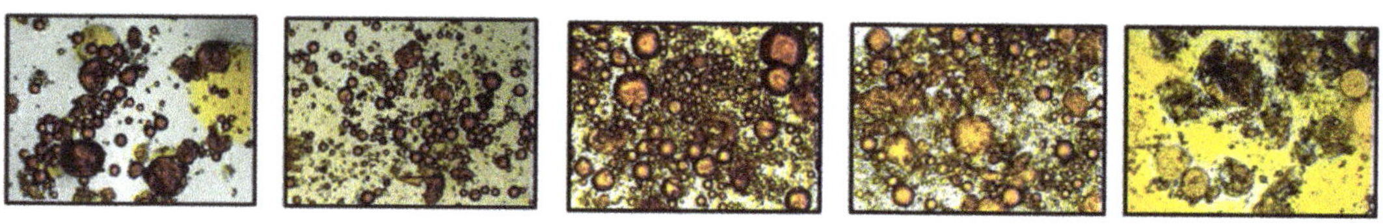

3/1 **4.5/1** **6/1** **7.5/1** **9/1**

Figure 3. (**A**) Reaction percent yield (%), the final mass of dried microcapsules (g), and the average microcapsule diameter (μM) for the five different core/shell ratios that were tested. (**B**) Optical microscopy images at 4x magnification of the microcapsules immediately after synthesis and before rinsing/filtration. The cargo is tagged in orange with DCM. In general, a core/shell ratio of 6/1 resulted in the highest reaction yield, as highlighted in the microscopy images by the increased density of microcapsules. When core/shell ratios exceeded this optimal value (7.5/1 and 9/1), the reaction medium contained an excess of free cargo, unbalancing the equilibrium between the phases and surpassing the concentration of shell polymer precursors required for forming polymeric shells. Conversely, at lower core/shell ratios (3/1 and 4.5/1), the microdroplets formed during the emulsification process were significantly larger, resulting in larger microcapsules. However, the yield was also decreased because the shell polymer precursors' encapsulation capacity was not fully utilized due to the lower concentration of oil-phase microdroplets.

Interestingly, core/shell ratios groups 3/1 and 4.5/1 resulted in larger microcapsules (104.5 ± 63.5 μm and 131.2 ± 97.3 μm, respectively) than groups 7.5/1 and 9/1 (62.3 ± 30.7 μm and 79.4 ± 61.4 μm, respectively). It is related to the fact that, at higher ratios such as those induced in groups 3/1 and 4.5/1, the surfactant molecules tend to orient themselves substantially parallel to each other. This behavior differs from their usual arrangement, where they straddle the interface with the polar group in the water phase and the hydrophobic tail in the cargo phase. This change affects the stability of the emulsion and the breakup of droplets, leading to the formation of larger droplets and, ultimately, larger microcapsules [19]. Regarding the reaction yields, 3/1 and 4.5/1 resulted in values as low as the groups 7.5/1 and 9/1. The low yield may be related to an extensive degree of demulsification, induced by the destabilization of the emulsion and the subsequent separation of oil and water phases [19,20]. At low concentrations in a system, the surfactant can adsorb onto the surfaces or interfaces and significantly alter their surface or interfacial free energies, as discussed previously. In addition, the increased water content leads to the external pressure of the water phase becoming lower than the internal pressure, which is translated into an increase in the interface film thinning and, consequently, the increased water droplet drawing and demulsification [19].

Therefore, for the system tested in this study, the core/shell ratio of 6/1 resulted in a more stable equilibrium between the oil and water phases among the tested concentrations. This ratio was selected for the next phases of the study.

3.2. Phase 2—Influence of Microemulsification Technique on Microcapsule Morphology and Reaction Percent Yield

Different techniques can be employed to promote the emulsification of a two-phase reaction. In this study, magnetic stirring (MA), ultrasonication (U), and mechanical stirring (ME) were compared. These techniques were employed to encapsulate two distinct cargo systems: the first composed of 100 wt.% TEGDMA, and the second composed of 80 wt.% TEGDMA + 20 wt.% DMAM (57 mol.% TEGDMA + 43 mol.% DMAM). DMAM is a low-molecular-weight tertiary acrylamide (~99.3 g/mol) and is consequently highly hydrophilic (logP = 0.3) [21]. The morphological characteristics of microcapsules, the size distribution, the averages of reaction percent yield (%), microcapsule diameter (μm), and the encapsulation efficiency (%) results are presented in Figure 4.

Ensuring that the diameter of the PUF microcapsules meets the requirements for practical applications is crucial. Excessively small capsules may contain a limited amount of cargo, while overly large capsules may lack stability, become fragile, and fail to resist handling. In general, the microemulsification technique played a pivotal role, with groups synthesized through mechanical stirring exhibiting a more uniform size distribution, as highlighted by the narrower profiles depicted in the histograms in Figure 4A. The capsule sizes for the 100T-ME group ranged from 50 to 225 μm (average size = 142.9 ± 12.1 μm), while for the 80T/20D-ME group, the range was from 25 to 200 μm (average size = 100.3 ± 16.3 μm). It is related to the fact that the shear stress generated by the impeller blades of mechanical stirrers is distributed more evenly throughout the solution, resulting in microdroplets with more consistent sizes and, consequently, a more uniform size distribution of microcapsule diameters [22]. On the other hand, groups synthesized using magnetic stirring yielded microcapsules with a broader size distribution. Capsule sizes for the 100T-MA group ranged from 50 to 550 μm (average size = 160.5 ± 88.0 μm), and for the 80T/20D-MA group, they spanned from 50 to 450 μm (average size = 158.9 ± 24.0 μm). In general, the magnitude of the shear forces generated by magnetic stirrers is highly heterogeneously distributed, with high intensity near the stir bar and becoming almost negligible towards the periphery of the reaction vial [23]. The scenario is even more critical when the viscosity of the emulsion is high because it imposes more resistance to the shear forces propagation. Therefore, magnetic stirring seems to be appropriate for emulsifying low-to-medium-viscosity solutions. In contrast, solutions with higher viscosity benefit from mechanical stirrers equipped with impellers due to the greater magnitude of the shear stress generated by the blades in comparison with magnetic stir bars [24].

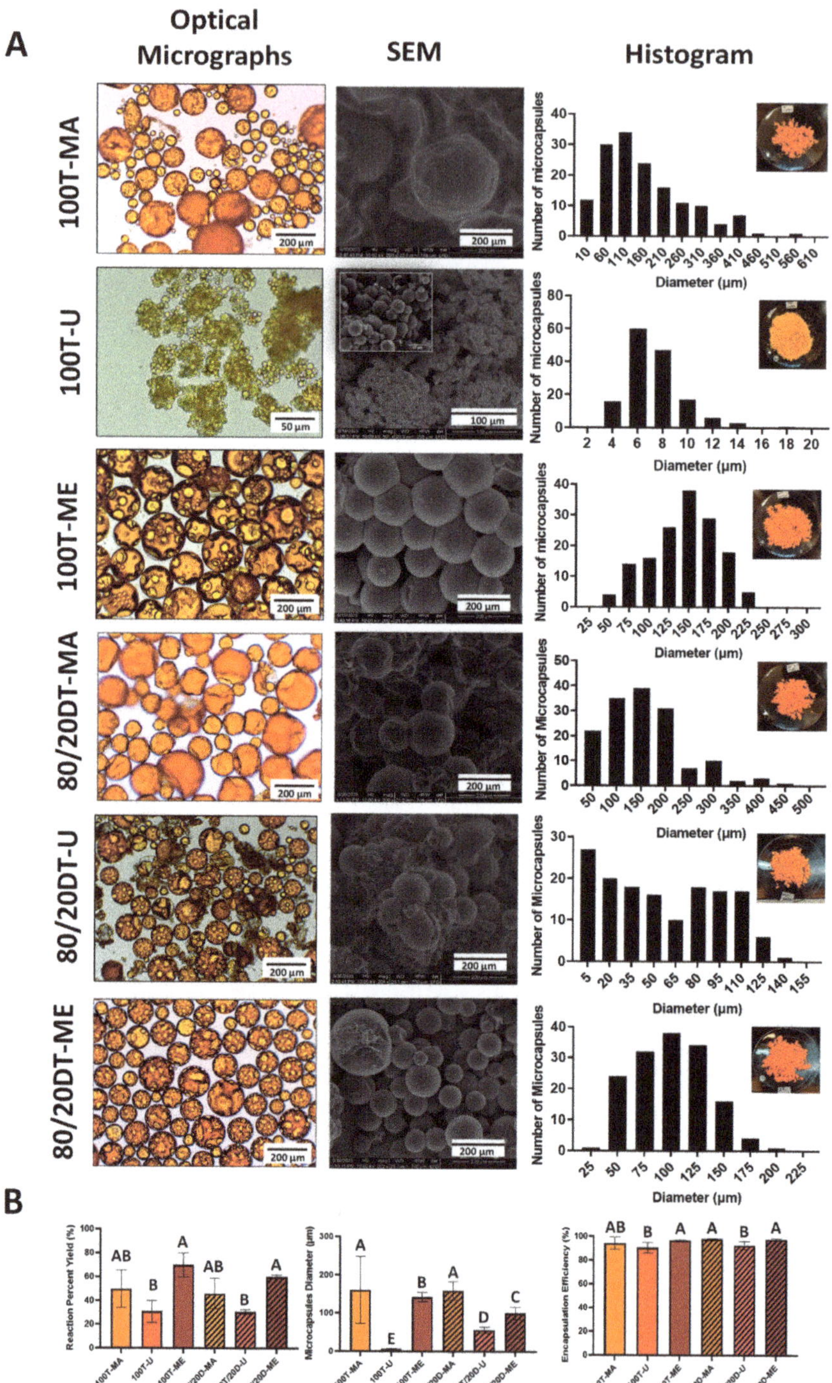

Figure 4. (**A**) Optical and scanning electron micrographs, along with a histogram displaying the size distribution of the tested experimental groups (n = 150 microcapsules from three independent

batches (50 microcapsules from each batch)). Optical micrographs were captured at 10× magnification for all groups except 100T-U, which required a magnification of 40× due to the significantly smaller size of microcapsules ranging from 4 to 14 μm. Scanning electron micrographs were taken at 200× magnification except for 100T-U (500×), low-vacuum mode, 10 kV voltage, and 10 mm working distance. (**B**) Graphical representations of the averages and standard deviations for all the tested experimental groups in terms of reaction percent yield (%), microcapsule diameter (μm), and encapsulation efficiency (%). Each experimental group was synthesized three times in independent chemical reactions, and the results shown in the graphs represent the averaged data. Bars with different letters indicate a statistically significant difference ($p < 0.05$).

While the composition of the cargo did not play a significant role in the microcapsule sizes of the mechanical and magnetic emulsification techniques, it had a substantial impact on ultrasonication. The 100T-U group exhibited a capsule size distribution ranging from 4 to 14 μm (average size = 6.5 ± 0.6 μm), whereas the 80T/20D group displayed a broader distribution, spanning from 15 to 135 μm (average size = 56.1 ± 8.05 μm) (Figure 4A). In ultrasonication, the horn-tip produces vibrations that generate ultrasonic waves. These waves lead to the formation of cavitation bubbles, which are ruptured upon contact with the dispersed phase [25]. This rupture process results in the formation of emulsions with smaller microdroplets compared to other methods, making it highly suitable for therapeutic applications that require low micro- or nano-sized capsules. The differences between the 100T-U and 80T/20D-U groups may be attributed to several challenges associated with the ultrasonication method. Firstly, an abundance of cavitation bubbles can lead to collisions among the bubbles, resulting in uneven bubble collapse, which affects the interaction between the bubbles and the cargo, thus disrupting the stability of microdroplets. Secondly, cavitation bubbles can accumulate around the ultrasonic probe, imposing a challenge for the uniform transmission of ultrasonic waves throughout the cargo [26]. This situation often leads to the formation of smaller microdroplets near the ultrasonic probe, with sizes increasing as the distance from the probe increases, which results in non-homogeneous microdroplet sizes. In fact, it has been shown that formation and cavitation collapse are the major contributing factors to the size and polydispersity index, which are affected by the cavitation threshold of the emulsion, the location at which the ultrasonic horn is placed during the reaction, the acoustic pressure at the oil–water interface, and the acoustic pressure in the continuous phase [27]. Since all the parameters were standardized and the only difference between the groups was the composition of the cargo, it is reasonable to hypothesize that the incorporation of DMAM (20 wt.% and 43 mol.%) increased the cavitation threshold of the emulsion due to the increased concentration of hydrogen bonding. The presence of strong hydrogen bonds creates strong intermolecular forces that hold the molecules of the emulsion together, which opposes the formation, propagation, and growth of the cavitation bubbles since additional energy is required to break these intermolecular forces [28]. Furthermore, hydrogen bonds play a role in diminishing the stability of cavitation bubbles. These bubbles become more susceptible to collapse because hydrogen bonds can easily reform after the expansion of the bubble, resulting in either the shrinkage or rupture of the bubble [28]. Therefore, DMAM-containing emulsions may have presented higher cavitation thresholds, leading to the formation of larger and more heterogenous emulsion droplets and, consequently, microcapsules [27]. In addition, oil phases composed of more than one compound are more susceptible to the Ostwald ripening phenomenon, which leads to a shift toward a broader size distribution with a higher average droplet size [29]. In summary, when the oil phase consists of two liquids, the more water-soluble compound can diffuse through the aqueous phase, leading to the coalescence of smaller droplets into larger ones [15,30]. This effect was more pronounced during ultrasonication in comparison to magnetic and mechanical stirring, possibly due to the generation of smaller microdroplets via this technique, as discussed earlier. Smaller droplets exhibit a higher curvature, resulting in increased Laplace pressure and, consequently, facilitating the migration of the cargo from smaller to larger droplets [30].

It is important to note that the clear circles in the core of the microcapsules observed in the optical micrographs (Figure 4A) are air microbubbles trapped within the cargo. The entrapment of air bubbles into the core of the microcapsules results from air being incorporated during the agitation process required to form the emulsion in the double-phase encapsulation technique [31]. The visibility of these bubbles varies depending on the focus on the core or shell during optical microscopy imaging. Over time, these bubbles are released, and the wrinkles on the microcapsule shells become more evident [31].

In terms of the physical aspect and morphological features, 100T-MA and 80T/20D-MA tended to form agglomerates, as evidenced via the SEM micrography (Figure 4A). The agglomerates were even resistant to the optimized rinsing and filtration procedures. It is important to note that the rinsing protocol was optimized and tailored to the different cargo systems encapsulated in this study. Standard procedures described in the literature involve rinsing the microcapsules with acetone. However, the acetone-based rinsing method in this study proved harmful, inducing a dramatic plasticizing effect on the polymeric shells, and leading to the premature rupture of the microcapsules (Figure 5). Although there are no specific studies that have investigated the impact of the acetone-based rinsing method on the physicochemical stability of the poly(urea-formaldehyde) networks, acetone is a well-known plasticizing agent that has the potential to cause the softening, smearing, or even dissolution of polymeric networks [32]. In the context of PUF microcapsules, the plasticizing effects resulting from the exposure to acetone may have adversely affected the shell's mechanical properties to a degree where the mild vacuum applied during filtration posed a more significant challenge than the polymeric network of the shells could withstand. Therefore, rinsing protocols with several different solvents were tested (data not presented here) and the integrity of the microcapsules was analyzed under optical microscopy after filtration. For the systems tested in this study, the optimal protocol consisted of the decantation of the microcapsules in distilled water at 10 times the volume of the reaction for 1 h, followed by rinsing with 200 mL of hexanes for 100T groups and 200 mL of hexanes + 100 mL of chloroform for 80T/20D groups. Decantation in water proved to be an effective strategy for physically separating the microcapsules, which tended to accumulate at the bottom of the vial, from the unreacted starting materials and solvents (Figure 5). This significantly reduced the volume of solvents required for the rinsing phase. Hexane-based rinsing was the optimal solvent for 100T systems, being capable of dissolving the unreacted compounds without compromising the physical stability of the polymeric shells and maintaining the integrity of the microcapsules. For the 80T/20D systems, in addition to the hexanes, an extra rinse with chloroform was required. This is related to the fact that due to the low relative polarity, hexanes can dissolve the unencapsulated TEGDMA but not DMAM, which is a highly polar compound (Figure 5).

Although the optimization and tailoring of the rinsing/filtration protocols resulted in a free-flowing, light, and dry appearance for most experimental groups, as mentioned earlier, the magnetic stirring groups, especially 100T-MA, exhibited an agglomerated and oily aspect, indicating cargo leakage. In addition, this group presented a significant amount of polymer sheets, which are essentially polymeric structures that did not transform into microcapsules or are residues of microcapsules ruptured during the synthesis. This may be due to the significantly larger microcapsule average size seen in this group in comparison to the other groups. Larger microcapsules are ruptured more easily than smaller microcapsules due to their lower stability, compromised shell stiffness, and greater hydrostatic pressure imposed by the higher volume of cargo [33]. Moreover, larger capsules are more susceptible to settling at the bottom of the reaction flask, where they are subjected to intense mechanical stress. The strong magnetic field created by the proximity of the stirrer bar and the magnets on the plate generates stronger shear and compressive forces, due to collisions of the microcapsules with the stirrer bar or other microcapsules in the reaction mixture [24]. These forces are particularly detrimental to the capsules because they are still undergoing thermopolymerization, which means that their shells have not reached the maximum crosslinking density yet and, consequently, present lower mechanical resistance to endure the mechanical challenge.

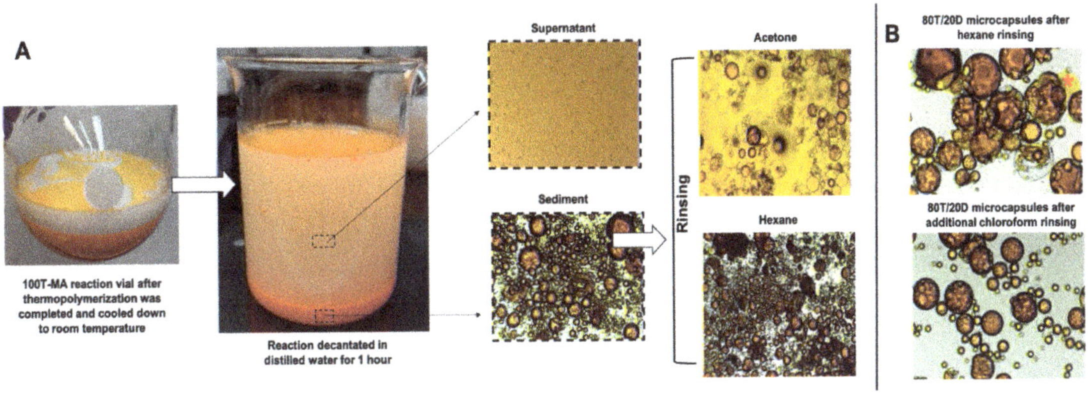

Figure 5. (**A**) Representative pictures and optical micrographs at 4× magnification of the 100T-MA synthesis reaction, illustrating the post-synthesis procedures. After thermopolymerization was completed and cooled from 55 °C to room temperature, the reaction mixture was dispersed in distilled water at a volume corresponding to 10 times the final reaction volume for 1 h. Optical micrographs of the supernatant and sediment layers reveal a notable concentration of microcapsules in the sediment layer. After discarding the supernatant, the microcapsules were rinsed with either acetone (following the standard procedure described in the literature) or hexane. The aliquot rinsed with acetone exhibited a dramatic rupture of the shells and leakage of the cargo, as evidenced by the bright yellow background in the optical micrograph. Conversely, the aliquot rinsed with hexane showed preserved integrity and the effective removal of unreacted starting materials, highlighted by the clear background in the optical micrograph. (**B**) Optical micrographs at 20× magnification of 80T/20D-MA, showing unencapsulated cargo dispersed around the microcapsules (indicated by the red *), which was completely removed after complementary chloroform rinsing.

In addition, given the lower and heterogeneous gradient of the shear forces magnitude generated by the magnetic stirring method, as discussed earlier, it is expected that the shell precursors were not homogeneously distributed into the reaction media. This non-uniform distribution may have resulted in a heterogeneous PUF polymeric network and, therefore, suboptimal mechanical responses. In fact, even the microcapsules that survived into the synthesis process started showing some level of cargo leakage after rinsing and filtration, evidenced by the oily physical aspect and the formation of microcapsule agglomerates. It may indicate that the high level of heterogeneity of the poly(urea-formaldehyde) network formed during the magnetic stirring. It is important to highlight that highly crosslinked polymeric networks, such as poly(urea-formaldehyde), are subject to experience heterogeneity due to several factors such as the randomness of chain compositions, the polydispersity of the polymer chains between reticulation nodes, the uneven distribution of the chemical crosslinkers leading to non-uniform reticulation nodes, random network topologies, and the lack of uniformity of the reticulation node density [34]. As heterogeneities are progressively introduced into these highly crosslinked networks, a dramatic impact on their topological structures and mechanical properties is observed [34]. Therefore, it seems that the high disparity in the shear forces distribution in the magnetic stirring contributed to the formation of a highly porous and stiff poly(urea-formaldehyde) network that allowed for the leakage of the cargo and eventual rupture of the microcapsule.

Interestingly, the 80T/20D-MA group exhibited better performance than the 100T-MA group, indicating that the composition of the cargo plays a crucial role in the stability and integrity of the microcapsules. The key role played by the cargo composition was also evidenced by the physical and morphological differences between the 100T-U and 80T/20D-U groups. While the 100T-U microcapsules were highly free-flowing, lightweight, and non-sticky, the 80T/20D-U capsules were sticky and exhibited some level of cargo leakage after drying (Figure 4A). As mentioned earlier, the introduction of a more hydrophilic compound into the cargo system is particularly challenging in ultrasonication oil-in-water emulsion. This challenge arises due to the magnification of the Ostwald ripening phenomenon, leading to a dramatic increase in the overall diameter of the microcapsules from 6.5 μm to 56.1 μm, and resulting in lower microcapsule stability.

However, a noticeable impact on the cargo composition was not observed when mechanical stirring was used as the microemulsification technique. This observation is attributed to the morphological similarities found between the 100T-ME and 80T/20D-ME microcapsules. In fact, the robustness of the mechanical stirring technique regardless of the cargo systems tested in this study is also reflected in the highest values of the reaction percent yield exhibited by 100T-ME and 80T/20D-ME, ranging from 69.9 ± 9.9% to 60.3 ± 1.7%, respectively (Figure 4B). The ultrasonication groups showed over 50% lower reaction percent yield compared to mechanical stirring, with values ranging from 30.7 ± 9.3% to 30.4 ± 1.94% for the 100T-U and 80T/20D-U groups, respectively (Figure 4B). For the 80T/20D-U group, it may be mainly related to some loss of DMAM as it may have diffused through the aqueous phase due to Ostwald ripening [35]. However, DMAM only accounts for 20 wt.% of the cargo composition, and even if all the DMAM was lost, it would not explain the 50% reduction in yield shown by this group. The explanation may rely on the impact on the core/shell ratio due to the reduction in the oil phase and the increase in the aqueous phase. If 25 wt.% of the DMAM was lost from the oil phase, the reaction ended up with a core/shell ratio of 4.5/1 instead of the optimal 6/1. As shown in the first phase of this study, this increase in the core/shell ratio impacts the equilibrium of the emulsion and leads to suboptimal reaction yield. However, Interestingly, 100T-U showed a similar yield to 80T/20D-U; therefore, DMAM loss is not the only reason for the lower percent yield in ultrasonication groups. It seems that TEGDMA, although more hydrophobic than DMAM, also lost some mass to the aqueous phase during ultrasonication. This may happen only in this technique because the droplets formed are at least one order of magnitude smaller than the ones formed in mechanical and magnetic stirring techniques, contributing to their coalescence and some loss of the cargo. Since the loss of TEGDMA may have increased the viscosity of the water phase, it may have reduced cavitation and, ultimately, the reaction yield [26]. While the microemulsification technique played a key role in the reaction percent yield, the differences in the cargo systems did not affect it significantly (Figure 4B). It is well known that the equilibrium between the oil and aqueous phases is a pivotal factor in determining the reaction yield of oil-in-water double emulsion reactions. Importantly, the replacement of 20 wt.% TEGDMA with DMAM seems not to have compromised this equilibrium. In terms of cargo encapsulation efficiency, the values ranged from 97.9 ± 0.4% to 90.5 ± 4.4%, with the lowest values presented by the ultrasonication groups (Figure 4B). This was anticipated, given the significantly smaller size of 100T-U and 80T/20D-U, implying a diminished capacity for carrying cargo. Nevertheless, it is crucial to highlight that achieving a 90% encapsulation efficiency is a remarkable outcome, indicating success in optimizing the microencapsulation reactions.

3.3. *Phase 3—Physicochemical Stability of the Microcapsules under Different Osmotic Pressures*

In the last phase of this study, the microcapsules synthesized in phase 2 were stored dry at 4 °C, in distilled water, or in 0.1 M of phosphate-buffered saline (PBS) for 24 h, 1 week, 2 weeks, or 4 weeks. The morphological changes in the microcapsules were monitored using optical microscopy, and the cargo volume variation was quantified using the acetone extraction technique. The objectives were to (1) identify the optimal conditions for the storage of the microcapsules to maximize their integrity; (2) understand how changes in the core composition impact the microcapsule responses; (3) probe the differences in microcapsules mechanical properties due to different microemulsification techniques; and

(4) gain insight into how the versatile PUF microcapsules can have their properties tailored for different purposes and therapeutic niches.

The results for 100T groups are depicted in Figures 6–8. In general, the microcapsules stored dry at 4 °C for 24 h, 1 week, and 2 weeks did not see a significant change in integrity and loss of cargo regardless of the microemulsification technique. These capsules showed the highest degrees of wrinkles on their shells and structural deformation from spherical round-shaped to a flattened oval format. After 4 weeks, there was a slight increase in the cargo loss that, although it was not statistically significant, led to microcapsules clumping, mainly for the 100T-MA group. It was anticipated that dry storage at low temperatures would result in the most stable behavior, as the capsules are subjected to much milder conditions. This expectation is based on the fact that, in a dry environment, morphological changes are mainly associated with the mechanical properties of the polymeric shell given the low hydrostatic and external pressures imposed by the liquid core and the environment, respectively [36]. In other words, the stability of the microcapsules will be mainly related to shell thickness, the polymeric features of the poly(urea-formaldehyde) networks, and the mechanical properties of the shells [37].

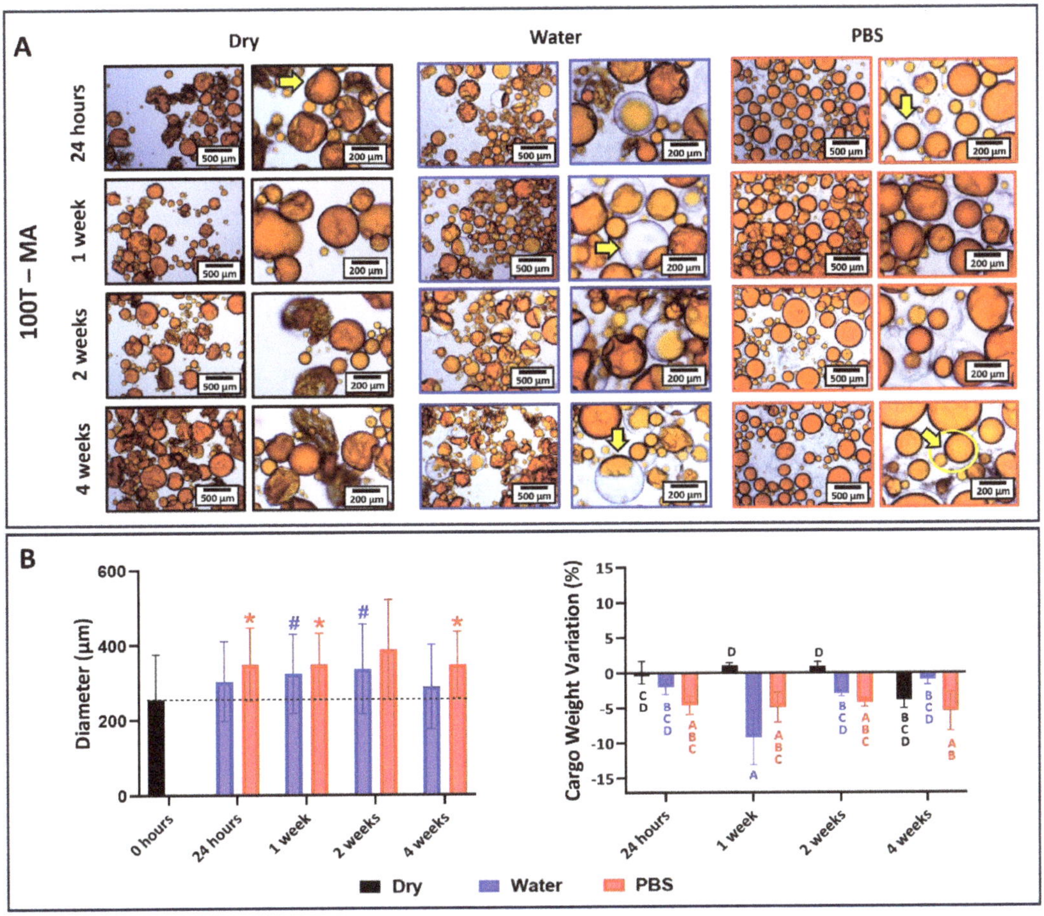

Figure 6. (**A**) Optical micrographs at 4× and 20× magnifications of 100T-MA microcapsules stored dry at 4 °C, in distilled water, or in PBS for 1 day, 1 week, 2 weeks, and 4 weeks. In the dry-stored

condition, the capsules showed deformation from spherical round-shaped to a flattened morphology, exhibiting a high degree of wrinkles (yellow arrow). In water, the microcapsules had their cargo replaced with water, leading to a significant increase in their diameter (yellow arrows). In PBS, the shells of the microcapsules seemed to have undergone swelling, forming a clear halo surrounding the healing agent (yellow arrow). Eventually, this led to the rupture of the weak shell spot and the release of the healing agent (yellow circle). (**B**) The average diameter of microcapsules as a function of the time points and incubation solution. The average diameter of the microcapsules immediately after drying and before incubation was used as the control and the groups were statistically compared to it. Bars with # (for water) or * (for PBS) indicate a significant difference in relation to the control group ($p < 0.05$). Percentage in cargo weight variation as a function of the time point and incubation condition. Bars with different letters indicate a statistically significant difference ($p < 0.05$). In general, there are statistically significant differences between the water group at 1 week and the dry group at 24 h, 1 week, and 2 weeks.

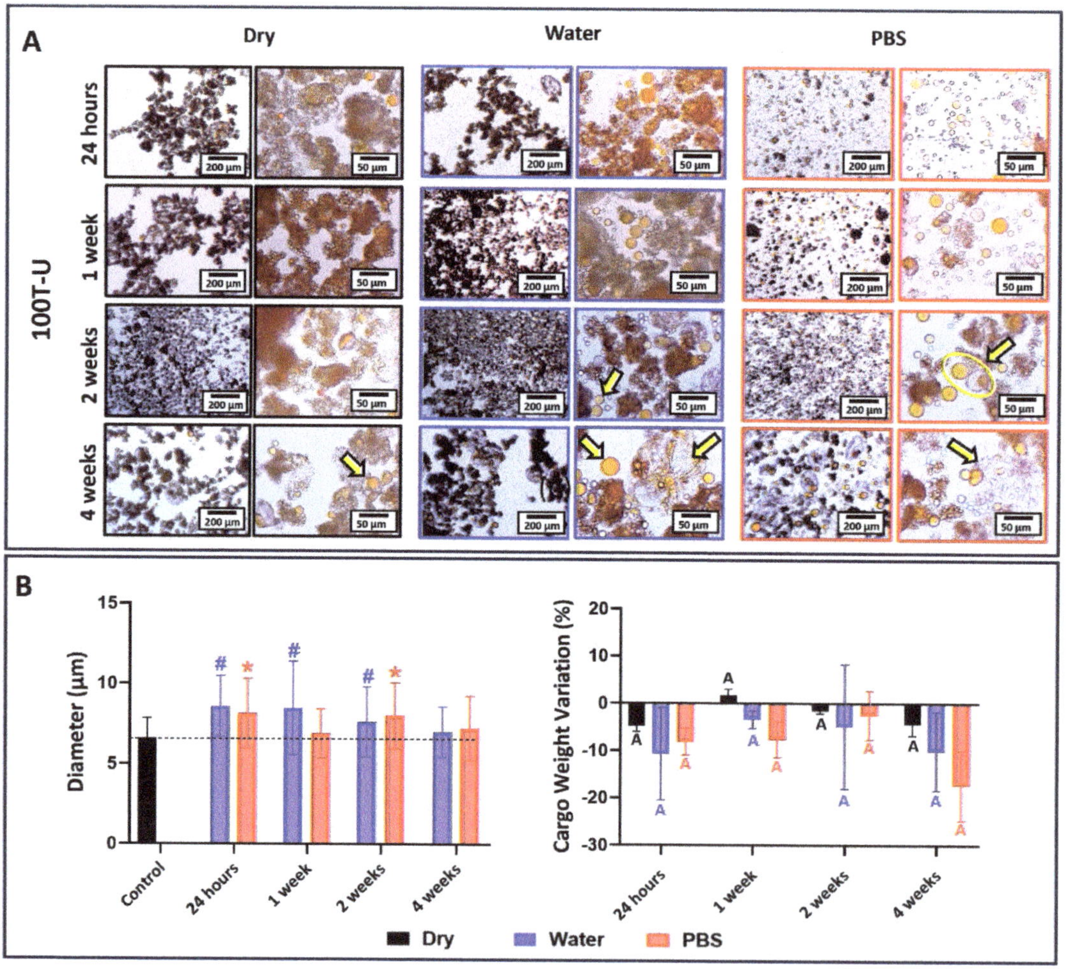

Figure 7. (**A**) Optical micrographs at 10× and 40× magnifications of 100T-U microcapsules stored dry at 4 °C, in distilled water, or in PBS for 1 day, 1 week, 2 weeks, and 4 weeks. We can observe that the microcapsules stored in dry conditions exhibited the maximum stability and the broken shells/leaked

cargo can be observed only after 4 weeks of incubation in dry conditions (yellow arrows). Meanwhile, when incubated in water or PBS, the 100T-U microcapsules started leaking after 2 weeks of incubation (yellow arrows). The yellow circle denotes actively leaking microcapsule after 2 weeks of incubation in PBS (**B**) The average diameter of microcapsules as a function of the time points and incubation solution. The average diameter of the microcapsules immediately after drying and before incubation was used as the control, and the groups were statistically compared to it. Bars with # (for water) or * (for PBS) indicate a significant difference in relation to the control group ($p < 0.05$). Percentage in cargo weight variation as a function of the time point and incubation condition. Bars with the same letter indicate no statistically significant difference ($p < 0.05$).

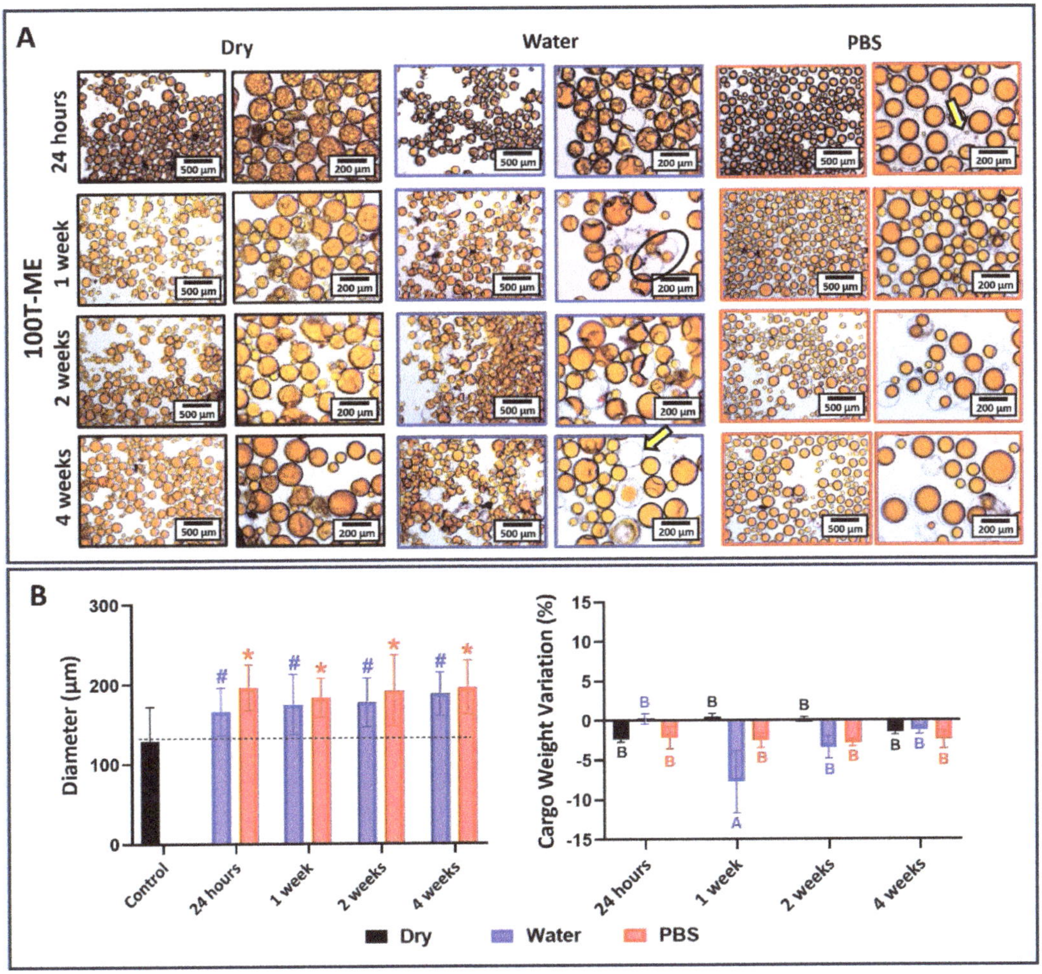

Figure 8. (**A**) Optical micrographs at 10× and 40× magnifications of 100T-ME microcapsules stored dry at 4 °C, in distilled water, or in PBS for 1 day, 1 week, 2 weeks, and 4 weeks. We can observe that the microcapsules stored in dry conditions exhibited maximum stability even after 4 weeks of incubation. The 100T-ME microcapsules incubated in water underwent an exchange of fluids after 1 week of incubation (black circle). After 4 weeks of incubation in water, we could observe multiple

empty shells (yellow arrow). The microcapsules incubated in PBS did not undergo fluid exchange, but the shells were swollen even after 24 h of incubation and a clear halo (yellow arrow) could be seen between the shell and the encapsulated cargo. (**B**) The average diameter of microcapsules as a function of the time points and incubation solution. The average diameter of the microcapsules immediately after drying and before incubation was used as the control, and the groups were statistically compared to it. Bars with # (for water) or * (for PBS) indicate a significant difference in relation to the control group ($p < 0.05$). Percentage in cargo weight variation as a function of the time point and incubation condition. Bars with different letters indicate a statistically significant difference ($p < 0.05$).

The flattening and wrinkling observed in these microcapsules seem to be mainly associated with the incomplete filling of the shells with core material or the loss of some core material over time [38]. Given the fact that the microcapsules did not form agglomerates or present an oily surface, it may mean that some residual solvent incorporated into the core during synthesis or rinsing and filtration procedures further evaporated over the storage time. Interestingly, the 100T-MA group started clumping, and some free cargo marked in orange was identified in the vial after 4 weeks, indicating core leaking. This observation corroborates with the suboptimal performance presented by this group in phase 2, which was mainly attributed to the low mechanical properties of their poly(urea-formaldehyde) network shells and the larger size of the microcapsules, making them more fragile. Although the magnitude of hydrostatic pressure imposed by the liquid core expected in microsystems is low, it seems that in cases where the shell properties are suboptimal, this pressure overwhelms the polymer resistance over time, making it incapable of maintaining a resistant physical barrier to keep the cargo restrained within the microcapsule core.

On the other hand, noticeable structural changes were seen in 100T microcapsules incubated in water and PBS. In water, the microcapsules showed significant swelling that led to a diameter increase at approximately 51%, 30%, and 46% for the magnetic, ultrasonication, and mechanical stirring groups, respectively. This was expected since interactions between poly(urea-formaldehyde) networks and water were anticipated due to the presence of amide and hydroxyl functional groups on the shells, which can form hydrogen bonding with water molecules [39]. The swelling increased significantly in the first 24 h and reached a plateau after that for 100T-U and 100T-ME, indicating that PUF microcapsules reached the equilibrium swollen size, a thermodynamically favorable condition, considerably fast. It is important to highlight the microcapsules swell in response to the differences in osmotic pressure across their shells, which becomes negligible as the capsule reaches the equilibrium swollen size [40]. It is also important to observe that the swelling process is a dynamic phenomenon characterized by the inward diffusion of water and the outward diffusion of cargo through the solvent-permeable shell. This is evidenced by the increase in the microcapsule diameter and the optical micrographs showing microcapsules with their core only partially filled with the cargo (marked in orange). The 100T-MA group reached the plateau a little later, with 1-week incubation, which is probably related to increased porosity in their shells due to heterogeneities in the polymeric network, as discussed earlier. In addition, all the groups experienced an increase in the microcapsule diameter but a decrease in cargo weight. This is because the density of water is approximately 10% lower than TEGDMA density (~1.092 g/mL at 25 °C). Altogether, these findings indicate that the osmotic pressure inside the capsule was significantly higher than the outer solution (hypotonic conditions), and the equilibrium was reached at the expense of water influx and cargo efflux through the solvent-permeable microcapsule shell [40,41]. The 100T-MA and 100T-U groups showed a significant rupture of microcapsules after 4 weeks of incubation, as evidenced by the presence of free orange drops of cargo and polymeric sheets dispersed into the background of the optical micrographs (Figures 6 and 7). This was expected, as the 4-week incubation reflects the cumulative effects of the water plasticizing effect during the entire incubation period. This also indicates that the larger swollen capsules did not withstand the deformation and burst after 3 weeks [41]. The burst of these microcapsules was caused when their internal pressure exceeded the failure strength of the shell material [41]. It is important to note that for both the 100T-MA and 100T-U groups, the diameters of their microcapsules after 4 weeks are like those of the control. Although some microcapsules are capable of deswelling, this is unlikely to be the case in this study. This similarity arises since the larger capsules, more susceptible to breaking, burst after 3 weeks, and the intact remaining capsules that could have their diameter assessed were the smaller ones. In general, 100T-ME microcapsules demonstrated higher stability and mechanical properties than 100T-MA and 100T-U, as shown through their physical integrity and the preservation of cargo highlighted in the optical micrographs and stable cargo weight variation profile. This underscores the superior mechanical properties of their polymeric shells and showcases their resilience against solvent effects [40].

In PBS, the swelling of the microcapsules was as noticeable as that seen in water incubation. However, differently from water-incubated groups, it was mainly related to the swelling of the shells rather than outer solution influx and cargo efflux. It is evidenced by the preservation of the shell core that, despite the capsule swelling, was maintained well delimited, regular, and spherical. Surrounding the undisturbed core there is a distinct asymmetrical clear halo, which is characteristic of shell swelling and typically seen in microcapsules with uneven shell thickness [40,41]. To confirm that the microcapsule expansion relied solely on the swelling of the shell, 10 mg of 100T-ME microcapsules was dispersed in 1 mL of 0.1 M PBS, and a single microcapsule with a diameter of 163 μm was observed to monitor its response in real time via optical microscopy (Figure 9A). After 2 min of incubation, a halo began forming on the bottom of the microcapsule and expanded quickly, reaching its maximum dimension after 15 min. During this time span, the microcapsule volume increased by about 12%, reaching a diameter of 185.5 μm. After 15 min, as the PBS evaporated, the halo experienced a decreasing change in volume, fading away after 50 min. Throughout the monitoring period, the cargo remained undisturbed, and no efflux was observed during the microcapsule shell expansion and regression processes. This experiment demonstrated that shell polymer is highly tough and capable of enduring a large level of mechanical strain [41]. It also suggested an unexpected degree of ionization occurring at the PUF network [40]. When dispersed in a polar solvent enriched with salt, such as PBS, an unbalanced concentration of ions is observed among the microcapsule core, the shell, and the outer solution. Under hypertonic conditions, where the osmotic pressure of the microcapsule inner core is lower than the salt-enriched external solution, the osmotic pressure difference across the shell should lead cargo to diffuse out of the microcapsules [41]. However, the experiments showed the opposite behavior. A possible explanation for this may be based on the ionic behavior of the PUF shells, which might become charged by dissociating counterions from the polymer backbones and swell by absorbing the solvent into the polymer network [42]. This redistribution of the mobile counterions of the shells and the co-ions of the outer solution affects the swelling behavior of the microcapsules until a local Donnan equilibrium is established among the core, shell, and external media [40]. While the PUF network and the PBS are individually neutral, their mixture results in a 0.5-unit drop in pH (Figure 9B). This observation suggests the potential transfer of ions between the microcapsule and the external media. It is important to highlight that the microcapsule swells to an equilibrium size because it is not capable of sustaining a non-neutral osmotic pressure. As the equilibrium swollen size is reached, thermodynamic equilibrium is achieved [40]. The leakage of the cargo, noticed in the optical micrographs, is the eventual result of the shell ruptured at its thinnest part, i.e., its weak spot [40]. The microcapsules most adversely affected by the incubation in PBS were the ones synthesized via the ultrasonication technique (Figure 7). This was expected given the significantly smaller size of the microcapsules, which means a higher surface area-to-volume ratio in comparison to the other two groups and, ultimately, more susceptibility to interact with the external solution.

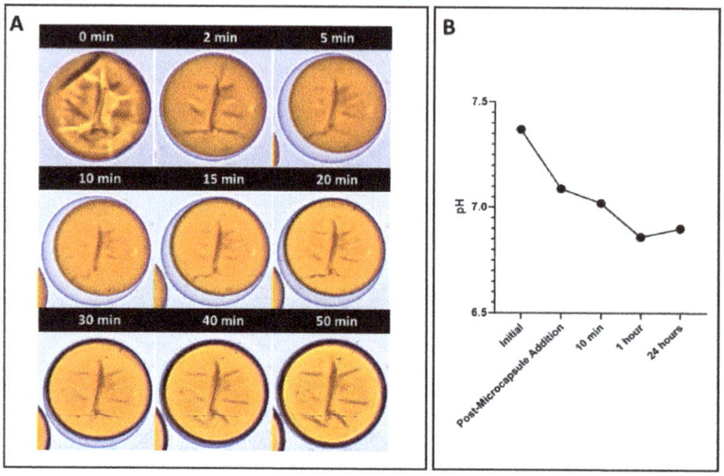

Figure 9. (**A**) Monitoring the microcapsule response incubated in a limited volume of PBS for up to 50 min via optical microscopy, showing shell swelling and deswelling as the PBS evaporates. (**B**) pH fluctuation of the PBS solution as microcapsules are added, showing a decrease of 0.5.

The results for 80T/20D groups incubated at different conditions are depicted in Figures 10–12. In general, the morphological changes as a function of the storage conditions followed the same trends observed in 100T groups. In other words, wrinkles and shrinkage are observed as the microcapsules are stored in dry conditions at 4 °C; the dynamic influx of water and the efflux of cargo are observed at water incubation; and shell swelling is observed at PBS incubation. However, the 80T/20D microcapsules demonstrated superior stability and resistance to incubation, irrespective of integrity preservation, diameter, and cargo weight variation. This is particularly evident when comparing the magnetically stirred groups (Figures 6 and 10). The anticipated increased stability in water or PBS can be attributed to the highly hydrophilic nature of DMAM. Beyond the advantages discussed earlier regarding microemulsification stability and encapsulation efficiency, DMAM may have diminished the permeability of the microcapsule shell to external media due to its water affinity. This may have posed a challenge for water penetration, ultimately minimizing cargo efflux and shell plasticization, hydrolysis, and swelling [43]. Furthermore, more hydrophilic cargo may act as stabilizing agents by preventing the coalescence and aggregation of microcapsules, thereby enhancing their stability in aqueous media. In fact, DMAM-containing microcapsules exhibited a more dispersed and free-flowing aspect compared to 100T microcapsules, which tended to form agglomerates. This phenomenon is linked to the water-attracting nature of the cargo, creating a barrier between adjacent microcapsules and increasing their dispersion. Lastly, acrylamides have been added into poly(urea-formaldehyde) polymeric networks as a strategy to increase mechanical strength and water resistance [44–46]. The DMAM that migrated to the water phase and dissolved with the shell precursors may have been incorporated into the shell networks, thereby enhancing their mechanical performance. This optimization might likely contribute to increased stability and resistance to incubation for these microcapsules. A comprehensive investigation of this potential phenomenon will be conducted in a separate study. In contrast to the magnetic and mechanically stirred groups, the 80T/20D-U microcapsules exhibited a significant number of empty and broken microcapsules and droplets of cargo, as evidenced by the optical micrographs (Figure 11A). The variation in size and cargo weight was also pronounced, as shown in Figure 11B. This group was the most affected by the Ostwald Ripening effect, which is related to shells with extensive variations in thickness, polymeric structural irregularities, increased porosity, and points of stress concentration [30]. It may have compromised the mechanical strength of the PUF polymeric networks, jeopardizing their stability and ability to withstand the osmotic challenge imposed by aqueous incubation.

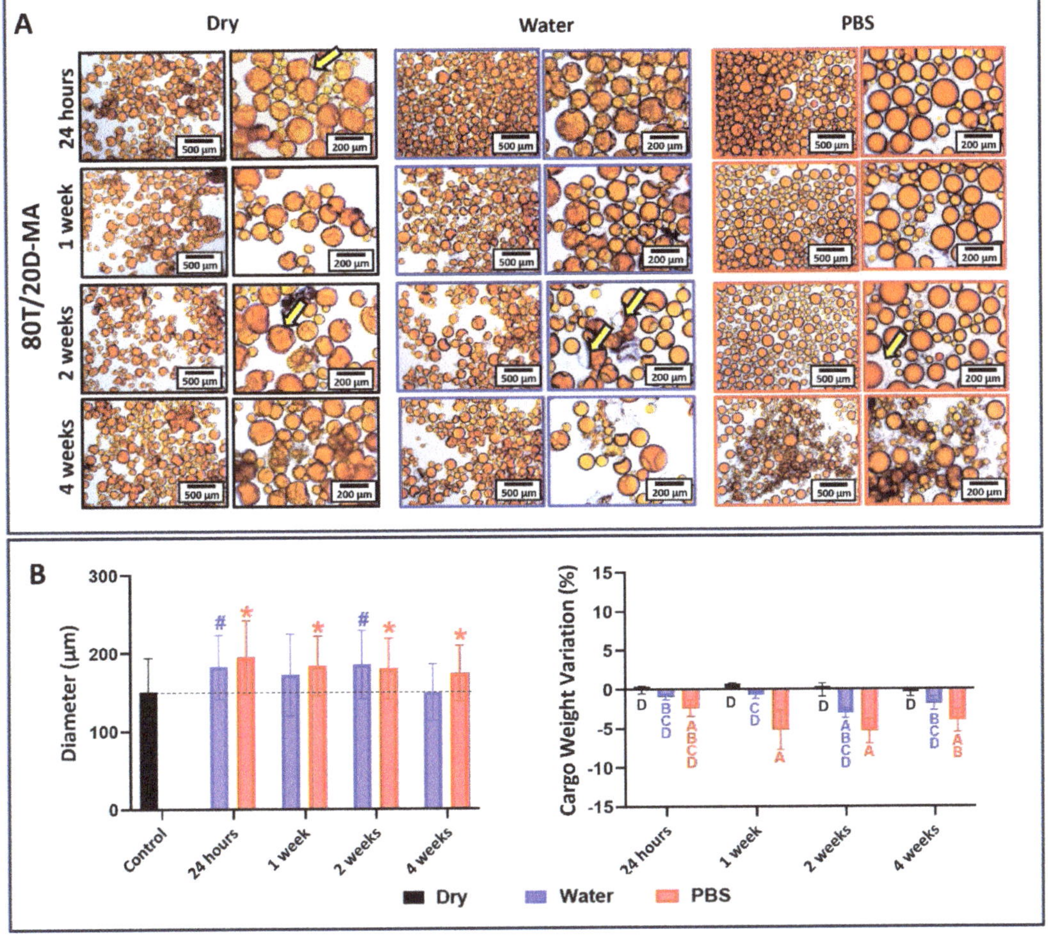

Figure 10. (**A**) Optical micrographs at 10× and 40× magnifications of 80T/20D-MA microcapsules stored dry at 4 °C, in distilled water, or in PBS for 1 day, 1 week, 2 weeks, and 4 weeks. The presence of wrinkles can be observed in all the time points when the microcapsules were stored in dry conditions (yellow arrows). Water-incubated microcapsules were stable until 2 weeks, after which a loss in cargo can be observed We can observe that the microcapsules stored in dry conditions exhibited the maximum stability even after 4 weeks of incubation (yellow arrows). When incubated in PBS, the microcapsules exhibited swelling and halo formation (yellow arrow). (**B**) The average diameter of microcapsules as a function of the time points and incubation solution. The average diameter of the microcapsules immediately after drying and before incubation was used as the control, and the groups were statistically compared to it. Bars with # (for water) or * (for PBS) indicate a significant difference in relation to the control group ($p < 0.05$). Percentage in cargo weight variation as a function of the time point and incubation condition. Bars with different letters indicate a statistically significant difference ($p < 0.05$).

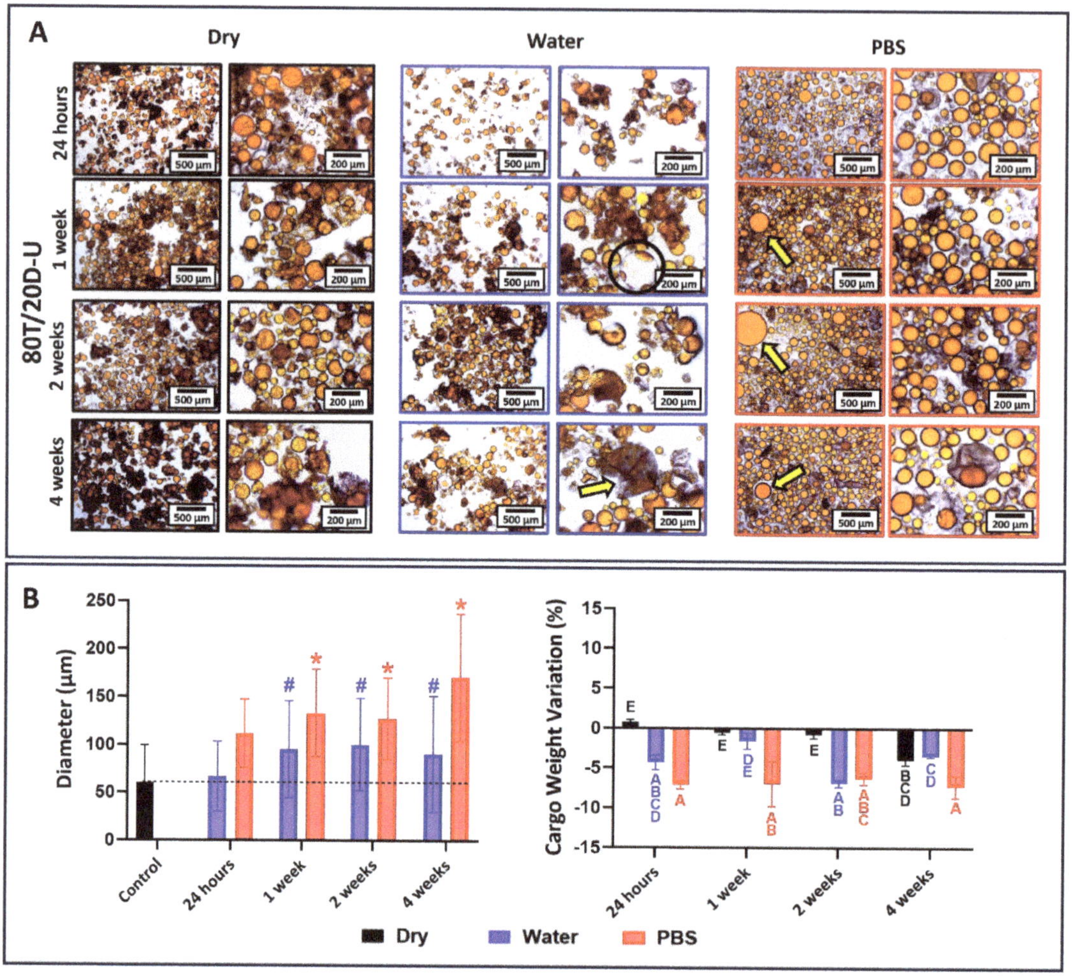

Figure 11. (**A**) Optical micrographs at 10× and 40× magnifications of 80T/20D-U microcapsules stored dry at 4 °C, in distilled water, or in PBS for 1 day, 1 week, 2 weeks, and 4 weeks. The 80T/20D-U microcapsules, when incubated in dry conditions, did not leak the cargo, and maintained their morphology. But when incubated in water, the loss of cargo was evident after 1 week of incubation (black circle) and empty shells can be observed after 4 weeks (yellow arrow). In the case of incubation in PBS, we can observe the leaked cargo from 1 week of incubation (yellow arrows). This shows that 80T/20D-U is the least stable group when compared to the 80T/20D magnetic and mechanical stirring ones. (**B**) The average diameter of microcapsules as a function of the time points and incubation solution. The average diameter of the microcapsules immediately after drying and before incubation was used as the control, and the groups were statistically compared to it. Bars with # (for water) or * (for PBS) indicate a significant difference in relation to the control group ($p < 0.05$). Percentage in cargo weight variation as a function of the time point and incubation condition. Bars with different letters indicate a statistically significant difference ($p < 0.05$).

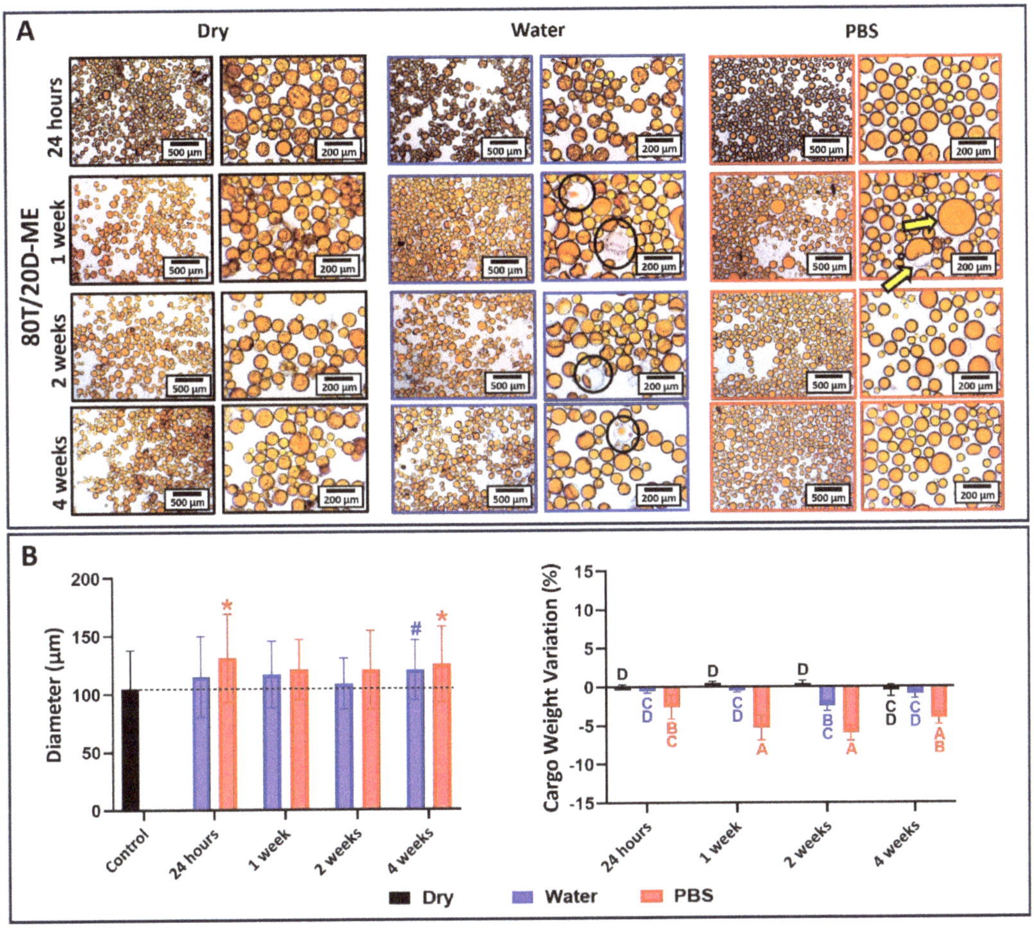

Figure 12. (**A**) Optical micrographs at 10× and 40× magnifications of 80T/20D-ME microcapsules stored dry at 4 °C, in distilled water, or in PBS for 1 day, 1 week, 2 weeks, and 4 weeks. In dry conditions, the microcapsules look stable through all the incubation time points. Meanwhile, when incubated in water, the loss of cargo could be observed after one week of incubation (black circles). In PBS, similar to other groups, shell swelling can be observed without the loss of encapsulated cargo (yellow arrow). (**B**) The average diameter of microcapsules as a function of the time points and incubation solution. The average diameter of the microcapsules immediately after drying and before incubation was used as the control, and the groups were statistically compared to it. Bars with # (for water) or * (for PBS) indicate a significant difference in relation to the control group ($p < 0.05$). Percentage in cargo weight variation as a function of the time point and incubation condition. Bars with different letters indicate a statistically significant difference ($p < 0.05$).

4. Conclusions

In summary, the microemulsification technique exerted a substantial impact on the morphology and physicochemical characteristics of the microcapsules. Magnetic stirring emerged as a suitable choice for less viscous emulsions. Ultrasonication demonstrated efficacy, particularly for hydrophobic and singularly composed cargo, especially when nano- or low micro-sized capsules are deemed optimal for the application. Mechanical stirring consistently yielded the most reliable results, exhibiting resilience to cargo compositions and establishing itself as a robust and versatile technique. Considering chemical stability across various scenarios, the PUF system exhibited distinct responses to diverse osmotic pressure conditions. It demonstrated an ability to retain the healing agent in dry conditions, releasing it only under mechanical stress. In aqueous environments, it functioned as a semi-permeable membrane, showcasing dynamic fluid exchange characterized by water influx and cargo efflux. In PBS, microcapsule shells exhibited uneven swelling, with cargo gradually released as the thinnest parts of the microcapsules ruptured, illustrating the system activation potential through osmotic shock. Finally, the incorporation of DMAM led to capsules with higher mechanical resistance and physicochemical stability. In conclusion, this study highlights the necessity of tailoring synthetic procedures to accommodate the unique characteristics of each system and their intended final applications.

Author Contributions: Methodology, A.P.P.F. and S.P.R.; conceptualization, A.P.P.F.; investigation, S.P.R. and B.H.; data curation, S.P.R. and B.H., writing—original draft preparation, S.P.R. and A.P.P.F.; writing—review and editing, A.P.P.F.; supervision, A.P.P.F.; visualization, S.P.R. and A.P.P.F.; funding acquisition, A.P.P.F. All authors have read and agreed to the published version of the manuscript.

Funding: This research was funded by the National Institutes of Health/National Institute of Dental and Craniofacial Research (NIH/NIDCR) R00 DE028876.

Data Availability Statement: The original contributions presented in the study are included in the article, further inquiries can be directed to the corresponding authors.

Conflicts of Interest: The authors declare no conflicts of interest.

References

1. Singh, M.; Hemant, K.; Ram, M.; Shivakumar, H. Microencapsulation: A promising technique for controlled drug delivery. *Res. Pharm. Sci.* **2010**, *5*, 65. [PubMed]
2. Khandbahale, S.V. Microencapsulation-A novel approach in drug delivery: A review. *Asian J. Res. Pharm. Sci.* **2020**, *10*, 39–50. [CrossRef]
3. Chuanjie, F.; Juntao, T.; Xiaodong, Z. Effects of process parameters on the physical properties of poly (urea–formaldehyde) microcapsules prepared by a one-step method. *Iran. Polym. J.* **2013**, *22*, 665–675. [CrossRef]
4. Kothari, J.; Iroh, J.O. Self-Healing Poly(urea formaldehyde) Microcapsules: Synthesis and Characterization. *Polymers* **2023**, *15*, 1668. [CrossRef] [PubMed]
5. Halász, G.; Gyüre, B.; Jánosi, I.M.; Szabó, K.G.; Tél, T. Vortex flow generated by a magnetic stirrer. *Am. J. Phys.* **2007**, *75*, 1092–1098. [CrossRef]
6. Kenneth, S.; Suslick, G.J.P. Applications of Ultrasound to Materials Chemistry. *Annu. Rev. Mater. Res.* **1999**, *29*, 295–326.
7. Jaszczur, M.; Młynarczykowska, A. A General Review of the Current Development of Mechanically Agitated Vessels. *Processes* **2020**, *8*, 982. [CrossRef]
8. Li, H.; Wang, R.; Hu, H.; Liu, W. Surface modification of self-healing poly (urea-formaldehyde) microcapsules using silane-coupling agent. *Appl. Surf. Sci.* **2008**, *255*, 1894–1900. [CrossRef]
9. Wu, J.; Weir, M.D.; Zhang, Q.; Zhou, C.; Melo, M.A.S.; Xu, H.H. Novel self-healing dental resin with microcapsules of polymerizable triethylene glycol dimethacrylate and N, N-dihydroxyethyl-p-toluidine. *Dent. Mater.* **2016**, *32*, 294–304. [CrossRef]
10. Fan, C.; Wei, T.; Hu, C.; Zhou, X. Preparation of GO/PUF hybrid shell microcapsules using GO sheets as the particulate emulsifier. *Micro Nano Lett.* **2016**, *11*, 207–211. [CrossRef]
11. Madelatparvar, M.; Hosseini, M.S.; Zhang, C. Polyurea micro-/nano-capsule applications in construction industry: A review. *Nanotechnol. Rev.* **2023**, *12*, 20220516. [CrossRef]
12. Althaqafi, K.A.; Satterthwaite, J.; Silikas, N. A review and current state of autonomic self-healing microcapsules-based dental resin composites. *Dent. Mater.* **2020**, *36*, 329–342. [CrossRef] [PubMed]
13. Fugolin, A.P.P.; Ferracane, J.L.; Pfeifer, C.S. Fatigue-Crack Propagation Behavior in Microcapsule-Containing Self-Healing Polymeric Networks. *Mater. Des.* **2022**, *223*, 111142. [CrossRef] [PubMed]
14. de la Paz Miguel, M.; Ollier, R.; Alvarez, V.; Vallo, C. Effect of the preparation method on the structure of linseed oil-filled poly(urea-formaldehyde) microcapsules. *Prog. Org. Coat.* **2016**, *97*, 194–202. [CrossRef]
15. Ollier, R.P.; Penoff, M.E.; Alvarez, V.A. Microencapsulation of epoxy resins: Optimization of synthesis conditions. *Colloids Surf. A Physicochem. Eng. Asp.* **2016**, *511*, 27–38. [CrossRef]
16. Zotiadis, C.; Patrikalos, I.; Loukaidou, V.; Korres, D.M.; Karantonis, A.; Vouyiouka, S. Self-healing coatings based on poly(urea-formaldehyde) microcapsules: In situ polymerization, capsule properties and application. *Prog. Org. Coat.* **2021**, *161*, 106475. [CrossRef]
17. Basuri, P.; Kumar, J.S.; Unni, K.; Manna, S.; Pradeep, T. Aggregation of molecules is controlled in microdroplets. *Chem. Commun.* **2022**, *58*, 12657–12660. [CrossRef] [PubMed]

18. Tadros, T.F. *Emulsion Formation, Stability, and Rheology*; Wiley-VCH Verlag GmbH & Co. KGaA: Weinheim, Germany, 2013; pp. 1–75.
19. Al-Sabagh, A.; Noor El-Din, M.; Abo-El Fotouh, S.; Nasser, N. Investigation of the demulsification efficiency of some ethoxylated polyalkylphenol formaldehydes based on locally obtained materials to resolve water-in-oil emulsions. *J. Dispers. Sci. Technol.* **2009**, *30*, 267–276. [CrossRef]
20. Telmadarreie, T.; Berton, P.; Bryant, S.L. Treatment of water-in-oil emulsions produced by thermal oil recovery techniques: Review of methods and challenges. *Fuel* **2022**, *330*, 125551. [CrossRef]
21. Albarghouthi, M.N.; Buchholz, B.A.; Huiberts, P.J.; Stein, T.M.; Barron, A.E. Poly-N-hydroxyethylacrylamide (polyDuramide): A novel, hydrophilic, self-coating polymer matrix for DNA sequencing by capillary electrophoresis. *Electrophoresis* **2002**, *23*, 1429–1440. [CrossRef]
22. Yom-Tov, O.; Neufeld, L.; Seliktar, D.; Bianco-Peled, H. A novel design of injectable porous hydrogels with in situ pore formation. *Acta Biomater.* **2014**, *10*, 4236–4246. [CrossRef] [PubMed]
23. Saberi, A.; Zhang, S.; van den Bersselaar, C.; Kandail, H.; den Toonder, J.M.; Kurniawan, N.A. A stirring system using suspended magnetically-actuated pillars for controlled cell clustering. *Soft Matter* **2019**, *15*, 1435–1443. [CrossRef] [PubMed]
24. Alshanski, I.; Bentolila, M.; Gitlin-Domagalska, A.; Zamir, D.; Zorsky, S.; Joubran, S.; Hurevich, M.; Gilon, C. Enhancing the Efficiency of the Solid Phase Peptide Synthesis (SPPS) Process by High Shear Mixing. *Org. Process Res. Dev.* **2018**, *22*, 1318–1322. [CrossRef]
25. Wang, X.; Wang, Z.; Guo, S.; Wang, G.; Xue, M. Sonochemical synthesis of protein microcapsules loaded with traditional Chinese herb extracts. *Green Process. Synth.* **2022**, *11*, 164–175. [CrossRef]
26. Zabot, G.L.; Vigano, J.; Silva, E.K. Low-Frequency Ultrasound Coupled with High-Pressure Technologies: Impact of Hybridized Techniques on the Recovery of Phytochemical Compounds. *Molecules* **2021**, *26*, 5117. [CrossRef] [PubMed]
27. Tiong, T.J.; Chu, J.K.; Lim, L.Y.; Tan, K.W.; Yap, Y.H.; Asli, U.A. A computational and experimental study on acoustic pressure for ultrasonically formed oil-in-water emulsion. *Ultrason. Sonochem.* **2019**, *56*, 46–54. [CrossRef]
28. Leong, T.S.; Martin, G.J.; Ashokkumar, M. Ultrasonic encapsulation—A review. *Ultrason. Sonochem.* **2017**, *35*, 605–614. [CrossRef] [PubMed]
29. Weerapol, Y.; Manmuan, S.; Chaothanaphat, N.; Okonogi, S.; Limmatvapirat, C.; Limmatvapirat, S.; Tubtimsri, S. Impact of fixed oil on Ostwald ripening of anti-oral cancer nanoemulsions loaded with Amomum kravanh essential oil. *Pharmaceutics* **2022**, *14*, 938. [CrossRef] [PubMed]
30. Taylor, P. Ostwald ripening in emulsions. *Adv. Colloid Interface Sci.* **1998**, *75*, 107–163. [CrossRef]
31. Blaiszik, B.; Caruso, M.; McIlroy, D.; Moore, J.; White, S.; Sottos, N. Microcapsules filled with reactive solutions for self-healing materials. *Polymer* **2009**, *50*, 990–997. [CrossRef]
32. Tong, X.-M.; Zhang, T.; Yang, M.-Z.; Zhang, Q. Preparation and characterization of novel melamine modified poly(urea–formaldehyde) self-repairing microcapsules. *Colloids Surf. A Physicochem. Eng. Asp.* **2010**, *371*, 91–97. [CrossRef]
33. Ning, K.; Loomans, B.; Yeung, C.; Li, J.; Yang, F.; Leeuwenburgh, S. Influence of microcapsule parameters and initiator concentration on the self-healing capacity of resin-based dental composites. *Dent. Mater.* **2021**, *37*, 403–412. [CrossRef] [PubMed]
34. Munoz, G.; Dequidt, A.; Martzel, N.; Blaak, R.; Goujon, F.; Devémy, J.; Garruchet, S.; Latour, B.; Munch, E.; Malfreyt, P. Heterogeneity Effects in Highly Cross-Linked Polymer Networks. *Polymers* **2021**, *13*, 757. [CrossRef] [PubMed]
35. Park, S.H.; Hong, C.R.; Choi, S.J. Prevention of Ostwald ripening in orange oil emulsions: Impact of surfactant type and Ostwald ripening inhibitor type. *LWT* **2020**, *134*, 110180. [CrossRef]
36. Zheng, S.; Huang, S.; Xiong, L.; Yang, W.; Liu, Z.; Xie, B.; Yang, M. Tunable wrinkle structure formed on surface of polydimethylsiloxane microspheres. *Eur. Polym. J.* **2018**, *104*, 99–105. [CrossRef]
37. Yuan, L.; Liang, G.; Xie, J.; Li, L.; Guo, J. Preparation and characterization of poly(urea-formaldehyde) microcapsules filled with epoxy resins. *Polymer* **2006**, *47*, 5338–5349. [CrossRef]
38. Riccobelli, D.; Al-Terke, H.H.; Laaksonen, P.; Metrangolo, P.; Paananen, A.; Ras, R.H.A.; Ciarletta, P.; Vella, D. Flattened and Wrinkled Encapsulated Droplets: Shape Morphing Induced by Gravity and Evaporation. *Phys. Rev. Lett.* **2023**, *130*, 218202. [CrossRef] [PubMed]
39. Qin, R.; Xu, G.; Guo, L.; Jiang, Y.; Ding, R. Preparation and characterization of a novel poly(urea–formaldehyde) microcapsules with similar reflectance spectrum to leaves in the UV–Vis–NIR region of 300–2500 nm. *Mater. Chem. Phys.* **2012**, *136*, 737–743. [CrossRef]
40. Alziyadi, M.O.; Denton, A.R. Osmotic pressure and swelling behavior of ionic microcapsules. *J. Chem. Phys.* **2021**, *155*, 214904. [CrossRef]
41. Zhang, W.; Qu, L.; Pei, H.; Qin, Z.; Didier, J.; Wu, Z.; Bobe, F.; Ingber, D.E.; Weitz, D.A. Controllable Fabrication of Inhomogeneous Microcapsules for Triggered Release by Osmotic Pressure. *Small* **2019**, *15*, e1903087. [CrossRef]
42. Jia, D.; Muthukumar, M. Theory of charged gels: Swelling, elasticity, and dynamics. *Gels* **2021**, *7*, 49. [CrossRef] [PubMed]
43. Akhmetzhan, A.; Myrzakhmetova, N.; Amangeldi, N.; Kuanyshova, Z.; Akimbayeva, N.; Dosmaganbetova, S.; Toktarbay, Z.; Longinos, S.N. A Short Review on the N,N-Dimethylacrylamide-Based Hydrogels. *Gels* **2021**, *7*, 234. [CrossRef] [PubMed]
44. Cui, J.; Mei, C.; Jia, C.; Zhou, Z.; Zhang, Y. Acrylamide–formaldehyde–urea copolymer as a novel compatibilizer for high density polyethylene/plant fiber composite. *Polym. Bull.* **2011**, *67*, 375–382. [CrossRef]

45. Avis, R. Glyoxal-Acrylamide-Formaldehyde-Urea Wet Strength Resin. U.S. Patent No 3,773,612, 20 November 1973.
46. Abdullah, Z.A.; Park, B.D. Influence of acrylamide copolymerization of urea–formaldehyde resin adhesives to their chemical structure and performance. *J. Appl. Polym. Sci.* **2010**, *117*, 3181–3186. [CrossRef]

Journal of
Functional Biomaterials

MDPI

Article

Nano-Reactors Based on Ovotransferrin Organic Skeleton through a Ferroptosis-like Strategy Efficiently Enhance Antibacterial Activity

Zihan Zhuo [1,†], Chunfang Yin [1,†], Zhenqing Zhang [1], Yumeng Han [1], Haoye Teng [1], Qi Xu [1,*] and Changming Li [1,2,*]

1 Institute of Advanced Cross-Field Science, College of Life Science, Qingdao University, Qingdao 266800, China; zhuo@qdu.edu.cn (Z.Z.); ycf1462722151@163.com (C.Y.); zhangzhenqing0330@163.com (Z.Z.); hanym0105@163.com (Y.H.); hy12122021@163.com (H.T.)

2 Institute of Materials Science and Devices, School of Materials Science and Engineering, Suzhou University of Science and Technology, Suzhou 215009, China

* Correspondence: xq@qdu.edu.cn (Q.X.); ecmli@usts.edu.cn (C.L.)

† These authors contribute equally to this work.

Abstract: The issue of bacterial resistance is an escalating problem due to the misuse of antibiotics worldwide. This study introduces a new antibacterial mechanism, the ferroptosis-like death (FLD) of bacteria, and an approach to creating green antibacterial nano-reactors. This innovative method leverages natural iron-containing ovotransferrin (OVT) assembled into an organic skeleton to encapsulate low-concentration adriamycin (ADM) for synthesizing eco-friendly nano-reactors. FLD utilizes the Fenton reaction of reactive oxygen species and ferrous ions to continuously produce ·OH, which can attack the bacterial cell membrane and destroy the cell structure to achieve bacteriostasis. The OVT@ADM nano-reactors are nearly spherical, with an average diameter of 247.23 nm and uniform particle sizing. Vitro simulations showed that Fe^{3+} in OVT@ADM was reduced to Fe^{2+} by glutathione in the bacterial periplasmic space, which made the structure of OVT loose, leading to a sustained slow release of ADM from OVT@ADM. The H_2O_2 continuously produced by ADM oxidized Fe^{2+} through the Fenton reaction to produce ·OH and Fe^{3+}. The results of the antibacterial assay showed that OVT@ADM had a satisfactory antibacterial effect against *S. aureus*, and the inhibition rate was as high as 99.3%. The cytotoxicity results showed that the mitigation strategy significantly reduced the cytotoxicity caused by ADM. Based on the FLD mechanism, OVT@ADM nano-reactors were evaluated and applied to bacteriostasis. Therefore, the novel antibacterial mechanism and OVT@ADM by the green synthesis method have good application prospects.

Keywords: ovotransferrin; nano reactors; antibacterial; ferroptosis-like death; green synthesis

1. Introduction

Antibiotics have revolutionized medicine, farming, and other fields with their powerful antibacterial effects, but their overuse has led to environmental concerns and an alarming rise in antibiotic-resistant bacteria [1]. This necessitates the development of alternative antimicrobial strategies. Currently, nonantibiotic antibacterials hold considerable promise, but they encounter significant barriers in practical applications due to issues like cytotoxicity, instability, and poor targeting, such as benzalkonium chloride (BKC), which has also been identified as an emerging pollutant with respiratory toxicity and neurotoxicity [2–4]. New antibacterial mechanisms are urgently needed to combat resistance and toxicity. Ferroptosis, a new form of iron-dependent cell death characterized by an iron-dependent accumulation of reactive oxygen species (ROS), is biochemically, genetically, and morphologically distinct from apoptosis, necrosis, and cellular autophagy, and it is now being demonstrated to be a potent pathway for killing cancer cells. Although the precise and complete role of iron in ferroptosis remains unclear, the iron-catalyzed ROS production, such as the Fenton reaction, has proven to be an important pathway for iron-induced ferroptosis [5]. At the same time, the onset of ferroptosis is often accompanied by the loss of plasma membrane integrity and the leakage of intracellular contents [6]. The precise mechanisms of ferroptosis are not fully understood, but a critical pathway involves iron-catalyzed ROS production, such as through the Fenton reaction [7–9]. The bacterial cell membrane contains unsaturated fatty acids, which play a crucial role in the physiological activity of the cell membrane and are prone to initiating free-radical reactions [10–12]. Notably, bacteria with low intracellular reducing substances are more vulnerable to ROS [13]. Based on the material basis and conditions described, this work proposes a novel antibacterial mechanism: the ferroptosis-like death for bacteria (FLD). FLD triggers the Fenton reaction by providing ROS and Fe^{3+}, destroying bacterial cell membranes.

Fe^{2+} exhibits dose-dependent cytotoxicity, where excessive levels can induce ROS and increase bacterial lipid peroxidation [14]. A previous study designed iron-loaded proteins loaded with Adriamycin (ADM) for cancer treatment and confirmed that cancer cell death was attracted by ferroptosis [15]. To improve the iron level around the bacteria, we skillfully used the natural iron-containing ovotransferrin (OVT), which is an iron-binding glycoprotein from egg white, with a variety of biological activities such as antibacterial, antioxidant, and other activities [16–18]. As the natural substrate of OVT, Fe^{3+} has a strong binding ability with OVT. After binding Fe^{3+}, the structure of OVT is closed and tight, and after Fe^{3+} is released, its structure becomes open and loose [16–19]. When OVT is used as a drug carrier, this property favors the release of drug pH responses in nanoparticles. Glutathione (GSH), a prominent antioxidant in organisms, exhibits diverse biological functions and is crucial in safeguarding cells against oxidative harm and upholding a stable redox milieu. The bacterial periplasm space contains GSH with a reducing effect, which can reduce Fe^{3+} to Fe^{2+}, laying the foundation for the occurrence of FLD [20].

In addition, the mechanism of ferroptosis is also affected by the insufficient supply of H_2O_2. ADM is an anthracycline antineoplastic drug that has been one of the most effective antineoplastic drugs used alone or in combination with other medications [21]. Low concentrations of ADM can induce the production of H_2O_2 [22]. The moiety of anthracene in the chemical structure of ADM can be converted into a semiquinone radical form, and, subsequently, nonenzymatic semiquinone radical can be converted into superoxide (O^{2-}) and hydrogen peroxide (H_2O_2) by molecular oxygen (O_2) re-oxidation and interact with various macromolecules [23,24]. Low-concentration ADM could not only compensate for the lack of H_2O_2 around the colony but also avoid the strong toxic side effects of ADM. Both OVT and ADM can induce the development of ferroptosis. Nanoparticles built from transferrin and ADM have been shown to induce ferroptosis in cancer cells [15,25,26].

Based on the above, we propose to use the FLD mechanism for antibacterial activity in this work. The FLD nano-reactors (OVT@ADM) were constructed here, which loaded ADM on natural iron-containing OVT by the green desolvation method. OVT@ADM nano-reactors did not need to add other auxiliary sterilization methods, such as photothermal and photodynamic treatment, to achieve good antibacterial effects. As shown in Scheme 1, OVT compensated for the lack of iron supply around the bacteria by carrying Fe^{3+} on its own, GSH in the bacterial periplasmic space could reduce Fe^{3+} to Fe^{2+}, and low concentrations of ADM were responsible for the production of H_2O_2, which underwent a Fenton reaction with Fe^{2+} to produce hydroxyl radicals, leading to FLD causing the bacteria to rupture and, thus, become antibacterial. The OVT@ADM nano-reactors are safe and controllable, could alleviate the adverse effects of antibiotic abuse or toxic agents, and provide an innovative strategy for future antibacterial research.

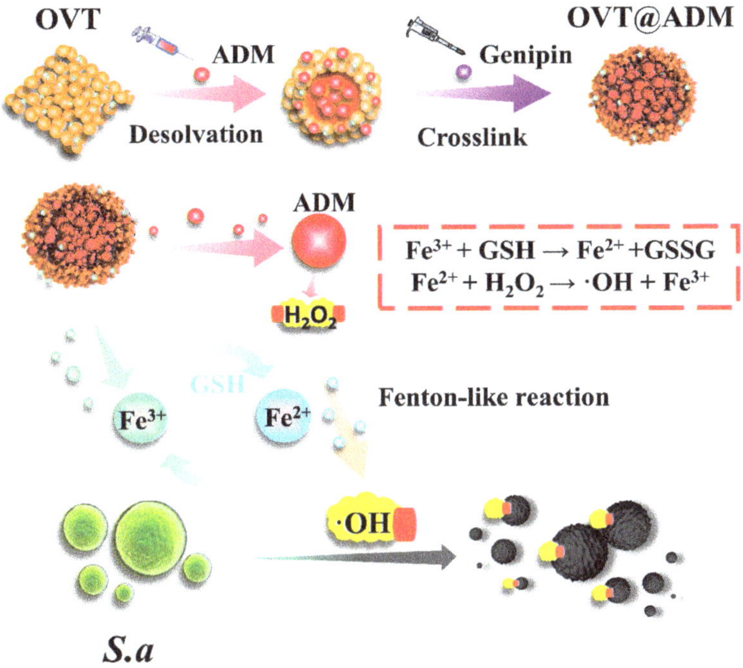

Scheme 1. The synthesis process and the antibacterial principle of OVT@ADM. OVT: ovotransferrin; ADM: adriamycin; GSH: glutathione; GSSG: oxidized glutathione; *S. a*: *Staphylococcus aureus*.

2. Materials and Methods

2.1. Materials

The following materials were purchased from commercial suppliers: OVT (extraction from egg white in the laboratory, purity ≥ 95%), ADM, genipin, and methylene blue (MB) were purchased from Macklin (Macklin Biochemical Co., Ltd., Shanghai, China). 1,10-Phenanthroline, Ammonium iron(II) sulfate hexahydrate, Hydroxylammonium chloride, and Glutathione (Reduced) (GSH) were purchased from Aladdin (Shanghai Aladdin Biochemical Technology Co., Ltd., Shanghai, China). OxoidTM yeast extract was obtained from (Thermo Fisher Scientific Co., Ltd., Shanghai, China), Agar from (Beijing Solarbio Science & Technology Co., Ltd., Beijing, China), and trypsin from (Qingdao Hope Bio-Technology Co., Ltd., Qingdao, China). Ultra-pure water was obtained from a Basic2002-UV ultrapure water system (Laibre, Qingdao, China). All other chemicals and solvents used in the study were analytical reagents.

The *Staphylococcus aureus* (ATCC25923) used in this study came from the −80 °C cryopreserved strain of the College of Life Sciences, Qingdao University. The mouse fibroblasts (L929) used in this study were provided by Future Testing Company (Qingdao, China).

2.2. Methods

2.2.1. Preparation of Nano-Reactors

OVT-NPs and OVT-ADM were prepared by the desolvent method and by adding genipin crossing [27]. OVT-NPs: OVT was dissolved in ultrapure water and prepared into a 5 mg/mL OVT solution, and insoluble impurities were removed from the filter membrane over 0.45 nm. Absolute ethanol was slowly added to the OVT solution using a syringe, and 5% (*w*/*w*) genipin was crosslinked to a 37 °C water bath and incubated for 4 h [28,29]. The reaction was terminated with glycine, and the ethanol unloaded drug was removed by dialysis.

OVT@ADM: OVT and ADM were dissolved into ultrapure water, respectively, prepared into 5 mg/mL and 3 mg/mL OVT solution and ADM solution, and the insoluble impurities were removed by the 0.45 μm filter membrane. Beyond these differences, the remaining steps align with the method described for OVT-NPs.

2.2.2. Particle Size and Zeta-Potential Measurements

After completing the preparation, the nano-reactors solution was sonicated for 15 s, and 1 mL of the sample was added to the cuvette; the bubbles were driven away and put into the sample pool, the outer cover of the instrument was closed, and the zeta-potential of the nano-reactors was determined. The particle size of nano-reactors was measured based on the principle of dynamic light scattering (DLS) using a nanoparticle-sized zeta-potential meter (Malvern Instruments, Worcestershire, UK). Determination conditions: 3 cycle scans; detection temperature: 25 °C.

2.2.3. Scanning Electron Microscopy (SEM)

The sample solution was lyophilized using a vacuum freeze dryer (ZEISS, Oberkochen, Germany), and a small amount was placed on the silicon wafer. Scanning electron microscopy (Jsm-780of, Nippon Electronics, Tokyo, Japan) was used to detect the surface morphology of lyophilized nano-reactors. All samples were covered with a gold layer before analysis.

2.2.4. Encapsulation Efficiency

First, most of the nano-reactors were separated by high-speed centrifugation (Sk-300, Sigma, Taufkirchen, Germany), and then ultrafiltration was performed at 4000 rpm. The lower solution was detected by a UV absorption value at 478 nm using a UV-spectrophotometer (UV-2600, Shimadzu, Kyoto, Japan) and replaced by the ADM standard curve (R^2 = 0.9995). The entrapment efficiency and drug loading capacity were calculated. The entrapment efficiency is calculated as follows:

$$\text{Drug loading capacity } (\%) = \frac{(M_0 - M_s)}{M_f} \times 100\%, \tag{1}$$

$$\text{Entrapment efficiency } (\%) = \frac{(M_0 - M_s)}{M_f} \times 100\%. \tag{2}$$

Here, M_0 refers to the initial weight of ADM, and M_f refers to the total weight of the nano-reactors; M_S refers to the weight of ADM in the supernatant.

2.2.5. UV–Visible Spectroscopy and Fluorescence Analysis

The sample solution was sonicated and dispersed, and then it was added to 2/3 of the height of the cuvette. Then, the sample tank was placed, and the instrument's outer cover was closed. The UV absorption spectrum of different samples at 350–700 nm was measured by a UV-spectrophotometer (UV-2600, Shimadzu, Japan).

Fluorescence measurements were performed using a fluorescence spectrometer (FS5, Edinburgh Instrument, Livingston, UK). The excitation bandwidth and emission bandwidth were 4.0 nm, and the excitation wavelength was 295 nm. It selectively excites the 214 residue of tryptophan, with an emission wavelength of 330 nm and an emission spectrum recording range of 300~750 nm.

2.2.6. Fourier Transform Infrared Spectroscopy (FTIR) Analysis

The sample solution was lyophilized using a freeze dryer, and the powder was placed on the sample table. Fourier transform infrared spectroscopy (Nicolet is50, Thermo Fisher Scientific Inc., Waltham, MA, USA) was used to obtain OVT-NPs, OVT@ADM, etc., to determine their molecular structure. The samples were scanned 32 times per spectrum.

2.2.7. X-ray Diffraction (XRD) Analysis

The powder X-ray diffraction (XRD) pattern of the samples was investigated (Bruker, Karlsruhe, Germany) using a diffractometer system with Cu-ka radiation in the scan range of 2θ from 10 to 50° and scan rate of 20°/min.

2.2.8. Simulated Release of ADM

In order to study the simulated release in vitro, OVT@ADM solution was reacted under three different conditions: pH 7.4 and GSH (−), pH 5.5 and GSH (−), pH 5.5 and GSH (+). The concentration of Nps was kept at 50 μg/mL, and the concentration of GSH was kept at 0.1 mmol/L. Three groups of mixed solutions were shaken at 5 min at 37 °C and incubated at 37 °C. The release of ADM at different reaction times was recorded by a UV-spectrophotometer.

2.2.9. Reduction of Fe^{2+}

OVT@ADM was mixed with GSH mother liquor (10 mM) and shaken for 5 min at 37 °C, and then it was incubated at 37 °C. It was taken out at 0, 30, 60, 90, and 120 min, respectively, and mixed with 0.15% 1,10-Phenanthroline. The UV absorbance of the mixed solution at 510 nm was recorded after a 20 min reaction.

2.2.10. OH Generate

OVT@ADM (50 μg/mL) and GSH mother liquor (2 mM) were mixed and diluted with PBS, shaken well for 5 min at 37 °C, mixed with H_2O_2 (100 mM) and MB (100 μg/mL), and incubated at 37 °C, and the UV absorption spectra of the mixed solution at different times were recorded. At the same time, a group of the mixed solution without GSH (PBS instead of GSH solution) was set up, where the other conditions were the same; it was incubated at 37 °C, and the UV absorption spectra of the mixed solution at different times were recorded.

2.2.11. Antibacterial Property Test

The antibacterial effect of OVT@ADM was evaluated by plate coating using *S. aureus* (ATCC25923) grown in the LB medium. In this study, a diluted bacterial suspension (10^7 CFU/mL) was mixed with ultrapure water (control), OVT-NPs, free ADM, and OVT@ADM, respectively. The concentration of OVT and OVT@ADM was 1 mg/mL and 1.02 mg/mL, respectively. The concentration of ADM was 18.5 and 8 μg/mL, and it was cultured in an incubator at 37 °C. Then, 100 μL of diluted bacterial solution was coated on the petri dish with an LB medium and incubated at 37 °C for 24 h. Here, we photographed plots of colonies on the dish.

In this study, we also observed the effect of no sample treatment on bacterial morphology by SEM. Firstly, the bacteria treated with ultra-pure water, free ADM, and OVT@ADM were collected by centrifugation, and the mixture was fixed overnight with glutaraldehyde at 4 °C. After fixation, the mixture was washed with ultrapure water, and then the bacteria were gradually dehydrated by successively treating them with a series of concentration gradients of ethanol. Finally, the bacterial solution was coated on the silicon dioxide wafer, dried, and sprayed with a gold layer, which was observed by a scanning electron microscope [30].

2.2.12. Cytotoxicity Assay

The L929 cell survival assay was used to test the toxicity of OVT@ADM. When the confluence of L929 cells in the culture bottle reached 80%, cells were digested with 0.25% trypsin and prepared as a cell suspension. Cells were counted, seeded at 6000 cells/well in 96-well cell culture plates, and incubated in a 37 °C cell incubator for 24 h. The 100 μL sample was mixed with a 900 μL culture medium, and the old medium in the 96-well plate was discarded. A volume of 300 μL of the mixture was added to each well, and 3 multiple holes were set up for each sample; the culture was continued for 24 h in a cell incubator at

37 °C. In 96-well plates, 100 μL of a new medium and 10 μL CCK-8 solution were added per well for 1–4 h for about 20 min to observe the degree of color development, and OD was read at 450 nm and 630 nm using a microplate reader.

3. Results and Discussion

3.1. Preparation and Characterization of the Nano-Reactors

3.1.1. Green Synthesis of Nano-Reactors

The OVT@ADM nano-reactors were constructed using renewable raw materials: leveraging OVT from egg white as the organic skeleton and genipin from gardenia fruit as the cross-linking agent to load ADM [16,31]. The synthesis process only involves ethanol, water, and glycine. The nanoparticles produced by this method do not generate heavy metal pollution, do not persist in the environment for a long time, and do not cause severe pollution to nature, thus achieving green synthesis.

3.1.2. Particle Size and Zeta-Potential Measurements

The mean hydration size and polymer dispersity index (PDI) of OVT-NPs, OVT@ADM are shown in Figure 1 and Table 1. From the particle size test results, the particle size of OVT-NPs was 256.57 ± 6.42 nm, but when ADM was loaded into OVT, the hydrodynamic diameter of OVT@ADM nano-reactors was slightly reduced to 247.23 ± 4.37 nm. The results show that the intermolecular cross-linking of OVT could prepare monodisperse nano-reactors, and the loading of ADM could make the OVT nanoparticles more compact. PDI was an important index to evaluate the size uniformity of nanoparticles [32]. The smaller the value, the more uniform the size distribution of nanoparticles. As shown in Table 1, the PDI was 0.283 ± 0.051 for OVT-NPs and the PDI for OVT@ADM was 0.223 ± 0.018, both with small PDI values, indicating the same size distribution of the nano-reactors. Zeta-potential is the electrostatic repulsion existing in the surface charge of suspended particles, which is an important index to evaluate the stability of particle suspension [33,34]. To investigate the changes in the zeta-potential of nano-reactors after ADM loading, the zeta-potentials of the OVT-NPs and OVT@ADM were tested. Due to the deprotonation of carboxyl groups, OVT has a negative charge in the range of pH 9–6.218. As shown in Table 1, OVT had a negative charge, and the potential of OVT-NPs and OVT@ADM was negative. After loading ADM, the potential of the OVT@ADM nano-reactors changed from −22.94 mV to −14.21 mV. This phenomenon might be caused by the attachment of ADM to the surface of nano-reactors rather than being completely encapsulated in NPs, and the interaction of OVT with genipin neutralizes some of the amino groups that also have an effect on it. As shown in Table 1, what is noteworthy is that the entrapment efficiency of ADM was 86.7%, indicating a strong OVT drug loading capacity. The results show that OVT@ADM had a narrow particle size distribution, high zeta-potential, and good entrapment efficiency, which provide conditions for its excellent bacteriostatic effect.

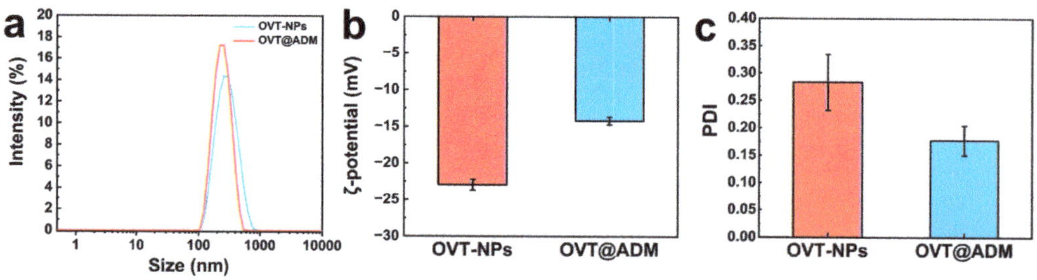

Figure 1. Particle size (**a**), zeta-potential (**b**), and PDI (**c**) of OVT-NPs and OVT@ADM.

Table 1. Characteristic data of OVT-NPs and OVT@ADM.

Sample	Size (nm)	Zeta-Potential (mV)	PDI	EE (%)
OVT-NPs	256.57 ± 6.42	−22.94 ± 0.73	0.283 ± 0.051	-
OVT@ADM	247.23 ± 4.37	−14.21 ± 0.533	0.223 ± 0.018	86.7

PDI: Polymer dispersity index; EE: Entrapment efficiency.

3.1.3. Scanning Electron Microscopy (SEM)

In Figure 2a, the morphology of the OVT-NPs and OVT@ADM nano-reactors are provided by field emission scanning microscopy (FE-SEM). Consistent with the particle size analysis, both particles show an approximate spherical morphology and similar dimensions. The OVT@ADM was regularly spherical and evenly dispersed. After loading ADM, the morphology of protein nanoparticles did not change significantly, indicating that the loading of ADM had no significant effect on the morphology of protein nanoparticles. Considering the shelf life, microbial contamination, convenience, and transportation cost, freeze-dried powder has advantages in transportation, storage, and distribution. Therefore, the freeze-drying of nanoparticles is very important in practical applications [35]. The morphology of freeze-dried OVT@ADM was tested here. As shown in Figure 2b, OVT@ADM maintained its physical properties in the drying process, indicating that it had good stability. At the same time, we also measured the iron on OVT@ADM by the EDS spectrum. As shown in Figure 2b (iron), after the formation of OVT@ADM nano-reactors by OVT, iron remained uniformly distributed on the surface of the OVT@ADM nano-reactors, which provided the conditions for the Fenton reaction to proceed.

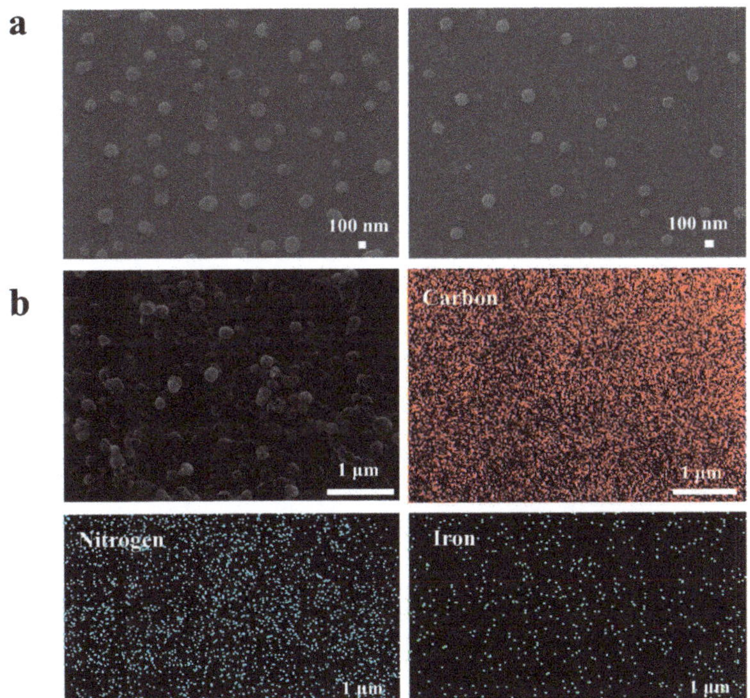

Figure 2. (**a**) FE-SEM images of OVT-NPs (left) and OVT@ADM (right), scale = 100 nm. (**b**) EDS of OVT@ADM, scale = 1 μm.

3.2. Structural Properties

3.2.1. UV–Visible Spectroscopy and Molecular Fluorescence Analysis

As shown by the UV–Vis absorption spectra (Figure 3a), both ADM and OVT@ADM had UV absorption characteristic peaks at 478 nm, while OVT-NPs had no absorption peak there, which proved that ADM had been successfully loaded into the OVT@ADM nano-reactors. Fluorescence spectroscopy is an effective method to explore the interaction between small molecules and macromolecules such as proteins, which provides valuable information for their binding mechanism. The inherent fluorescence of proteins may be caused by three aromatic amino acid residues—tryptophan, tyrosine, and phenylalanine19. It can be seen from Figure 3b that both free OVT and OVT@ADM had characteristic peaks at 330 nm. When free OVT was changed to OVT-NPs, the intensity of the fluorescence emission peak at 330 nm decreased, but the shape of the peak remained unchanged, showing a typical fluorescence-quenching phenomenon. When ADM was encapsulated in OVT@ADM nano-reactors, the intensity of the fluorescence emission peak at 330 nm was further weakened, and the shape of the peak remained unchanged, indicating that there was an interaction between ADM and OVT. As can be seen in Figure 3a,b, ADM was successfully loaded into the OVT@ADM nano-reactors and caused a change in the tertiary structure of the protein.

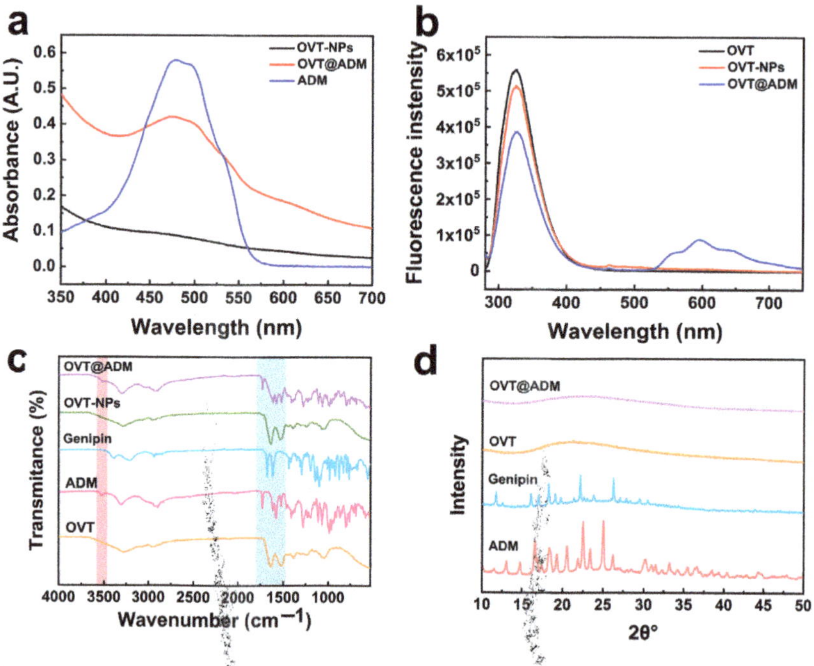

Figure 3. UV–Vis absorption spectra (**a**), fluorescence spectrogram (**b**), FT-IR spectra (**c**), and XRD patterns (**d**) of different samples.

3.2.2. Fourier Transform Infrared Spectroscopy (FTIR) and X-ray Diffraction (XRD) Analysis

To evaluate the effect of ADM addition on the OVT@ADM nano-reactors, the FTIR spectra of different samples were compared. The amide I region was more suitable for determining the secondary structure of the protein than the other amide regions because compared to the other amide regions, its vibration comes from an amide functional group [36]. As shown in Figure 3c, the absorption peak of OVT was at 1644.16 cm^{-1}, which represents the amide I region formed by the stretching vibration of the C=O stretching of the amide group and the action of a part of C-N [37]. After free OVT was transformed into OVT-NPs, the absorption peak changed from 1644.16 cm^{-1} to 1640.39 cm^{-1}. And the peak intensities of α-helix (1651 cm^{-1}) and β-turns (1669 cm^{-1}) decreased, indicating that the secondary structure of OVT changed [37]. After the nano-reactors were loaded with ADM, the absorption peak was at 1615.91 cm^{-1}, indicating that the secondary structure of OVT had further changed after the formation of nanoparticles. ADM had a characteristic absorption peak at 3526.46 cm^{-1}, attributed to N-H expansion vibration, and this characteristic peak also existed in OVT@ADM and was blue-shifted to 3522.67 cm^{-1}, proving that ADM was successfully loaded on OVT@ADM nano-reactors.

Figure 3d shows the X-ray diffraction spectra (X-ray diffraction profile) of pure OVT, pure ADM, genipin, and OVT@ADM at 2θ at 10–50. It can be observed that there were many obvious reflections in the diffraction patterns of ADM and genipin, indicating that they had crystalline properties. In contrast, OVT was a colloidal material that exhibited patterns of amorphous polymers. As shown in Figure 3d, the distinctive sharp reflections of ADM and genipin disappeared in the XRD patterns of OVT@ADM.

3.3. In Vitro Release Analysis

3.3.1. Simulated Release of ADM

H_2O_2 production was controlled by ADM, and a low concentration of ADM can effectively produce H_2O_2, while a high concentration of ADM will lead to high cytotoxicity, so the release of ADM is very important. As can be seen from Figure 4a,b, the changes in pH alone had no significant effect on the release of ADM, and there was almost no release of ADM in the first 12 h. However, after adding GSH under acidic conditions, 5% of ADM was released within 12 h and 8% of ADM was released within 24 h (Figure 4c), which is equivalent to twice the release rate of the control group (Figure 4a). Within 72 h, three groups of different treatments of OVT@ADM released 55% of ADM. As shown in Figure 4c, the release efficiency of ADM was significantly increased by the combined effect of acidic conditions and GSH compared with the other two groups.

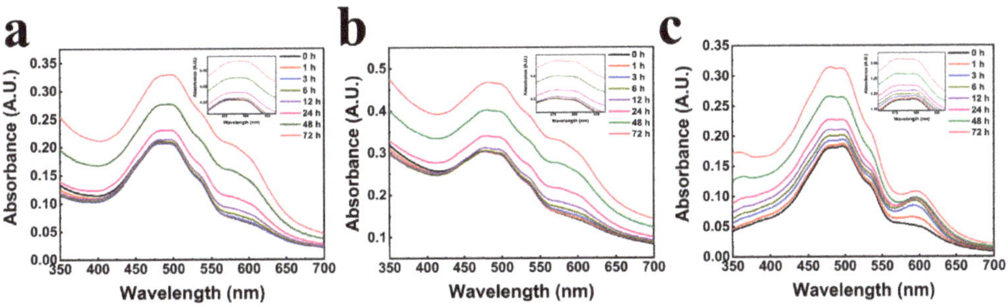

Figure 4. The in vitro drug release curve of OVT@ADM under the condition of pH 7 (**a**), pH 5.5 (**b**), and pH 5.5 + GSH (**c**).

A total of 46% of ADM was loaded on the OVT@ADM surface, which made the surface potential of OVT@ADM lower than that of the nanoparticles without ADM, which is consistent with the result of the zeta-potential of OVT@ADM being lower than that of OVT-NPs in Figure 1b. This is because in a neutral environment, the nucleophilic amino group (nucleophilic amino groups) in OVT attacked olefinic carbon atom at C-3 in genipin of the olefin carbon atom of genipin at C-3, opened the dihydropyran ring dihydropyran ring, and made the ester group in the genipin replace nucleophilic substitution, forming a secondary amide secondary amide with OVT [29]. ADM also contained the amino group, which reacted with the olefinic carbon atoms at the C-3 position of genipin, and could also cross-link with genipin. Therefore, part of the ADM was cross-linked on the surface or inside of the OVT@ADM nano-reactors, and part of the ADM was not cross-linked and was wrapped in the OVT@ADM nano-reactors due to the protein tertiary structure. When the OVT structure became loose, the uncross-linked ADM was released, while the ADM cross-linked to the interior could not be released rapidly. The results show that ADM had a slow-release effect, which both avoided the rapid drug depletion due to burst release and provided a low concentration of ADM to compensate for the insufficient supply of H_2O_2.

3.3.2. Reduction of Fe^{2+}

The existence of Fe^{2+} is very important in the process of FLD, and it participates in the production of ·OH, which is essential for inducing FLD. Phenanthrolines is a class of multifunctional chelating agents, which are well known for their formation of non-fluorescent complexes with Fe^{2+}, and it is very important in coordination chemistry. 1,10-Phenanthroline is the parent compound of the phenanthroline [38]. 1,10-Phenanthroline and its derivatives have been widely used as analytical probes [39]. 1,10-Phenanthroline reacted with Fe^{2+} to produce an orange-red complex with a maximum absorption peak at 510 nm without such a complex with Fe^{3+} [40]. GSH could reduce Fe^{3+} to Fe^{2+}, and Fe^{2+} reacted with 1,10-Phenanthroline to form an orange-red complex. After the reaction of the sample with GSH for a period of time, the mixed solution was mixed with 1,10-Phenanthroline, and the absorbance value of the product at 510 nm was measured. Figure 5 shows the concentration change curve of Fe^{2+} at different times. According to Figure 5a, the Fe^{2+} concentration of OVT-NPs in 120 min increased from 0.476 μg/mL to 1.65 μg/mL, and the Fe^{2+} concentration increased by 247% (1.2 μg/mL). The UV absorption characteristic peak of ADM was at 478 nm, which is close to the UV absorption characteristic peak of the orange-red complex, and had influence on its UV absorption value. But as shown in Figure 4, ADM was hardly released within 120 min, so the rise in UV absorption values at 510 nm is attributed to the generation of Fe^{2+}; the Fe^{2+} concentration of OVT@ADM was increased by 144% (1.25 μg/mL). The Fe^{2+} concentrations of OVT-NPs and OVT@ADM both increased by about 1.2 μg/mL within 120 min, indicating that the addition of ADM would not have a significant impact on the production and release of Fe^{2+}. The Fe^{3+} carried in OVT could be successfully reduced to Fe^{2+} by GSH, which provides a prerequisite for the smooth progress of the Fenton reaction.

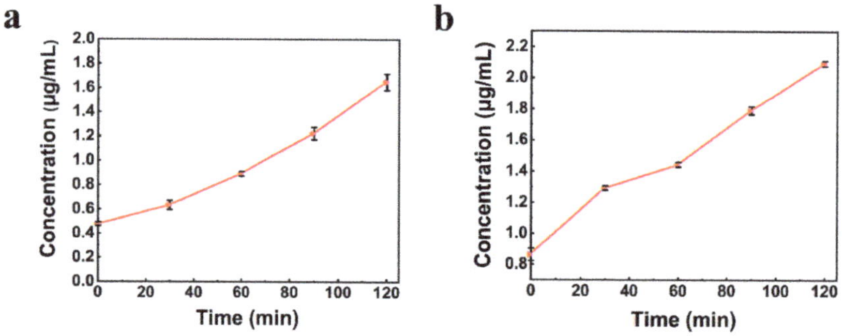

Figure 5. The Fe^{2+} release curves of OVT-NPs (**a**) and OVT@ADM (**b**) in the external environment at 37 °C.

3.3.3. ·OH Generation

Hydroxyl radicals (·OH) play an important role in the process of FLD. It is mainly produced by the Fenton reaction between H_2O_2 and Fe^{2+}, which further induces FLD. H_2O_2 could be converted to more toxic hydroxyl radicals by undergoing a Fenton reaction with Fe^{2+}. To prove that OVT@ADM had the ability to produce ·OH, we used a specific indicator of ·OH: methylene blue (MB) [41]. MB showed strong absorption at 664 nm and could bleach in the action of ·OH. As shown in Figure 6a, the typical absorption of MB was gradually decreased after incubation of OVT@ADM in solutions containing H_2O_2 and GSH, indicating that OVT@ADM exhibited good ·OH generation capacity. In the group without GSH reaction, the absorption of MB did not decrease, indicating that without the participation of GSH, Fe^{3+} could not be transformed into Fe^{2+}, and ·OH could not be produced by a Fenton reaction, resulting in MB not being degraded (Figure 6b). As shown in Figure 6d, the addition of GSH prompted a Fenton reaction that could significantly degrade MB and lead to MB discoloration compared to the system without GSH addition.

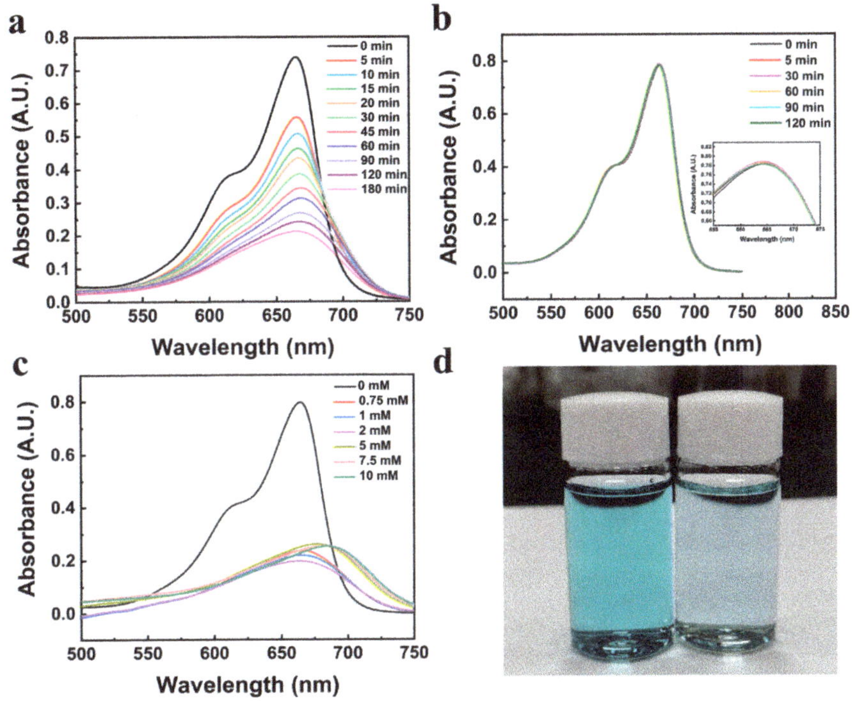

Figure 6. (**a**) Changes in MB uptake at different time points in solutions containing OVT@ADM (50 µg/mL), GSH (0.1 mM), and H_2O_2 (25 mM). (**b**) Changes in MB absorption at different time points in solutions containing OVT@ADM (50 µg/mL) and H_2O_2 (25 mM). (**c**) In the presence of H_2O_2 (20 mmol/L), the effect of different GSH concentrations on the absorption peak of MB. (**d**) Intuitive diagram of adding MB to the mixed solution; no GSH was added on the left, and GSH was added to the right to react. MB: Methylene blue; GSH: Glutathione.

Since GSH had antioxidant effects that inhibited the occurrence of FLD, the effect of GSH concentration in the periplasmic space on ·OH production was evaluated here [42]. The Fe^{3+} contained in OVT@ADM could effectively reduce the concentration of GSH and make the bacteria more sensitive to FLD. As shown in Figure 6c, the typical absorption peak of MB decreased with the increase in GSH concentration in the system. When the GSH concentration reached 5 mM, the characteristic absorption peak increased slightly, but it was still significantly lower than that of the control group. Moreover, when the concentration of GSH was as high as 10 mM, the characteristic peak of MB was still significantly decreased, indicating that a high concentration of GSH could be reduced to generate more Fe^{2+} and then generate ·OH in a Fenton reaction with H_2O_2 to degrade more MB. When the concentration of GSH increased to 10 mM, MB could still be degraded effectively, indicating that even if there was a high concentration of GSH, the system could still produce ·OH efficiently. The above results show that OVT@ADM could effectively produce ·OH after reducing Fe^{3+} to Fe^{2+} by GSH. This laid a foundation for inducing FLD.

3.4. Anti-Bacterial Properties

3.4.1. The Antibacterial Properties

The results of the above in vitro simulations show that OVT@ADM could successfully perform the Fenton reaction. Here, we used the plate coating method to analyze the antibacterial activity of OVT@ADM. The number of colony-forming units (CFUs) is shown in Figure 7b. The control group was *S. aureus* incubated with ultrapure water, and the control group had dense colonies with a colony count of 296, indicating that *S. aureus* grew well on the LB medium. There was no obvious difference between the OVT-NPs group and the control group. The colony number was 292, and the concentration of the OVT-NPs group was much lower than its minimum inhibitory concentration, so it did not show an antibacterial effect. The results of the in vitro release experiments showed that ADM was not released from OVT@ADM during incubation time (Figure 4); 30% of the loaded ADM existed on the surface of the OVT@ADM nano-reactors, and the rest was wrapped inside the OVT@ADM nano-reactors. Therefore, two different concentrations of pure ADM were set up: the concentration of ADM loaded on the surface of the OVT@ADM nano-reactors (8 μg/mL) and the concentration of all ADM loaded on the OVT@ADM nano-reactors (18.5 μg/mL). The colony number of the pure ADM group (8 μg/mL and 18.5 μg/mL) was 137 and 38, respectively, indicating that ADM itself had a certain antibacterial effect. It is worth noting that the antibacterial effect of OVT@ADM was very obvious, only two colonies were found, and the inhibition rate was up to 99.3%. This indicates that the ADM in the OVT@ADM nano-reactors, although mostly encapsulated inside the nano-reactors and unable to be released, was conducive to its rapid Fenton reaction with Fe^{2+} in the system to produce ·OH. The antibacterial ability of OVT@ADM is attributed to the Fenton reaction of iron carried in OVT with H_2O_2 produced by ADM to produce ·OH, and a portion of ADM's own antibacterial ability, both of which acted synergistically to exert antibacterial effects.

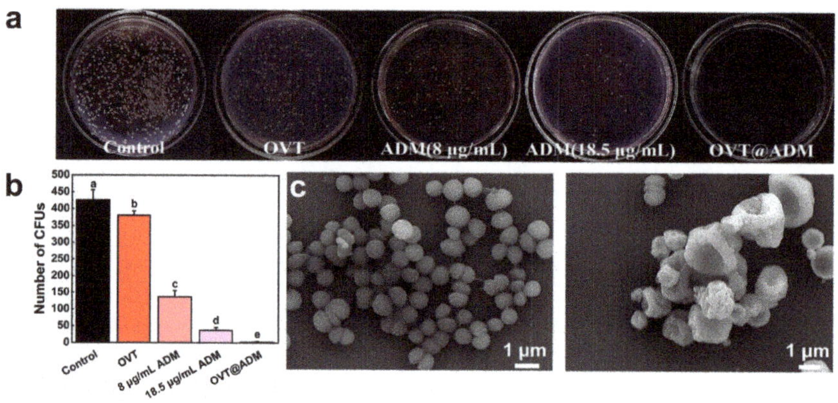

Figure 7. (**a**) Representative images of *S. aureus* grown on different samples after 24 h of culture; from left to right: control group, OVT group, ADM group (8 μg/mL), ADM group (18.5 μg/mL), and OVT@ADM group. (**b**) *S. aureus* colonies on different samples were cultured for 24h and counted. (c) SEM images of *S. aureus* under normal conditions (left) and treated with OVT@ADM (right). Letters (a–e) that are different in this figure indicate the significant difference between different series of concentration levels ($p < 0.001$).

After *S. aureus* was fixed with glutaraldehyde and dehydrated from ethanol, the surface morphology was observed using scanning electron microscopy. According to Figure 4c, the surface of normal *S. aureus* was smooth, and *S. aureus* was uniformly distributed spherically. After OVT@ADM, the morphology of *S. aureus* changed significantly, the cell surface became rough, the cells were deformed, and the surface underwent shrinkage. This might be caused by a distortion of the cell membrane as well as a leakage of intracellular material [43]. From this, we infer that the antibacterial activity of OVT@ADM was synergized by the antibacterial activity of ADM itself as well as by FLD. Among these, the antibacterial mechanism of FLD was cellular damage caused by an imbalance between reactive oxygen species and the antioxidant system within the biomolecule. FLD killed cells through iron-dependent accumulation of ·OH and could reduce the concentration of GSH in bacteria, making the bacteria less antioxidant and more susceptible to attack by ·OH. At the same time, OVT@ADM killed the bacteria by disrupting the cell membrane of *S. aureus*, causing cellular crumpling and possibly leading to leakage of cellular contents. This shows that FLD is expected to be an effective mechanism for killing Gram-positive bacteria in the future.

3.4.2. Cytotoxicity Analysis

As shown in Figure 8a–c, there was a dose-dependent cytotoxicity of OVT, ADM, and OVT@ADM on L929 cells at all concentrations tested. The cell viability after a low concentration of OVT treatment was greater than 90%, indicating low cytotoxicity. When the concentration reached 1.5 mg/mL, the cell viability was still maintained at about 88%, indicating the low toxicity of OVT to L929 cells. However, the cell viability decreased to 70% after treatment with a low concentration of ADM (5 μg/mL) and was only 50% when the concentration was increased to 40 μg/mL, indicating that ADM was strongly cytotoxic. As shown in Figure 8c, when ADM was loaded into the OVT@ADM nano-reactors, cell viability was significantly increased after a series of concentration treatments, indicating that loading ADM into the nano-reactors could significantly reduce the cytotoxicity of ADM. This may be related to the incomplete release.

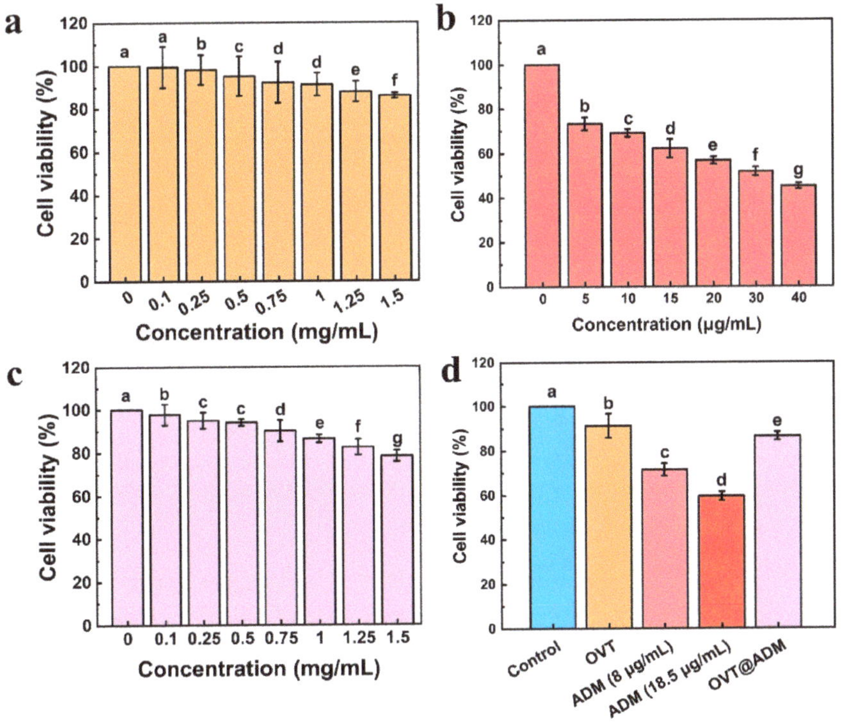

Figure 8. The cell viability of L929 cells treated with different concentrations of (**a**) OVT, (**b**) ADM, (c) OVT@ADM, and (**d**) samples used in the bacteriostatic experiment. Letters (a–g) that are different in this figure indicate the significant difference between different series of concentration levels ($p < 0.05$).

Further, the cytotoxicity of OVT@ADM at antibacterial concentrations and its corresponding concentrations of free OVT and free ADM were evaluated. Since ADM was not released during the incubation time of the antimicrobial assay, the cytotoxicity of free ADM equivalent to the concentration of ADM loaded on the surface of 1 mg/mL OVT@ADM nano-reactors (8 μg/mL) and the concentration of free ADM loaded in the OVT@ADM nano-reactors in its total concentration (18.5 μg/mL) were compared here. As shown in Figure 8d, the cell viability decreased to 71.5% and 59.5% after 8 μg/mL and 18.5 μg/mL ADM treatment, respectively, indicating that ADM had strong cytotoxicity at this concentration. The cell viability increased to 86.47% after treatment with the same concentration of OVT@ADM (1 mg/mL), indicating that OVT@ADM could effectively reduce the cytotoxicity caused by ADM. Therefore, the OVT@ADM nano-reactors could significantly reduce the cytotoxicity of the drug while exerting its good antibacterial effect. This indicates that OVT@ADM had significantly enhanced antibacterial activity and high security as a practical biomaterial.

4. Conclusions

In conclusion, OVT@ADM nano-reactors were synthesized through green methods using renewable resources. The experiments proved that OVT@ADM had excellent antibacterial effect and could significantly reduce the cytotoxicity of ADM. By using scanning electron microscopy, the OVT@ADM nano-reactors were found to be spherical; the average hydrodynamic diameter of OVT@ADM was 247.23 ± 4.37 nm, and it had a small PDI and a zeta-potential of −14.21 ± 0.533 mV. The material has good stability and prospects for application in different systems. The zeta-potential showed that OVT@ADM could successfully convert Fe^{3+} to Fe^{2+} in the presence of GSH and further reacted with H_2O_2 produced by ADM to generate ·OH, which eventually induced FLD and caused the bacteria to crumple and die. Notably, the OVT@ADM nano-reactors exhibited favorable biocompatibility and maintained robust antibacterial activity, underscoring their potential for medical applications. Importantly, the OVT@ADM nano-reactors represent a novel, green, and eco-friendly approach to antimicrobial strategies. The FLD mechanism exerts its antibacterial effects, showing potential for infection control and the creation of sterile cell systems. This discovery introduces a pioneering approach to the development of sustainable bacteriostatic materials, offering a fresh perspective for future research in the field of environmentally benign antimicrobial agents.

Author Contributions: Conceptualization, Z.Z. (Zihan Zhuo) and C.Y.; methodology, Z.Z. (Zihan Zhuo) and H.T.; software, C.Y. and Z.Z. (Zhenqing Zhang); validation, Z.Z. (Zihan Zhuo); formal analysis, Z.Z. (Zhenqing Zhang); investigation, C.Y.; resources, H.T.; data curation, C.Y.; writing—original draft preparation, Z.Z. (Zihan Zhuo) and C.Y.; writing—review and editing, Q.X. and C.L; visualization, Y.H.; supervision, Q.X.; project administration, Q.X. and C.L.; funding acquisition, Q.X. and C.L. All authors have read and agreed to the published version of the manuscript.

Funding: This work was supported by the Natural Science Foundation of Shandong Province (ZR2023QC037) and Qingdao Municipal Science and Technology Commission (DC1900013623).

Institutional Review Board Statement: Not applicable.

Informed Consent Statement: Not applicable.

Data Availability Statement: The data presented in this study are available on request from the corresponding author.

Conflicts of Interest: The authors declare no conflicts of interest.

Abbreviations

Abbreviation	Meaning
FLD	ferroptosis-like death
BKC	benzalkonium chloride
OVT	ovotransferrin
ADM	adriamycin
ROS	reactive oxygen species
GSH	glutathione
GSSG	oxidized glutathione
S. a	*Staphylococcus aureus*
NP	nanoparticle
SEM	scanning electron microscopy
FTIR	Fourier transform infrared spectroscopy
XRD	X-ray diffraction
PDI	Polydispersity
MB	methylene blue
CFU	colony forming units

References

1. de Sousa, J.M.; Balbontín, R.; Durao, P.; Gordo, I. Multidrug-resistant bacteria compensate for the epistasis between resistances. *PLoS Biol.* **2017**, *15*, 24. [CrossRef] [PubMed]
2. Choi, H.Y.; Lee, Y.H.; Lim, C.H.; Kim, Y.S.; Lee, I.S.; Jo, J.M.; Lee, H.Y.; Cha, H.G.; Woo, H.J.; Seo, D.S. Assessment of respiratory and systemic toxicity of Benzalkonium chloride following a 14-day inhalation study in rats. *Part. Fibre Toxicol.* **2020**, *17*, 19. [CrossRef] [PubMed]
3. Kwon, Y.S.; Jung, J.W.; Kim, Y.J.; Park, C.B.; Shon, J.C.; Kim, J.H.; Park, J.W.; Kim, S.G.; Seo, J.S. Proteomic analysis of whole-body responses in medaka (*Oryzias latipe*) exposed to benzalkonium chloride. *J. Environ. Sci. Health Part A-Toxic/Hazard. Subst. Environ. Eng.* **2020**, *55*, 1387–1397. [CrossRef] [PubMed]
4. Herron, J.M.; Hines, K.M.; Tomita, H.; Seguin, R.P.; Cui, J.Y.; Xu, L.B. Multiomics Investigation Reveals Benzalkonium Chloride Disinfectants Alter Sterol and Lipid Homeostasis in the Mouse Neonatal Brain. *Toxicol. Sci.* **2019**, *171*, 32–45. [CrossRef] [PubMed]
5. Wan, X.Y.; Song, L.Q.; Pan, W.; Zhong, H.; Li, N.; Tang, B. Tumor-Targeted Cascade Nanoreactor Based on Metal-Organic Frameworks for Synergistic Ferroptosis-Starvation Anticancer Therapy. *ACS Nano* **2020**, *14*, 11017–11028. [CrossRef] [PubMed]
6. Tang, D.; Kroemer, G. Ferroptosis. *Curr. Biol.* **2020**, *30*, R1292–R1297. [CrossRef] [PubMed]
7. Zheng, D.W.; Lei, Q.; Zhu, J.Y.; Fan, J.X.; Li, C.X.; Li, C.; Xu, Z.S.; Cheng, S.X.; Zhang, X.Z. Switching Apoptosis to Ferroptosis: Metal-Organic Network for High-Efficiency Anticancer Therapy. *Nano Lett.* **2017**, *17*, 284–291. [CrossRef] [PubMed]
8. Shen, Z.Y.; Song, J.B.; Yung, B.C.; Zhou, Z.J.; Wu, A.G.; Chen, X.Y. Emerging Strategies of Cancer Therapy Based on Ferroptosis. *Adv. Mater.* **2018**, *30*, 15. [CrossRef] [PubMed]
9. Rishi, G.; Huang, G.; Subramaniam, V.N. Cancer: The role of iron and ferroptosis. *Int. J. Biochem. Cell Biol.* **2021**, *141*, 5. [CrossRef]
10. Crompton, M.J.; Dunstan, R.H. Evaluation of in-situ fatty acid extraction protocols for the analysis of staphylococcal cell membrane associated fatty acids by gas chromatography. *J. Chromatogr. B* **2018**, *1084*, 80–88. [CrossRef]
11. Blevins, M.S.; James, V.K.; Herrera, C.M.; Purcell, A.B.; Trent, M.S.; Brodbelt, J.S. Unsaturation Elements and Other Modifications of Phospholipids in Bacteria: New Insight from Ultraviolet Photodissociation Mass Spectrometry. *Anal. Chem.* **2020**, *92*, 9146–9155. [CrossRef] [PubMed]
12. Lin, T.Y.; Weibel, D.B. Organization and function of anionic phospholipids in bacteria. *Appl. Microbiol. Biotechnol.* **2016**, *100*, 4255–4267. [CrossRef] [PubMed]
13. Zhou, Y.; Cai, C.Y.; Wang, C.; Hu, G.M.; Li, Y.T.; Han, M.J.; Hu, S.; Cheng, P. Ferric-loaded lipid nanoparticles inducing ferroptosis-like cell death for antibacterial wound healing. *Drug Deliv.* **2023**, *30*, 1–8. [CrossRef] [PubMed]
14. Shen, X.; Ma, R.; Huang, Y.; Chen, L.; Xu, Z.; Li, D.; Meng, X.; Fan, K.; Xi, J.; Yan, X.; et al. Nano-decocted ferrous polysulfide coordinates ferroptosis-like death in bacteria for anti-infection therapy. *Nano Today* **2020**, *35*, 14. [CrossRef]
15. Yang, R.L.; Li, Y.Q.; Wang, X.Y.; Yan, J.J.; Pan, D.H.; Xu, Y.P.; Wang, L.Z.; Yang, M. Doxorubicin loaded ferritin nanoparticles for ferroptosis enhanced targeted killing of cancer cells. *RSC Adv.* **2019**, *9*, 28548–28553. [CrossRef] [PubMed]
16. Wang, X.; Wei, Z.H.; Xue, C.H. The past and future of ovotransferrin: Physicochemical properties, assembly and applications. *Trends Food Sci. Technol.* **2021**, *116*, 47–62. [CrossRef]
17. Legros, J.; Jan, S.; Bonnassie, S.; Gautier, M.; Croguennec, T.; Pezennec, S.; Cochet, M.F.; Nau, F.; Andrews, S.C.; Baron, F. The Role of Ovotransferrin in Egg-White Antimicrobial Activity: A Review. *Foods* **2021**, *10*, 21. [CrossRef] [PubMed]
18. Wei, Z.H.; Zhu, P.; Huang, Q.R. Investigation of ovotransferrin conformation and its complexation with sugar beet pectin. *Food Hydrocoll.* **2019**, *87*, 448–458. [CrossRef]
19. Santos, F.C.; Costa, P.J.; Garcia, M.H.; Morais, T.S. Binding of RuCp complexes with human apo-transferrin: Fluorescence spectroscopy and molecular docking methods. *Biometals* **2021**, *34*, 1029–1042. [CrossRef]

20. Cassier-Chauvat, C.; Marceau, F.; Farci, S.; Ouchane, S.; Chauvat, F. The Glutathione System: A Journey from Cyanobacteria to Higher Eukaryotes. *Antioxidants* **2023**, *12*, 1199. [CrossRef]
21. Carvalho, C.; Santos, R.X.; Cardoso, S.; Correia, S.; Oliveira, P.J.; Santos, M.S.; Moreira, P.I. Doxorubicin: The Good, the Bad and the Ugly Effect. *Curr. Med. Chem.* **2009**, *16*, 3267–3285. [CrossRef] [PubMed]
22. Cao, R.; Sun, W.; Zhang, Z.; Li, X.J.; Du, J.J.; Fan, J.L.; Peng, X.J. Protein nanoparticles containing Cu(II) and DOX for efficient chemodynamic therapy via self-generation of H_2O_2. *Chin. Chem. Lett.* **2020**, *31*, 3127–3130. [CrossRef]
23. Menna, P.; Recalcati, S.; Cairo, G.; Minotti, G. An introduction to the metabolic determinants of anthracycline cardiotoxicity. *Cardiovasc. Toxicol.* **2007**, *7*, 80–85. [CrossRef] [PubMed]
24. Simunek, T.; Sterba, M.; Popelová, O.; Adamcová, M.; Hrdina, R.; Gersl, V. Anthracycline-induced cardiotoxicity: Overview of studies examining the roles of oxidative stress and free cellular iron. *Pharmacol. Rep.* **2009**, *61*, 154–171. [CrossRef] [PubMed]
25. Xu, R.; Yang, J.; Qian, Y.; Deng, H.; Wang, Z.; Ma, S.; Wei, Y.; Yang, N.; Shen, Q. Ferroptosis/pyroptosis dual-inductive combinational anti-cancer therapy achieved by transferrin decorated nanoMOF. *Nanoscale Horiz.* **2021**, *6*, 348–356. [CrossRef] [PubMed]
26. Chen, W.; Xie, L.; Lv, C.; Song, E.; Zhu, X.; Song, Y. Transferrin-Targeted Cascade Nanoplatform for Inhibiting Transcription Factor Nuclear Factor Erythroid 2-Related Factor 2 and Enhancing Ferroptosis Anticancer Therapy. *ACS Appl. Mater. Interfaces* **2023**, *15*, 28879–28890. [CrossRef] [PubMed]
27. Tacias-Pascacio, V.G.; García-Parra, E.; Vela-Gutiérrez, G.; Virgen-Ortiz, J.J.; Berenguer-Murcia, A.; Alcántara, A.R.; Fernandez-Lafuente, R. Genipin as an Emergent Tool in the Design of Biocatalysts: Mechanism of Reaction and Applications. *Catalysts* **2019**, *9*, 19. [CrossRef]
28. Sentoukas, T.; Charitou, G.; Wagner, J.; Wagemans, A.M.; Moschakis, T.; Papagiannopoulos, A. Formation of nanoparticles from ethanol-denatured whey proteins. *Food Struct.* **2023**, *37*, 100337. [CrossRef]
29. Wei, Z.H.; Cheng, Y.J.; Zhu, J.Y.; Huang, Q.R. Genipin-crosslinked ovotransferrin particle-stabilized Pickering emulsions as delivery vehicles for hesperidin. *Food Hydrocoll.* **2019**, *94*, 561–573. [CrossRef]
30. Ge, L.M.; Xu, Y.B.; Li, X.Y.; Yuan, L.; Tan, H.; Li, D.F.; Mu, C.D. Fabrication of Antibacterial Collagen-Based Composite Wound Dressing. *ACS Sustain. Chem. Eng.* **2018**, *6*, 9153–9166. [CrossRef]
31. Bryś, M.; Urbańska, K.; Olas, B. Novel Findings regarding the Bioactivity of the Natural Blue Pigment Genipin in Human Diseases. *Int. J. Mol. Sci.* **2022**, *23*, 902. [CrossRef] [PubMed]
32. Silvestre, A.L.P.; dos Santos, A.M.; de Oliveira, A.B.; Ferrisse, T.M.; Brighenti, F.L.; Meneguin, A.B.; Chorilli, M. Evaluation of photodynamic therapy on nanoparticles and films loaded-nanoparticles based on chitosan/alginate for curcumin delivery in oral biofilms. *Int. J. Biol. Macromol.* **2023**, *240*, 13. [CrossRef] [PubMed]
33. Ribeiro, E.F.; de Barros-Alexandrino, T.T.; Assis, O.B.G.; Cruz, A.; Quiles, A.; Hernando, I.; Nicoletti, V.R. Chitosan and crosslinked chitosan nanoparticles: Synthesis, characterization and their role as Pickering emulsifiers. *Carbohydr. Polym.* **2020**, *250*, 10. [CrossRef] [PubMed]
34. Wei, Z.H.; Huang, Q.R. In vitro digestion and stability under environmental stresses of ovotransferrin nanofibrils. *Food Hydrocoll.* **2020**, *99*, 14. [CrossRef]
35. Abdelwahed, W.; Degobert, G.; Stainmesse, S.; Fessi, H. Freeze-drying of nanoparticles: Formulation, process and storage considerations. *Adv. Drug Deliv. Rev.* **2006**, *58*, 1688–1713. [CrossRef] [PubMed]
36. Surewicz, W.K.; Mantsch, H.H.; Chapman, D. Determination of protein secondary structure by fourier-transform infrared-spectroscopy—A critical-assessment. *Biochemistry* **1993**, *32*, 389–394. [CrossRef] [PubMed]
37. Acero-Lopez, A.; Ullah, A.; Offengenden, M.; Jung, S.; Wu, J.P. Effect of high pressure treatment on ovotransferrin. *Food Chem.* **2012**, *135*, 2245–2252. [CrossRef] [PubMed]
38. Arachchi, D.H.T.; Wijesekera, G.I.P.; De Costa, M.D.P.; Senthilnithy, R. Amino and chloro derivatives of 1,10-phenanthroline as turn-off fluorescence sensors for selective and sensitive detection of Fe(II). *J. Photochem. Photobiol. A-Chem.* **2020**, *402*, 8. [CrossRef]
39. Accorsi, G.; Listorti, A.; Yoosaf, K.; Armaroli, N. 1,10-Phenanthrolines: Versatile building blocks for luminescent molecules, materials and metal complexes. *Chem. Soc. Rev.* **2009**, *38*, 1690–1700. [CrossRef]
40. Sarzehi, S.; Chamani, J. Investigation on the interaction between tamoxifen and human holo-transferrin: Determination of the binding mechanism by fluorescence quenching, resonance light scattering and circular dichroism methods. *Int. J. Biol. Macromol.* **2010**, *47*, 558–569. [CrossRef]
41. Cao, S.H.; Fan, J.L.; Sun, W.; Li, F.H.; Li, K.X.; Tai, X.S.; Peng, X.J. A novel Mn-Cu bimetallic complex for enhanced chemodynamic therapy with simultaneous glutathione depletion. *Chem. Commun.* **2019**, *55*, 12956–12959. [CrossRef] [PubMed]
42. Guo, D.; Li, C.; Liu, G.Y.; Luo, X.G.; Wu, F.S. Oxidase Mimetic Activity of a Metalloporphyrin-Containing Porous Organic Polymer and Its Applications for Colorimetric Detection of Both Ascorbic Acid and Glutathione. *ACS Sustain. Chem. Eng.* **2021**, *9*, 5412–5421. [CrossRef]
43. Xue, Y.; Zhang, L.; Liu, F.W.; Dai, F.; Kong, L.; Ma, D.Y.; Han, Y. Alkaline "Nanoswords" Coordinate Ferroptosis-like Bacterial Death for Antibiosis and Osseointegration. *ACS Nano* **2023**, *14*, 2711–2724. [CrossRef]

Journal of
Functional Biomaterials

MDPI

Article

Curcumin and Metformin Infinite Coordination Polymer Nanoparticles for Combined Therapy of Diabetic Mice via Intraperitoneal Injections

Siwei Sun [1,2,†], Xinyi Hou [2,3,†], Ke Li [1,2], Chenqi Huang [4], Yu Rong [1,2], Jiao Bi [1,2], Xueping Li [2,5,*] and Daocheng Wu [4,*]

1 Institute of Basic and Translational Medicine, Xi'an Medical University, Xi'an 710021, China; bs1808008@sust.edu.cn (S.S.)
2 Xi'an Key Laboratory for Prevention and Treatment of Common Aging Diseases, Translational and Research Centre for Prevention and Therapy of Chronic Disease, Xi'an Medical University, Xi'an 710021, China
3 School of Pharmacy, Xi'an Medical University, Xi'an 710021, China
4 Key Laboratory of Biomedical Information Engineering of the Ministry of Education, School of Life Science and Technology, Xi'an Jiaotong University, Xi'an 710049, China
5 School of Clinical Medicine, Xi'an Medical University, Xi'an 710021, China
* Correspondence: lxp86@xiyi.edu.cn (X.L.); wudaocheng@mail.xjtu.edu.cn (D.W.)
† These authors contributed equally to this work.

Abstract: Metformin (Met) is one of the most commonly prescribed first-line drugs for diabetes treatment. However, it has several issues, including low bioavailability, therapeutic platform, and side effects at high doses. In order to improve the therapeutic efficiency of Met, this study proposes a strategy of using Met and curcumin (Cur) to prepare Cur-Zn(II)-Met infinite coordination polymer nanoparticles (CM ICP NPs), and combining this with intraperitoneal injections, for the treatment of diabetic mice. Fourier transform infrared (FTIR) spectroscopy, X-ray photoelectron spectroscopy (XPS), transmission electron microscopy (TEM), nanoparticle analysis, cytotoxicity experiments, and mice experiments were used to investigate structure, properties, and application effects. The results showed that CM ICP NPs exhibit a high drug encapsulation rate (100%), good stability, and an absence of in vivo and in vitro toxicity. The blood glucose level of diabetic mice after treatment was reduced to 6.7 ± 0.65 mmol/L at the seventh week. In terms of therapeutic mechanism, it appears that Met and Cur can synergistically regulate blood glucose in mice from multiple paths. This study provides a promising method for the treatment of diabetes using Met and other drugs.

Keywords: infinite coordination polymer; nanoparticles; metformin; curcumin; diabetes; combination therapy

1. Introduction

Diabetes is one of the leading causes of death, second only to cardiovascular disease and cancer [1]. With the increase in high-calorie diets and unhealthy lifestyles, such as being sedentary, the number of diabetic patients worldwide has increased dramatically. Currently, there are over 400 million people with diabetes worldwide, and this number is expected to reach 700 million by 2030, accounting for 10.9% of the global population [2,3]. Due to its complex pathogenesis, involving multiple mechanisms such as insulin resistance and β-cell dysfunction, and its chronic nature, patients often require long-term use of hypoglycemic drugs to control their blood glucose levels [4]. Metformin (Met) is a commonly prescribed first-line drug for the treatment of diabetes, with a history of widespread use for over 40 years [5]. However, its oral bioavailability is only 50% to 60% [6]. Ordinary tablets are absorbed through the small intestine and have a plasma half-life of 1.5–5.0 h. It is circulated unbound in plasma and cleared, unchanged, by the kidneys [7]. The biphasic technique is used to reduce the loss of Met during circulation [8]. As the disease progresses, it often becomes necessary to continuously increase the dosage. When the daily oral dosage exceeds 2000 mg, a plateau period of hypoglycemic effect may occur [9]. Additionally, accumulation of the drug in the intestine can lead to serious gastrointestinal diseases, lactic acidosis, poor absorption of vitamin B12, and other side effects [10]. Furthermore, individual differences may result in some patients having a lower sensitivity to Met, leading to unsatisfactory hypoglycemic effects when used alone [11,12]. Therefore, improving the utilization of the drug and exploring alternative treatment pathways have become crucial in enhancing the efficacy of Met.

In recent years, the combination of available anti-diabetes drugs and traditional Chinese medicine (phytochemicals with pharmacological properties) has emerged as a significant treatment strategy for hyperglycemia and other diabetes-related conditions [13–15]. Curcumin (Cur) is a kind of natural effective ingredient with a β-diketone structure, extracted from the natural medicine Curcuma turmeric, turmeric, and other ginger plants. Cur can play an anti-diabetes role by regulating oxidative stress, inflammatory reaction, pancreatic islet cell function, and more [16]. A study found that Cur is 400 times more effective than metformin (Met) in activating AMPK enzymes (AMPK activation is the "therapeutic target" of diabetes) [17]. In addition, Cur can also mediate FGF23 to affect the blood glucose of diabetes patients through calcium and phosphorus regulation [18,19]. Combining Cur and Met can provide multiple benefits in treating diabetes. Hassan et al. [20] used Cur silver nanoparticles to enhance the efficacy of Met. Roxo et al. [21] used Cur and Met to reduce blood sugar and lipids in diabetic rats. However, combination therapy often involves direct fractional application or nanotechnology encapsulation, and still acts independently when entering the body for absorption and metabolism, resulting in low drug utilization, poor compatibility, mutual influence of action spaces, and poor stability [22–24]. In recent years, there has been rapid development in the field of infinite coordination polymer (ICP) drug delivery systems. These systems have the ability to simultaneously possess multiple drug characteristics, achieve multi-channel combined effects of different drugs, enhance drug efficacy, reduce adverse reactions, expand the scope of applicability, and reduce drug dosage [25–27]. ICPs are typically supramolecular polymer amorphous nanomaterials formed by the repeated coordination and self-assembly of organic ligands and inorganic metal ions [28]. Due to their high cutting ability, flexible selection of raw materials, controllable material size, and ease of deeper processing, they are widely used in drug delivery systems [29]. Our research group [30] formed ICPs by coordination with doxorubicin, gossypol, and Fe^{3+}, which achieved the targeted delivery and graded treatment of various drugs to tumors. Huang et al. [31] constructed a novel radiosensitizer based on ICPs using hemoglobin, disodium 5′-guanylate, and Gd^{3+} to simultaneously perform X-ray deposition and glutathione depletion, promoting radiation-induced immunogenic cell death. ICPs have the ability to modify the interaction between metal ions and ligands as needed. Through a simple "one-step" reaction, multifunctional complexes with adjustable properties can be obtained. These composite ICPs have the capability to read data from multiple channels and utilize the stimulus response mechanism of binding bonds to the external environment. This allows for the creation of novel targeted functional drugs with ultra-small size and high dispersibility, enabling precise drug delivery and synergistic enhancement [32–34]. ICPs provide a feasible pathway for the combined delivery of Cur and Met [29]. In addition, injection administration can avoid first pass effects in the gastrointestinal tract or liver, and has the characteristics of low dosage, fast response, and minimal side effects [35]. Hyldbakk et al. [36] also used intraperitoneal injection to control the delivery pathway of cabozantine in mice. This also has advantages in the precise delivery of low-dose drugs.

Therefore, this research is the first to apply infinite coordination technology in the preparation of diabetes combination drugs. Through a simple one-step reaction, Met and Cur are coordinated with Zn^{2+} to form a closely linked infinite coordination polymer (CM ICP), which is enveloped by Pluronic F127 to prepare infinite coordination polymer nanoparticles (CM ICP NPs). At the same time, intraperitoneal injection is used. It aims to build solutions to the problems of low bioavailability, therapeutic platform, and side effects at high doses that are commonly encountered during the medication process of Met. The therapeutic effect on diabetic mice was evaluated by measuring the sample structure, in vitro release performance, in vivo and in vitro toxicity of different treatments, and hypoglycemic performance. Additionally, the mechanism of action was further revealed by examining its effects on insulin resistance, lipid metabolism, and liver and kidney function (Figure 1). This study introduces a promising advancement in combination therapy for diabetes using coordination polymer dual-drug nanoparticles. This method provides synergistic therapeutic benefits, effectively addressing issues of drug utilization, compatibility, and stability in diabetes management.

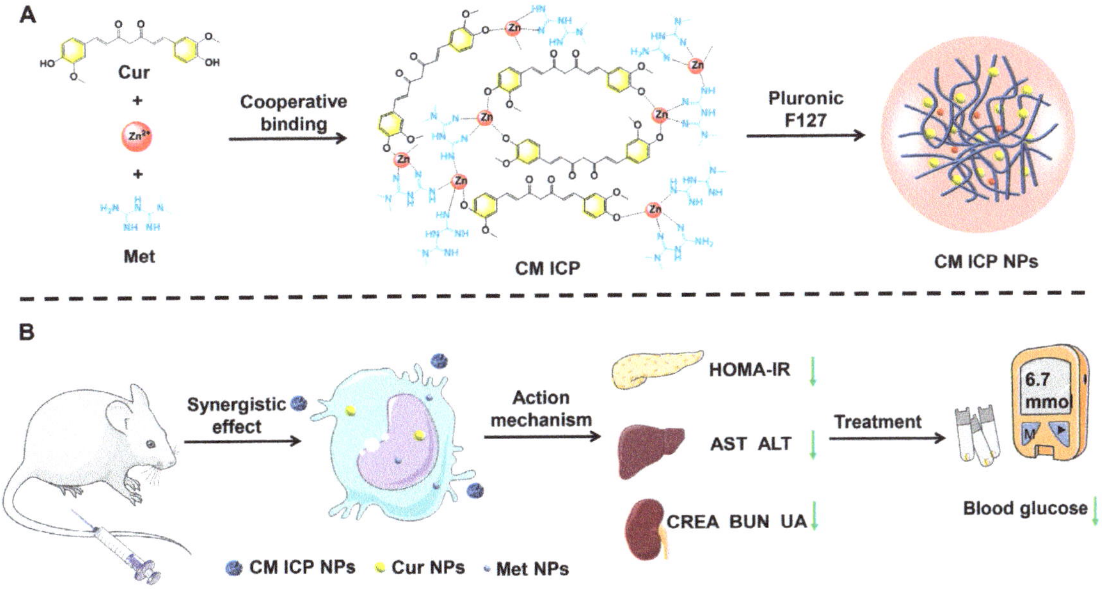

Figure 1. Synthetic route of CM ICP NPs (**A**) and their application in diabetes mice (**B**). (Curcumin, Cur; Metformin, Met; infinite coordination polymer, CM ICP; infinite coordination polymer nanoparticles, CM ICP NPs; Curcumin nanoparticles, Cur NPs; Metformin nanoparticles, Met NPs; insulin resistance index, HOMA-IR; aspartate aminotransferase, AST; alanine aminotransferase, ALT; creatinine, CREA; blood urea nitrogen, BUN; uric acid, UA; The green downward arrow indicates a decrease in the level of the indicator).

2. Materials and Methods

2.1. Materials

Metformin hydrochloride (Met·HCl, purity > 97%), curcumin (Cur, purity > 98%), Zinc(II) acetylacetonate ($Zn(C_5H_7O_2)_2$), and trihydroxymethamine (Tris) were purchased from Shanghai Macklin Biochemical Technology Co., Ltd. (Shanghai, China). Sodium chloride, Triton X-100, Pluronic F127, methanol, ethanol, and dimethyl sulfoxide (DMSO) were obtained from Shanghai Aladdin Biochemical Technology Co., Ltd. (Shanghai, China). Normal Cell Line 3T3 (Mouse Embryonic Fibroblasts), RSC96 (Rat Schwann Cells), HT22 (Mouse Hippocampal Neuron Cell Line), and Sheep Erythrocyte (6%) were provided by Servicebio Biological Technology Co., Ltd. (Wuhan, China). Beyotime Biological Technology Co., Ltd. (Shanghai, China) provided Dulbecco's modified Eagle's medium (DMEM) and a CCK-8 reagent kit. All in vivo tests were authorized by the Biomedical Research Ethics Committee of Xi'an Jiaotong University, and conducted according to the Guidelines for Use and Care at Xi'an Jiaotong University.

2.2. Preparation of CM ICP NPs

Met (72.8 mg) and Cur (7.28 mg) were dissolved in 1820 μL. These two solutions were combined and sonicated at 50 kHz for 10 min to prepare Solution A. Subsequently, 100 μL of a $Zn(C_5H_7O_2)_2$ (4.368 mg) ethanol solution (10 mg/mL) was added dropwise to Solution A at a rate of 100 drops per minute. After the addition was complete, the mixture was stirred for an additional 10 min at 600 rpm, resulting in Solution B. Solution B was added to a mixture of Pluronic F127 (14.56 mg) and Tris-alkaline buffer solution in 80 μL DMSO, followed by stirring for 30 min at 1800 rpm, and maintaining a pH of 7.4, to obtain CM ICP NPs. The final product concentrations were adjusted to 3.64 mg/mL for Cur and 36.4 mg/mL for Met.

2.3. Chemical Structural of CM ICP NPs

Ultraviolet-visible absorption spectroscopy (UV-Vis) was conducted using a Lambda 950 spectrophotometer (Perkin Elmer, New York, NY, USA), with a scanning range of 200 to 800 nm. The functional groups of the samples were analyzed using an FTIR spectrometer (Bruker Optik GmbH, Ettlingen, Germany) with a scanning range of 400–4000 cm^{-1}. X-ray photoelectron spectroscopy (XPS) was performed using an AXIS SUPRA instrument (Kratos, Manchester, UK), equipped with a water-cooled, focused monochromatic Al Kα radiation source. The Zn2p, N1s, C1s, and O1s peaks of the sample were analyzed, and data processing was carried out using Avantage software (version 5.9). The C1s energy was calibrated based on a binding energy of 284.8 eV. X-ray diffraction (XRD) analysis was performed using a D/max 2200PC instrument (Rigaku, Tokyo, Japan), with a scanning speed of 2°/min and a scanning angle range of 25° to 60°.

2.4. Characterization of Morphology and Release

The morphology, particle size, elemental distribution, and zeta potential of the CM ICP NP samples were analyzed using transmission electron microscopy (TEM, JEM-F200, JEOL Japan Electronics Co., Ltd., Tokyo, Japan), an energy dispersive spectroscopy (EDS) system (FEI Tecnai F20, FEI, Hillsboro, NJ, USA), and dynamic light scattering (DLS) with a Malvern Nano-ZS90 instrument (Malvern Instruments, Birmingham, UK). The particle size stability of the CM ICP NPs was monitored over a period of 40 days.

Additionally, the drug release profiles of the CM ICP NPs were evaluated. The CM ICP NPs were encapsulated in dialysis bags with a cut-off molecular weight of 3.5 kDa, and then immersed in PBS solutions with pH values of 7.4, 6.5, and 5.2, respectively. The dialysis process was conducted for 65 h at 25 °C by magnetic stirring with 30 rpm. The dialysate was collected at different time points, and the concentration of Cur was measured by UV-Vis at $\lambda = 427$ nm.

2.5. Animal Experiments

We confirm that we adhered to the guidelines for the use of animals in bioscience research as outlined in China. All ethical considerations were taken into account according to the appropriate standards in China. All animal experiments were approved by the Laboratory Animal Ethics Committee of Xi'an Medical University, with approval number XYLS2021209.

All animals were of specific-pathogen-free grade. 14 days of health observation and adaptive feeding were conducted before the experiment, while environmental conditions and care that are consistent with those for future feeding were provided. Furthermore, we employed an appropriate experimental design to minimize the harm and number of animals as much as possible, while ensuring the repeatability of our treatments within a margin of error. During the experiment, scientific and proficient operating techniques and prompt pacification were employed.

2.6. Toxicity In Vitro and In Vivo

2.6.1. In Vitro Toxicity Tests (CCK-8 Experiment)

Since CM ICP NPs are administered with intraperitoneal injections, and Met and Cur differ greatly in water, the same dose of intraperitoneal injections for the drug as for the CM ICP NPs could not be achieved. Therefore, we made Pluronic F127 nanoparticles loaded with Met and Cur (curcumin nanoparticles: Cur NPs, and metformin nanoparticles: Met NPs), as well as mixed Cur and Met nanoparticles (Cur–Met NPs), thus using the same dose of Met NP and Cur NP intraperitoneal injections as a control. Future biological experiments will be carried out according to this. The preparations of Cur NPs, Met NPs and Cur–Met NPs are provided in the Supplementary Information.

Cell line mouse embryonic fibroblasts (3T3), rat Schwann cells (RSC96), and mouse hippocampal neurons (HT22) were seeded into a 96-well plate at a density of 8000 cells per well. Subsequently, CM ICP NPs, Cur NPs, and Met NPs were added at concentrations of 1 μg/mL, 3 μg/mL, and 9 μg/mL, respectively. The cells were incubated at 37 °C in a 5% CO_2 environment. Once the cells in the control wells reached 90% confluency, the culture medium was replaced with a colorless medium containing 10% CCK-8 reagent. After a 2 h incubation period, the absorbance of each well was measured at 450 nm, using an enzyme-linked immunosorbent assay (ELISA) reader (Multiskan SkyHigh, Thermo Fisher Scientific, Waltham, MA, USA), to assess cell viability.

2.6.2. In Vivo Hemolysis Test

CM ICP NPs, Cur NPs, Met NPs, Saline, and Triton X-100 were added to Eppendorf tubes containing a 2% red blood cell suspension (6% Sheep Erythrocyte was diluted with saline solution), with each component making up 15% of the total solution volume. The mixtures were incubated at 37 °C for 2 h, after which the sedimentation of red blood cells was observed. The absorbance of the supernatant was measured at 490 nm using an ELISA reader, and the hemolysis rate was calculated.

2.6.3. In Vivo Toxicity Test

C57 mice (balanced for sex, approximately 25 g each) were randomly divided into three groups (n = 13 per group): a CM ICP NPs group, a mixed Cur–Met NPs group (the preparation of Cur–Met NPs is provided in the Supplementary Information), and a Saline group. The mice were intraperitoneally injected with the corresponding treatments, with all dosages adjusted to 30 mg/kg for Cur and 300 mg/kg for Met. The mice were prohibited from eating and drinking for 6 h before injection, and allowed to resume after 2 h. At the 24th hour, three individuals were randomly selected from each group to collected their eyeball blood. The mice were then monitored daily for their behavioral habits and mental state, including the conditions of insanity, messy hair, difficulty breathing, cachexia, astasia, fighting, and coma, over a 14-day period. Their survival rate was calculated. On the 14th day, the surviving mice were euthanized. Three mice were randomly selected from each group for eyeball blood collection. Blood samples were used to assess key indicators of liver function, including aspartate aminotransferase (AST), alanine aminotransferase (ALT), and total bilirubin (TBIL), as well as kidney function markers such as creatinine (CREA), blood urea nitrogen (BUN), and uric acid (UA). Their livers, kidneys, hearts, lungs, and spleens were taken for hematoxylin and eosin (H&E) staining, and pathological sections were made.

After fasting and water deprivation for 4 h, eye blood was collected from each group of experimental mice using the orbital blood collection method. After standing for 2 h, the eyeball blood was centrifuged for 15 min, at 3000 rpm, at 4 °C. The supernatant was taken for packaging, and the specimen was stored at −20 °C or −80 °C before being tested. To induce anesthesia, the experimental mice were place into an anesthesia tank connected to an anesthesia machine. The induction anesthesia concentration of isoflurane is usually adjusted to 4–5%, and the oxygen flow rate is controlled at 1 L/min. The mice faint after 2–3 min. To maintain anesthesia, after inducing anesthesia, the experimental mice were covered with a mask, and made to continuously inhale isoflurane. The concentration of isoflurane was controlled at 2–3%, and the flow rate was controlled at 0.2–0.4 L/min.

2.7. Hypoglycemic Effect

The db/db diabetic mouse model was used for this experiment. The mice had an initial blood glucose level of approximately 7 mmol/L and a weight of around 25 g. Their normal diet was replaced with a high-fat diet, and their blood glucose was measured every other day. After two weeks of continuous feeding, mice with blood glucose levels $\geq$ 11.1 mmol/L were considered successfully models for diabetes. The mice were then randomly divided into five groups (n = 6 per group): a CM ICP NPs group (30 mg/kg Cur and 300 mg/kg Met), a mixed Cur–Met NPs group (30 mg/kg Cur and 300 mg/kg Met), a Cur NPs group (30 mg/kg Cur), a Met NPs group (300 mg/kg Met), and a Saline group. Starting from the following day, the mice were intraperitoneally injected with the corresponding treatments for a duration of 7 weeks. The mice were then monitored daily for behavioral habits and mental state, including conditions of insanity, messy hair, difficulty breathing, cachexia, astasia, fighting, and coma. Their body weight and blood glucose levels were recorded weekly. Blood glucose levels were measured using a blood glucose meter (Yuyue, Shanghai, China) with tail vein blood samples. At the end of the therapeutic period, blood samples were collected via orbital sampling to assess glycated serum protein (GSP), insulin resistance index (HOMA-IR), free fatty acids (NEFA), blood lipids (cholesterol [CHO], low-density lipoprotein cholesterol [LDL-C], and high-density lipoprotein cholesterol [HDL-C], as well as key indicators of liver function (ALT, AST, TBIL) and kidney function (CREA, BUN, UA). Finally, the liver, kidney, and pancreas were harvested for H&E staining analysis (n = 3 per group). The methods of environmental adaptation, eyeball blood collection, serum procession, and anesthesia for mice are as described above in Section 2.6.3.

2.8. Statistical Analysis

All the data were exhibited as the average plus or minus the standard deviation (mean $\pm$ SD). Upon juxtaposing the experimental groups, it was revealed through the utilization of Student's t-test or one-way analysis of variance that the results exhibited statistical significance if p values were less than 0.05. Statistical analyses were performed using the SPSS 22.0 software. A data graph was drawn using Origin 2018.

3. Results and Discussion

3.1. Chemical Structure of CM ICP NPs

As Figure 2A shows, the results from the UV-Vis analysis indicate that Met exhibits a characteristic absorption peak at 249 nm, while Cur displays peaks at 217 nm, 264 nm, and 427 nm. Additionally, CM ICPs show characteristic peaks at 240 nm and 424 nm, with peak separation near 269 nm. These peak positions are similar to those of Met and Cur, albeit slightly shifted due to coordination, which also causes a superposition of peak shapes. As shown in Figure 2B, the infrared spectrum of Cur reveals an O-H stretching vibration peak at 3505 cm^{-1}, a C=O peak at 1601 cm^{-1}, a C=C peak at 1523 cm^{-1}, and a C-O peak at 1150 cm^{-1}. In contrast, Met exhibits an N–H stretching vibration peak at 3147 cm^{-1}, a C=N peak at 1546 cm^{-1}, and a C–N peak at 1058 cm^{-1}. The CM ICPs synthesized from these two materials display a C=C stretching vibration peak at 1340 cm^{-1}, corresponding to curcumin, and a C–N peak at 1086 cm^{-1}, characteristic of metformin. Notably, the C=C peak of raw curcumin and the C–N peak of raw metformin undergo a blue shift and a red shift, respectively, in CM ICPs. This suggests that these shifts may be attributed to the formation of a Zn coordination bond. These findings suggest that CM ICPs incorporate both Cur and Met. The XPS full spectrum and high-resolution spectra of CM ICPs (Figure 2C–F) reveal binding energy characteristic peaks for C 1s (284.0 eV), N 1s (401.09 eV), O 1s (531.0 eV), and Zn 2p (1019.73 eV), confirming the presence of carbon, nitrogen, oxygen, and zinc in the sample. The binding energies of these elements are detailed in Table S1 and Figure S1. Notably, the binding energy of O 1s in CM ICPs (532.80 eV) is higher than that in pre-coordination Cur (531.70 eV), and the binding energy of N 1s in CM ICPs (398.74 eV) is also higher than in pre-coordination Cur (397.56 eV). The Zn 2p spectrum of $C_{10}H_{14}ZnO_4$ displays two spin-orbitals: 2p3/2 (1019.90 eV) and 2p1/2 (1042.80 eV), corresponding to U and V, respectively. In the XPS spectrum of CM ICPs, the Zn 2p binding energy is split into two peaks: 1020.80 eV and 1043.83 eV. Based on these XPS results and covalent bond theory, it can be inferred that Zn (II) likely accepts lone pairs of electrons from O and N in the coordinated drug molecular chain (Figure 2G). Consequently, the electron transfer behavior during the coordination process is N $\rightarrow$ Zn and O $\rightarrow$ Zn, leading to the formation of CM ICPs through coordination.

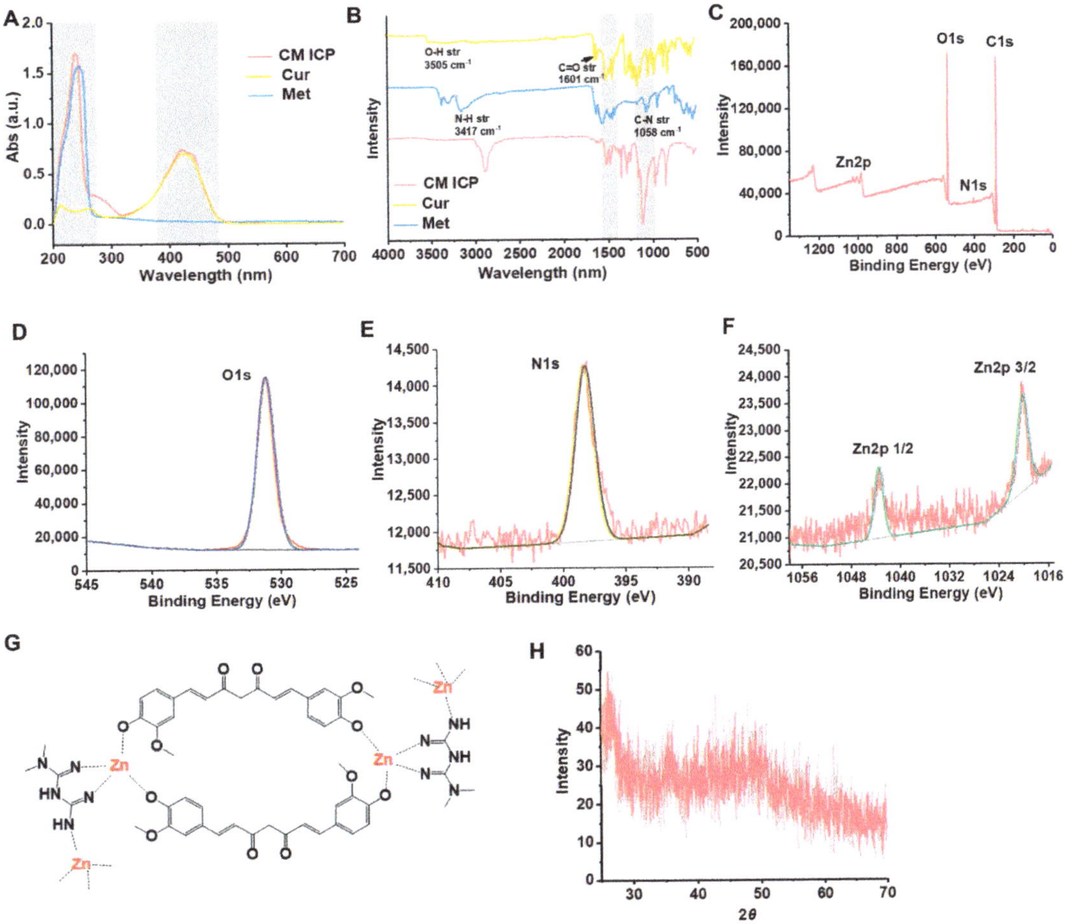

Figure 2. UV-Vis (**A**) and FTIR (**B**) of CM ICPs, Cur, and Met; XPS full spectrum (**C**), XPS high-resolution spectrum (O 1s, (**D**); N 1s, (**E**); Zn 2p, (**F**)), structure (**G**), and XRD spectrum (**H**) of CM ICPs.(The red line represents the original data, while the other colored lines represent the peak fitted data in (**E**,**F**)).

The preparation of CM ICPs was achieved using the solvent-induced precipitation method, which, due to its inability to crystallize slowly, results in the formation of an amorphous structure distinctly different from MOF crystals. The absence of prominent peaks in the XRD pattern (Figure 2H) further confirms that CM ICPs are amorphous supramolecular polymers with high structural flexibility. This is consistent with the structure of ICPs in paper [25]. Consequently, CM ICPs with infinite coordination structure characteristics were successfully synthesized from Cur, Met, and $Zn(C_5H_7O_2)_2$, effectively achieving the encapsulation and binding of Cur and Met. This is owing to the fact that CM ICP NPs are formed by directly coordinating Cur and Met with Zn^{2+} without the use of any carrier material, thus achieving a high encapsulation rate of 100%.

3.2. Morphology and Release of CM ICP NPs

The particle size of nanomedicines is critical for drug delivery and absorption in vivo [37]. Figure 3A–E illustrate the morphology, particle size, and elemental distribution of CM ICP NPs. The findings indicate that CM ICP NPs are uniformly dispersed within the system, forming aggregates in the core of the nanoparticles, with an average particle size of approximately 52 nm. The C, O, and N elements from Cur and Met, along with the coordinated metal Zn^{2+}, are densely and uniformly distributed throughout the nanoparticles, confirming the successful encapsulation of Cur, Met, and Zn. In Figure 3F, the addition of Pluronic F127 surfactant during the preparation process resulted in the formation of extensive hydration layers in the liquid. Therefore, the hydration particle size measured by DLS (107 ± 20.24 nm) was larger than that observed by TEM. The particle size of CM ICP NPs is conducive to their circulation within the body and absorption by cells [38]. Met primarily exists as a hydrophilic cation at physiological pH and has low fat solubility, making it unlikely for the drug to rapidly and passively diffuse through cell membranes [39,40]. Additionally, the zeta potential of CM ICP NPs is neutral, which is advantageous for in vivo absorption and metabolism, as well as for maintaining stability in vitro [41]. Furthermore, Figure 3G shows that after 40 days of storage at 4.0 °C, there was no significant change in the particle size and drug loading of CM ICP NPs, which remained in the range of 106–116 nm, indicating excellent storage stability in vitro. Met accumulates in the intestines, which makes it difficult for a large proportion of patients to tolerate sufficient amounts. Up to 25% of patients suffer from gastrointestinal side effects related to Met, and about 5% of patients simply cannot tolerate Met [42]. There is an effective method for controlling drug metabolism and improving bioavailability through the controlled release of drugs, which is based on changes in environmental pH [43]. To mimic the acidity and alkalinity in different environments of the body, the drug release characteristics in vivo of CM ICP NPs were investigated. The results are shown in Figure 3H. When pH = 6.5, the CM ICP NPs rapidly release 25% within 10 h, then slowly release, and the release amount gradually increases to around 45% after 30 h. This indicates that the CM ICP NPs can remain in the intestinal fluid for an extended period of time [44]. This can avoid adverse gastrointestinal reactions caused by the accumulation of Met in the intestine. At a pH of 5.2, 80% of the nanoparticles are rapidly released within 10 h, suggesting that they can be effectively released within cells. In an acidic environment, Cur can be rapidly released from CM ICP NPs, but as the pH increases to 7.4, the rate of drug release significantly decreases, and almost no drug release is detected. This indicates that CM ICP NPs have excellent stability in the intraperitoneal pathway and blood circulation. This is because ICP is more sensitive to acidic conditions due to the coordination binding between metals and organic compounds. Therefore, the CM ICP NPs can achieve controlled drug release in vivo.

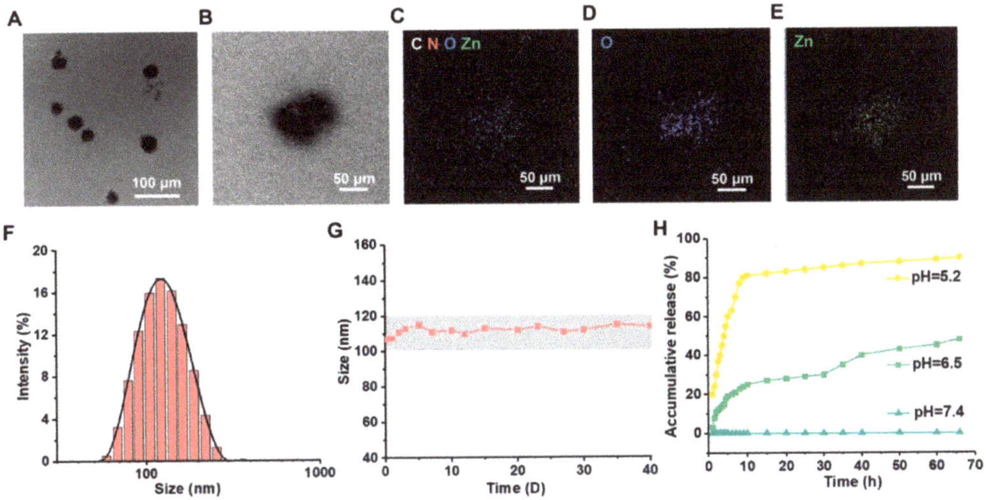

Figure 3. TEM (**A**) and EDS (**B**); (**C**): C, N, O, Zn; (**D**): O; (**E**): Zn; particle size distribution (**F**), stability (**G**), The gray area is between the maximum and minimum values of particle size.), and in vivo drug release (**H**) of CM ICP NPs.

3.3. In Vitro Toxicity of CM ICP NPs

Toxicity testing is a critical prerequisite for ensuring the safe application of drugs. Fibroblasts are widely distributed and abundant in organisms, with advantages such as rapid division and proliferation. Mouse embryonic fibroblasts (3T3) are multipotent mesenchymal cells that can differentiate into different tissues in various culture environments. Therefore, in this paper, 3T3 cells were used to investigate the effects of CM ICP NPs on embryonic toxicity, developmental toxicity, and overall cytotoxicity in diabetic mice. Additionally, two neural cell lines, Schwann cells (RSC96) and mouse hippocampal neurons (HT22), were included to examine the neurotoxicity from different perspectives [45–47]. In this study, these three cell lines were employed to assess the in vitro toxicity of CM ICP NPs. As shown in Figure 4A–C, Cur exhibits a slight inhibitory effect on the proliferation of HT22 and RSC96 cells at low concentrations. At a concentration of 9 μg/mL, Cur significantly inhibits the proliferation of all three cells. This could be attributed to Cur inhibiting cell proliferation by suppressing the MAPK/ERK signaling pathway [16]. Met functions by inhibiting mitochondrial respiration [48]. The proliferation rates of both 3T3 and HT22 cell lines were consistently below 100% at all concentrations of Met. However, CM ICP NPs have a minimal impact on cell proliferation within this range, only slightly affecting the viability of RSC96 cells at 9 μg/mL (the proliferation rate is 83.60 $\pm$ 5.48%). A cell proliferation rate greater than 100% means that the drug is non-toxic [49]. This suggests that CM ICP NPs are non-cytotoxic at the applied dose. CM ICPs reduce the dosage of Cur and Met, while affecting their coordination and integration structure with cells, diminishing their cytotoxicity. The interaction between CM ICP NPs and cells may have enhanced the cytocompatibility of the compounds due to the influence on the coordination and integration structure of Cur and Met. Table S2 shows that the combination index (CI) of CM ICP NPs is 0.43. The significant synergistic effect between Cur and Met in CM ICP NPs was further confirmed. In the hemolysis assay (Figure 4D,E), the hemolysis rate of the positive control group was 100%, whereas CM ICP NPs and their primary components, Cur NPs and Met NPs, did not cause significant red blood cell lysis. This indicates that CM ICP NPs are safe for intravenous administration.

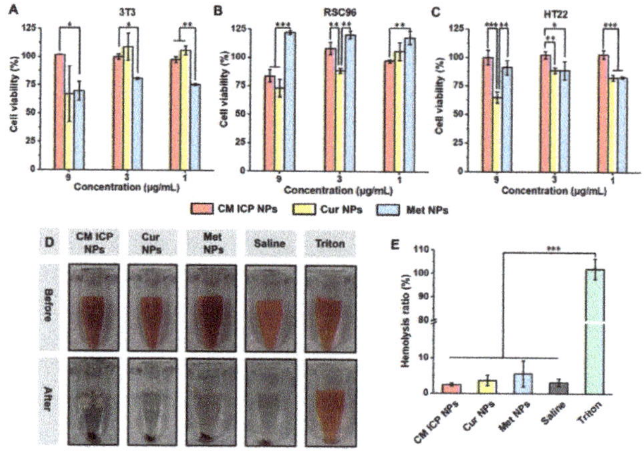

Figure 4. The inhibitory effects of CM ICP NPs, Cur NPs, and Met NPs on three cell lines (3T3) (**A**); RSC96 (**B**); and HT22 (**C**). CM ICP NPs, Cur NPs, and Met NPs were added at concentrations of 1 μg/mL, 3 μg/mL, and 9 μg/mL in vitro; picture (**D**) and numerical (**E**) of hemolysis test results for CM ICP NPs, Cur NPs, Met NPs, Saline, and Triton (they are 15% of the total solution volume). * $p < 0.05$; ** $p < 0.01$; *** $p < 0.001$.

3.4. In Vivo Toxicity of CM ICP NPs

The in vivo acute toxicity of CM ICP NPs was evaluated using C57 mice. Cur and Met are known for their ability to enhance insulin sensitivity, promote glucose utilization, and regulate fat metabolism [50]. Over a 14-day period, two mice in the mixed Cur–Met NPs group exhibited adverse symptoms of cachexia, and five mice died. In contrast, neither the CM ICP NPs group nor the Saline group showed these adverse symptoms or experienced any fatalities (Figure S2 and Table S3). This suggests that CM ICP NPs effectively load and release Cur and Met in a controlled manner, mitigating the risk of uncontrollable, wasteful, and harmful side effects that may arise from directly mixing the drugs.

As shown in Figure S3, there was no significant change in the body weight of mice in any group from 0 to 3 days post injection. However, beginning on day 5, the weight of the mice in the Saline group increased significantly compared to the CM ICP NPs and mixed Cur–Met NPs groups. The body weight of the CM ICP NPs group remained relatively stable, while the mixed Cur–Met NPs group showed a downward trend in weight. These results indicate that CM ICP NPs slowed down weight gain in mice without causing weight loss, suggesting a milder effect on the animals.

Aspartate aminotransferase (AST), alanine aminotransferase (ALT), and total bilirubin (TBIL) are important indicators reflecting liver function. As shown in Figure 5A–C, for mice injected with CM ICP NPs, mixed Cur–Met NPs, and saline separately, it was shown that the levels of AST in the mice increased on day 14 compared to 24 h post injection. There were no significant differences in ALT and TBIL levels between 24 h and 14 days post injection. Meanwhile, the mice injected with CM ICP NPs had higher levels of these indicators than the mixed Cur–Met NPs group and the Saline group. However, the main indicators of liver function in each group remained within the normal range, with no significant pathological changes observed in liver tissue (Figure 5G). This indicates that CM ICP NPs do not cause significant liver damage during metabolism. Kidney function markers such as creatinine (CREA), an indicator of kidney excretion function, showed no significant changes across the groups within the 14-day period, and remained within the normal range (Figure 5D). Although CREA levels only rise significantly when more than 70% of kidney function is compromised [51], other kidney function indicators, such as blood urea nitrogen (BUN) and uric acid (UA), provide additional insights. As shown in Figure 5E,F, BUN levels in mice injected with mixed Cur–Met NPs were significantly higher than those injected with saline, and reached the critically high value of the normal range. The UA levels initially increased and then decreased over time. Pathological analysis revealed lymphocyte infiltration in the kidneys of the mixed Cur–Met group (Figure 5G). In contrast, the UA value of the CM-ICP NPs group was lower than that of the mixed Cur–Met group. The indicators in the CM ICP NPs group were similar to those of the control group, and remained within the normal range. No significant pathological changes were observed in the major organs, including the heart, kidneys, lungs, and spleen (Figure 5G). These findings suggest that the mixed Cur–Met drug injection may cause mild kidney damage during metabolism, while the CM ICP NPs, formed through coordination binding, reduce this damage, and do not harm the major organs during the metabolic process.

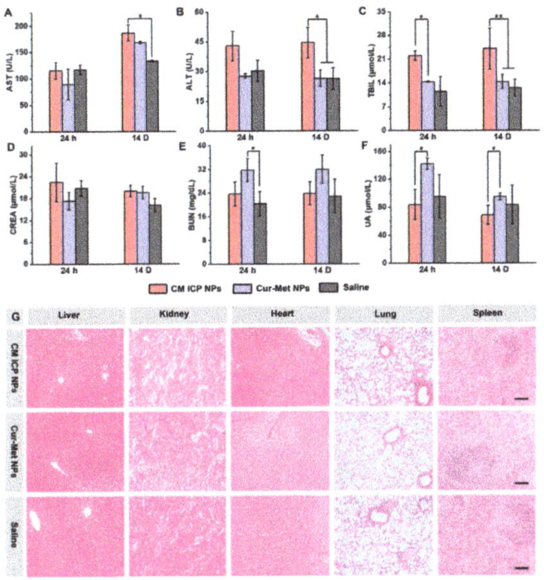

Figure 5. The main biochemical indicators of liver function (AST (**A**); ALT (**B**); TBIL (**C**)) and kidney function (CREA (**D**); BUN (**E**); UA (**F**)) of mice treated with CM ICP NPs, Cur-Met NPs, and saline at 24 h and 14 d (30 mg/kg for Cur and 300 mg/kg for Met). The pathological effects of heart, liver, kidney, spleen, and lungs (**G**) in mice treated with CM ICP NPs, Cur–Met NPs, and saline at 14 d. The dimensions of the scale bar is 100 μm. * $p < 0.05$; ** $p < 0.01$.

3.5. Hypoglycemic Performance of CM ICP NPs

Persistent hyperglycemia in diabetes patients can lead to various organ damages and complications. The effectiveness of blood glucose control is the primary indicator for evaluating hypoglycemic drugs [47]. Therefore, we tested the random blood glucose levels of each group of mice; the experimental mouse design is shown in Figure 6A, and the results are shown in Table S4 and Figure 6B–E. During the experiment, no adverse conditions were observed in any of the groups of mice. Due to the absence of drug interference, the blood glucose levels of the Saline group of mice remained elevated. The blood glucose levels of the Cur NPs group of mice showed a trend of initial decrease, then increase, and then decrease again. This indicates that although Cur NPs can quickly reduce blood glucose in mice, it may rebound in a short period of time, making their hypoglycemic effect unstable. This is due to the fast metabolism, low absorption, and low bioavailability of Cur NPs when used alone in an organism [52]. In Figure 6B, the blood glucose levels of mice injected with Met NPs steadily decreased from the third week onwards, and dropped below 11.1 mmol/L by the fourth week (the cumulative dosage of Met injected is

4200 mg/kg). In most research works, Met intake is carried out through gastric irrigation, enema, or drinking water. When using similar amounts of Met, even if the treatment time is prolonged, the blood glucose levels of mice cannot be reduced to a safe range. For example (see Figure 6C), Silamiķele et al. [53] dissolved Met in drinking water and fed mice for ten weeks. After that, the blood glucose levels of the mice remained at 15.01 mmol/L (the cumulative dosage of Met injected is 3500 mg/kg). Similarly, Tian et al. [54]. found that the blood glucose levels of mice remained above 11.1 mmol/L (the cumulative dosage of Met injected is 6300 mg/kg). In order to achieve therapeutic effects, the dosage and treatment time of Met were increased. For instance, Nahar et al. [55] used a dosage of 18,200 mg/kg and administered gastric irrigation continuously for 13 weeks, while Han et al. [56] even administered gastric irrigation continuously for 24 weeks to mice (the cumulative dosage of Met injected is 33,600 mg/kg). Therefore, intraperitoneal injection can effectively reduce the dosage of Met and achieve ideal therapeutic effects. However, the mixed Cur–Met NPs group of mice showed a continuous increase in blood glucose levels, before a gradually decrease after 3 weeks, but their blood glucose levels remained significantly higher than those of the other groups. This suggests that the pure mixed administration of Cur–Met NPs not only fails to exhibit synergistic effects, but may even lead to a phenomenon of $1 + 1 < 2$, due to the mutual interference of the action pathways. It is worth noting that the blood glucose levels of mice treated with CM ICP NPs decreased to below 11 mmol/L in the second week, and then continued to decrease over time, reaching 6.7 ± 0.65 mmol/L by 7 weeks. Additionally, the GSP indicators, which reflect long-term blood glucose control levels, also showed that the CM ICP NPs group had significantly lower levels than the other groups (Figure 6D). This demonstrates that the ICP nanoparticles formed by Cur and Met can effectively solve the problem of pathway interference caused by the simple drug mixture, improve its utilization rate, regulate the hypoglycemic action mode of both drugs in diabetic mice, and can achieve excellent hypoglycemic and glucose control effects. Furthermore, CM ICP NPs can also slow down the weight growth rate of diabetic mice (Figure 6E). The unique physicochemical properties of nanoparticles (NPs) confer significant advantages in terms of biocompatibility, target specificity, cellular uptake, and bioavailability. This provides a promising strategy for combined treatment with diabetes drugs [57].

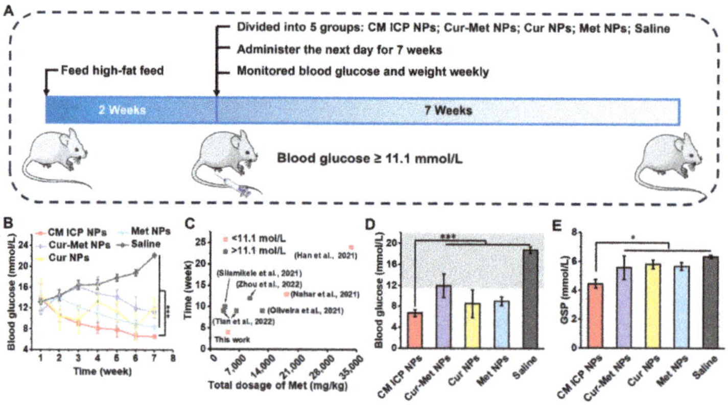

Figure 6. Experimental design of mice (**A**), effects on continuous blood glucose (**B**), The dosage and treatment duration of Met (**C**) [11,40,53–56], blood glucose at seventh week (**D**), The gray area represents the blood glucose level greater than 11.1 mmol/L), and GSP (**E**) in diabetic model mice of CM ICP NPs, Cur-Met NPs, Cur NPs, Met NPs, and Saline group (30 mg/kg for Cur and 300 mg/kg for Met); * $p < 0.05$; *** $p < 0.001$.

3.6. Mechanism of Action of CM ICP NPs

3.6.1. Effects of CM ICP NPs on Insulin Resistance

Diabetes is a metabolic disease caused by insufficient insulin secretion or utilization. Insulin plays a crucial role in promoting glucose utilization, which is converted into glycogen and stored in the body for energy. When insulin utilization decreases and cannot effectively control blood sugar, this results in insulin resistance. This condition is usually asymptomatic, and is often diagnosed through insulin index [50,58]. In Figure 7A, the insulin resistance values of the CM ICP NPs group have returned to normal levels, while the other groups still show varying degrees of insulin resistance. Compared with the normal pancreatic tissue (Figure S5), the H&E staining results of the pancreas in Figure 7F reveal that the Saline group has significantly reduced islet numbers, atrophied islets with a loose and irregular structure, and disordered cell arrangement. In comparison, the islet morphology in each treatment group has significantly improved. The CM ICP NPs group shows round and regular islets with clear boundaries, and a tight and neat cell arrangement. Wang et al. [59] found that improving insulin resistance can be beneficial in treating type 2 diabetes mellitus (T2DM). CM ICP NPs effectively improve pancreatic islet atrophy and structural lesions, significantly reduce systemic insulin resistance in mice, and restore normal glucose regulation.

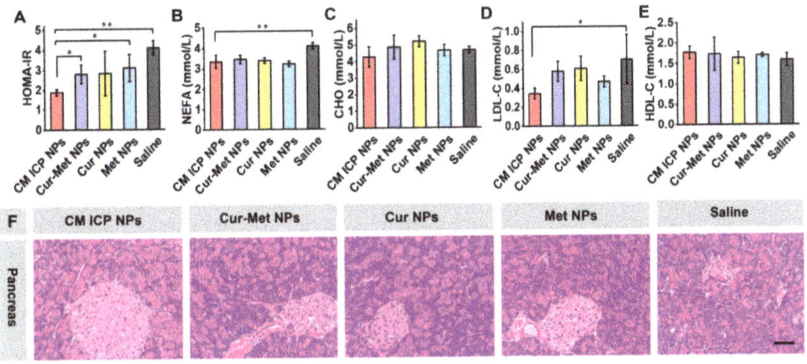

Figure 7. HOMA-IR (**A**), NEFA (**B**), CHO (**C**), LDL-C (**D**), HDL-C (**E**), and pancreatic tissue (**F**) in diabetic model mice of CM ICP NPs, Cur–Met NPs, Cur NPs, Met NPs, and Saline group (30 mg/kg for Cur and 300 mg/kg for Met). The dimensions of the scale bar is 100 μm. * $p < 0.05$; ** $p < 0.01$.

Met and Cur can improve insulin resistance by promoting the recovery of β-cell function, inhibiting liver glucose production, and increasing peripheral tissue utilization of glucose. Metformin achieves this effect through direct and indirect effects on mediators from the initial stages of the insulin signaling pathway, AMPK activation, GLUT4 trafficking and translocation mediators, and complex AMPK-dependent and -independent epigenetic modifications [60]. The action mechanism of Cur may increase pancreatic islet activity by inhibiting poly ADP-ribose polymerase-1 activation, as well as increasing the number of small islets by enhancing HSP-70 and HO-1 [61]. These two act from different pathways and targets. It is obvious that simple drug mixing provides little help in terms of complementing or synergizing with each other. However, the CM ICP NPs showed lower insulin resistance. This may be due to the coordination and combination changes in their pharmacokinetics, which enhance the synergistic effect.

3.6.2. Effects of CM ICP NPs on Lipid Metabolism

Free fatty acids (NEFA) are lipids present in the human body, and are substances broken down from neutral fats. NEFA can affect glucose metabolism through the glucose fatty acid cycle [62]. Increase in NEFA is a common lipid metabolism disorder in T2DM, which can inhibit the uptake and utilization of glucose in body tissues and provide raw materials for gluconeogenesis. From Figure 7B, it can be observed that the NEFA of the CM ICP NPs group is lower than that of the Saline group. CM ICP NPs can improve lipid metabolism in mice. Therefore, the blood lipids of each group of mice were further examined, and the results are shown in Figure 7C–E. CHO refers to the total amount of cholesterol carried by all the lipoproteins in the blood. Although there is no significant difference between the groups of mice, they are all higher than the normal range, indicating a certain degree of lipid metabolism disorder in all the groups of mice. However, it is worth noting that the LDL-C of the CM ICP NPs group is lower than that of the other groups, and the HDL-C is higher than that of the Saline group. This shows that CM ICP NPs can improve lipid metabolism disorder to a certain extent, and reduce the risk of atherosclerotic angiopathy and other diseases in diabetic mice.

3.6.3. Effects of CM ICP NPs on the Liver

Both sugar metabolism and lipid metabolism are inseparable from the metabolic effects of the liver and kidneys. Therefore, the characteristic indicators of liver and kidney function, as well as histopathology of each group, were analyzed. From Figure 8A,B, it was found that the mean values of AST in the CM ICP NPs group, mixed Cur–Met NPs group, Cur NPs group, and Met NPs group were all lower than those in the Saline group, but there was no significant difference among the groups. The ALT levels in the CM ICP NPs group were significantly lower than those in the Saline group, (92.20 $\pm$ 17.23, near the critical high value). The liver tissue slices of the Saline group in Figure 5G show the normal image of a liver with H&E staining. In Figure 8F, the Saline group showed significant liver tissue lesions with severe steatosis, abundant lipid vacuoles in the cytoplasm, and swollen and disorderly arrangement of liver cells. After administration, some liver cell morphology in the Cur NPs group, Met NPs group, and mixed Cur–Met NPs group returned to normal. The liver cell swelling and fat vacuoles were partially improved. The liver cell morphology in the CM ICP NPs group basically returned to normal, with only a small number of liver cells exhibiting lipid degeneration and disordered arrangement. The above results indicate that other groups had improved liver cell steatosis, but not significantly, while the CM ICP NPs group had a significantly better improvement in liver cell steatosis than the other groups, and experienced a certain regulatory effect on their renal metabolism.

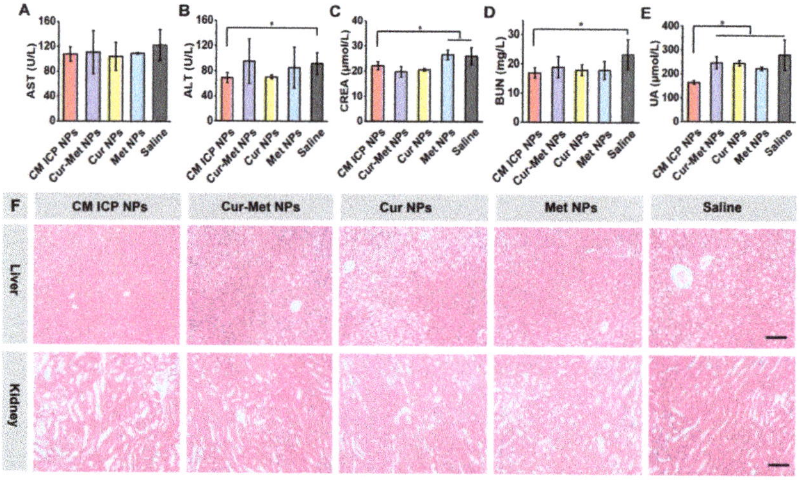

Figure 8. AST (**A**), ALT (**B**),CREA (**C**), BUN (**D**), UA (**E**), and liver and kidney tissue (**F**) in diabetic model mice of the CM ICP NPs, Cur–Met NPs, Cur NPs, Met NPs, and Saline groups (30 mg/kg for Cur and 300 mg/kg for Met). The dimensions of the scale bar is 100 μm. * $p < 0.05$.

3.6.4. Effects of CM ICP NPs on the Kidneys

The CREA of the CM ICP NPs group was lower than that of the Met NPs group and Saline group, but higher than that of the mixed Cur–Met NPs group and Cur NPs group (Figure 8C). Their BUN and UA were significantly lower than other groups (Figure 8D,E). The H&E stained sections of normal mouse kidney tissue (Figure 5G) were used as positive controls. The results of kidney pathological sections (Figure 8F) show that in the Saline group, the number of glomeruli decreased, the structure was scattered and irregular, and there was tearing of the cystic cavity of Baumann's with a small amount of inflammatory cell infiltration; there was distortion of the renal tubular morphology accompanied by swelling and hypertrophy, and compression of the official cavity; and they had a blurred renal interstitium. Compared with the Saline group, the number of glomeruli in each treatment group increased to varying degrees, and the degree of renal lesions improved. The CM ICP NPs group showed the most significant therapeutic effect, with regular glomerular morphology and almost no inflammatory cell infiltration in the renal tissue. The morphology of the Baumann's capsule was regular, and the renal tubular lumen was normal. This indicates that the improvement of renal lesions in the CM ICP NPs group was significantly better than that in other groups.

Met does not undergo changes in the body, and remains unchanged when secreted through rapid kidney excretion [61]. Impaired kidney function can slow down elimination and may lead to accumulation of Met [63]. Curcumin can restore renal integrity by increasing blood urea nitrogen, decreasing levels of albuminuria and enzymuria, and normalizing glutathione [64–66]. These mechanisms may be due to Cur-mediated activation of AMP, which reduces the expression of VEGF and VEGF receptor, diminishes the activities of PKC-α and PKC-β, and suppresses sterol regulatory element-binding protein (SREBP)-1c [67,68]. Clinical trials have further shown that Cur is beneficial for the treatment of end-stage renal disease [69]. ICP technology enhances the efficacy of Cur, which has a certain protective effect on the kidneys of T2DM mice.

To sum up, CM ICP NPs can regulate insulin resistance and improve lipid metabolism and glucose metabolism though the synergistic effects of multiple paths. They have a certain effect on the treatment of diabetic mice by improving the pancreas, liver, kidney and other tissues.

4. Conclusions

In order to improve the diabetic therapeutic efficiency of Met, a tightly bound infinite coordination polymer, CM ICP NP, was prepared by coordinating Met and Cur with Zn^{2+}. These nanoparticles exhibit a high drug encapsulation rate (100%) and stable dispersion in aqueous systems, with a controlled release profile in acidic environments, and a particle size of 107 $\pm$ 20.24 nm. The chemical structure and coordination state of the nanoparticles were characterized using FTIR spectroscopy, XPS, and XRD. Toxicity assessments in both cell and mouse models confirmed the absence of in vivo and in vitro toxicity. Diabetic mice treated with intraperitoneal injections of CM ICP NPs demonstrated significantly improved glucose control, with blood glucose levels reduced to 6.7 $\pm$ 0.65 mmol/L by the seventh week, markedly lower than in those treated with a mixture of the drugs or saline. The therapeutic mechanism appears to involve the restoration of normal glucose regulation in diabetic mice by improving insulin resistance, lipid metabolism, and liver and kidney function under the synergistic effects of Cur and Met. This study provides a promising approach for the combination therapy of diabetes using dual-drug coordination polymer nanoparticles. Further research is needed to explore the multiple paths mechanism of the synergistic effect, to provide theoretical support for drug development.

Supplementary Materials: The following supporting information can be downloaded at https://www.mdpi.com/article/10.3390/jfb15120388/s1. Table S1: Electron binding energies of key elements in CM ICP and Cur, Met, $Zn(C_5H_7O_2)_2$. Table S2: The IC50 value of CM ICP NPs; Table S3: Mice status treated with CM ICP NPs, mixed Cur-Met NPs, and Saline after 14 days; Table S4: Mice status treated with CM ICP NPs, mixed Cur-Met NPs, Cur NPs, Met NPs, and Saline after 7 weeks; Figure S1: The O 1s XPS fine spectrum of Cur (A); The N 1s XPS fine spectrum of Met (B); The Zn 2p XPS fine spectrum of $Zn(C_5H_7O_2)_2$ (C); Figure S2: The survival rate of mice treated with CM ICP NPs, mixed Cur-Met NPs, and Saline; Figure S3: The weight of mice treated with CM ICP NPs, mixed Cur-Met NPs, and Saline. ** $p < 0.01$; *** $p < 0.001$; Figure S4: The body weight in diabetes model mice of CM ICP NPs and Saline group. ** $p < 0.01$; *** $p < 0.001$; Figure S5: The image of pancreatic tissue stained with hematoxylin and eosin in normal db/db mouse [58].

Author Contributions: S.S., conceptualization, data curation, and writing-original draft preparation; X.H., methodology and validation; K.L., conceptualization and methodology; C.H., validation and investigation; Y.R., software and data curation; J.B., formal analysis and investigation; X.L., project administration and funding acquisition; D.W., project administration and writing—review and editing. All authors have read and agreed to the published version of the manuscript.

Funding: We thank the Research and Development Program of the Innovation Chain for Key industries in Shaanxi Province (NO: 2021ZDLSF02-09, Project leader: X.L.), Natural Science Basic Research Key Program of Shaanxi Province (NO: 2023-JC-ZD-53, Project leader: K.L.), and the Special Research Program Project of the Shaanxi Provincial Department of Education (NO: 23JK0653, Project leader: S.S.) for the financial support of our research, and the University level Research Fund (Doctoral Project) of Xi'an Medical University (NO: 2023DS08, Project leader: S.S.).

Institutional Review Board Statement: The animal study protocol was approved by the Ethics Committee of Xi'an Medical University (protocol code XYLS2021209 and date of approval 15 June 2021).

Informed Consent Statement: Not applicable.

Data Availability Statement: The original contributions presented in the study are included in the article/supplementary material, further inquiries can be directed to the corresponding authors.

Conflicts of Interest: The authors declare no conflicts of interest.

References

1. Zhao, J.Q.; Fan, H.X.; Wang, T.; Yu, B.; Mao, S.B.; Wang, X.; Zhang, W.J.; Wang, L.G.; Zhang, Y.; Ren, Z.Y.; et al. TyG index is positively associated with risk of CHD and coronary atherosclerosis severity among NAFLD patients. *Cardiovasc. Diabetol.* **2022**, *21*, 123. [CrossRef] [PubMed]
2. Awad, S.F.; Al-Mawali, A.; Al-Lawati, J.A.; Morsi, M.; Critchley, J.A.; Abu-Raddad, L.J. Forecasting the type 2 diabetes mellitus epidemic and the role of key risk factors in Oman up to 2050: Mathematical modeling analyses. *J. Diabetes Invest.* **2021**, *12*, 1162–1174. [CrossRef] [PubMed]
3. Hua, J.C.; Huang, B.F.; Liu, S.S.; Sun, Z.H. Trends in the burden of type 2 diabetes and its risk factors in Saudi Arabia. *J. Endocrinol. Metab. Diabetes S. Afr.* **2024**, *29*, 30–36. [CrossRef]
4. Kahn, S.E. The relative contributions of insulin resistance and beta-cell dysfunction to the pathophysiology of Type 2 diabetes. *Diabetologia* **2003**, *46*, 3–19.
5. "Metformin clinical application expert consensus" update expert group. Expert consensus on the clinical application of metformin. *Int. J. Endocrinol. Metab.* **2023**, *43*, 345–356.
6. Kirpichnikov, D.; McFarlane, S.I.; Sowers, J.R. Metformin: An update. *Ann. Intern. Med.* **2002**, *137*, 25–33. [CrossRef]
7. Ilias, I.; Rizzo, M.; Zabuliene, L. Metformin: Sex/Gender differences in its uses and effects-narrative review. *Medicina* **2022**, *58*, 430. [CrossRef] [PubMed]
8. Mariano, F.; Biancone, L. Metformin, chronic nephropathy and lactic acidosis: A multi-faceted issue for the nephrologist. *J. Nephrol.* **2021**, *34*, 1127–1135. [CrossRef] [PubMed]
9. Song, J.; He, G.N.; Dai, L. A comprehensive review on celastrol, triptolide and triptonide: Insights on their pharmacological activity, toxicity, combination therapy, new dosage form and novel drug delivery routes. *Biomed. Pharmacother* **2023**, *162*, 114705. [CrossRef]
10. Triggle, C.R.; Mohammed, I.; Bshesh, K.; Marei, I.; Ye, K.; Ding, H.; MacDonald, R.; Hollenberg, M.D.; Hill, M.A. Metformin: Is it a drug for all reasons and diseases? *Metabolism* **2022**, *133*, 155223.
11. Oliveira, W.H.; Braga, C.F.; Lós, D.B.; Araújo, S.M.R.; França, M.R.; Duarte-Silva, E.; Rodrigues, G.B.; Rocha, S.W.S.; Peixoto, C.A. Metformin prevents p-tau and amyloid plaque deposition and memory impairment in diabetic mice. *Exp. Brain Res.* **2021**, *239*, 2821–2839. [CrossRef] [PubMed]
12. Cai, Z.X.; Wu, X.T.; Song, Z.J.; Sun, S.M.; Su, Y.X.; Wang, T.Y.; Cheng, X.H.; Yu, Y.Y.; Yu, C.; Chen, E.; et al. Metformin potentiates nephrotoxicity by promoting NETosis in response to renal ferroptosis. *Cell Discovry* **2023**, *9*, 104. [CrossRef] [PubMed]
13. Chen, Y.; Huang, G.D.; Qin, T.; Zhang, Z.C.; Wang, H.L.; Xu, Y.T.; Shen, X.N. Ferroptosis: A new view on the prevention and treatment of diabetic kidney disease with traditional Chinese medicine. *Biomed. Pharmacother.* **2024**, *170*, 115952. [CrossRef]

14. Chen, J.; Ni, Y.D.; Yao, W.H.; Ding, X.S. Clinical observations and mechanistic insights of traditional Chinese medicine in the management of diabetic retinopathy. *Pharm. Biol.* **2024**, *62*, 529–543. [CrossRef]
15. Xue, C.X.; Chen, Y.; Bi, Y.T.; Yang, X.F.; Chen, K.Y.; Tang, C.; Tong, X.L.; Zhao, L.H.; Wang, H. Dilemmas in elderly diabetes and clinical practice involving traditional chinese medicine. *Pharmaceuticals* **2024**, *17*, 953. [CrossRef] [PubMed]
16. Kim, T.; Davis, J.; Zhang, A.J.; He, X.M.; Mathews, S.T. Curcumin activates AMPK and suppresses gluconeogenic gene expression in hepatoma cells. *Biochem. Biophys. Res. Commun.* **2009**, *388*, 377–382. [CrossRef] [PubMed]
17. Joshi, T.; Singh, A.K.; Haratipour, P.; Sah, A.N.; Pandey, A.K.; Naseri, R.; Juyal, V.; Farzaei, M.H. Targeting AMPK signaling pathway by natural products for treatment of diabetes mellitus and its complications. *J. Cell. Physiol.* **2019**, *234*, 17212–17231. [CrossRef]
18. Jin, T.; Feng, J.N.; Shao, W.; Yang, L.; Pang, J.; Ling, W.H.; Liu, D.H.; Wheeler, M.; He, H.S. Hepatic fibroblast growth factor 21 is required for curcumin or resveratrol in exerting their metabolic beneficial effect in male mice. *Nutr. Diabetes* **2024**. [CrossRef]
19. Bi, J.; Zheng, M.; Li, K.; Sun, S.W.; Zhang, Z.H.; Yan, N.N.; Li, X.P. Relationships of serum FGF23 and α-klotho with atherosclerosis in patients with type 2 diabetes mellitus. *Cardiovasc. Diabetol.* **2024**, *23*, 128. [CrossRef] [PubMed]
20. Hassan, I.; Al-Tamimi, J.; Ebaid, H.; Habila, M.A.; Alhazza, I.M.; Rady, A.M. Silver nanoparticles decorated with curcumin enhance the efficacy of metformin in diabetic rats via suppression of hepatotoxicity. *Toxics* **2023**, *11*, 867. [CrossRef]
21. Roxo, D.F.; Arcaro, C.A.; Gutierres, V.O.; Costa, M.C.; Oliveira, J.O.; Lima, T.F.O.; Assis, R.P.; Brunetti, I.L.; Baviera, A.M. Curcumin combined with metformin decreases glycemia and dyslipidemia, and increases paraoxonase activity in diabetic rats. *Diabetol. Metab. Syndr.* **2019**, *11*, 33. [CrossRef] [PubMed]
22. Naghdi, A.; Goodarzi, M.T.; Karimi, J.; Hashemnia, M.; Khodadadi, I. Effects of curcumin and metformin on oxidative stress and apoptosis in heart tissue of type 1 diabetic rats. *J. Cardiovasc. Thoracic.* **2022**, *14*, 128–137. [CrossRef]
23. Jin, H.; Wang, L.; Bernards, R. Rational combinations of targeted cancer therapies: Background, advances and challenges. *Nat. Rev. Drug Discov.* **2023**, *22*, 213–234. [CrossRef] [PubMed]
24. Yang, J.; Dai, D.H.; Zhang, X.; Teng, L.S.; Ma, L.J.; Yang, Y.W. Multifunctional metal-organic framework (MOF)-based nanoplatforms for cancer therapy: From single to combination therapy. *Theranostics* **2023**, *13*, 295–323. [CrossRef] [PubMed]
25. Zhang, S.; Zhang, S.; Luo, S.Y.; Wang, R.; Di, J.R.; Wang, Y.; Wu, D.C. Four-component of double-layer infinite coordination polymer nanocomposites for large tumor trimodal therapy via multi high-efficiency synergies. *J. Colloid. Interf. Sci.* **2024**, *666*, 259–275. [CrossRef] [PubMed]
26. Wang, T.M.; Hu, J.; Xu, J.Y.; Li, R.J. Self-calibrating Lanthanide infinite coordination polymer constructs fluorescent probes: A sensitive approach for early diagnosis of hepatocellular carcinoma and environmental analysis. *ACS Appl. Mater. Interfaces* **2023**, *15*, 51823–51832. [CrossRef] [PubMed]
27. Murphy, J.N.; Kobti, J.L.; Dao, M.; Wear, D.; Okoko, M.; Pandey, S.; Vukotic, V.N. Therapeutic coordination polymers: Tailoring drug release through metal-ligand interactions. *Chem. Sci.* **2024**, *15*, 7041–7050. [CrossRef] [PubMed]
28. Kothawade, S.; Shende, P. Coordination bonded stimuli-responsive drug delivery system of chemical actives with metal in pharmaceutical applications. *Coordin. Chem. Rev.* **2024**, *510*, 215851. [CrossRef]
29. Arroyos, G.; Campanella, J.E.M.; Silva, C.M.D.; Frem, R.C.G. Detection of anthrax biomarker and metallic ions in aqueous media using spherical-shaped lanthanide infinite coordination polymers. *Spectrochim. Acta A* **2023**, *286*, 122033. [CrossRef]
30. Zhu, H.R.; Huang, C.Q.; Di, J.G.; Chang, Z.P.; Li, K.; Zhang, S.; Li, X.P.; Wu, D.C. Doxorubicin-Fe(III)-gossypol infinite coordination polymer@PDA:CuO_2 composite nanoparticles for cost-effective programmed photothermal chemodynamic-coordinated dual drug chemotherapy trimodal synergistic tumor therapy. *ACS Nano* **2023**, *17*, 12544–12562. [CrossRef] [PubMed]
31. Huang, Z.S.; Wang, Y.X.; Yao, D.; Wu, J.H.; Hu, Y.Q.; Yuan, A. Nanoscale coordination polymers induce immunogenic cell death by amplifying radiation therapy mediated oxidative stress. *Nat. Commun.* **2021**, *12*, 145. [CrossRef]
32. Rams, M.; Lohmiller, T.; Bohme, M.; Jochim, A.; Foltyn, M.; Schengg, A.; Plass, W.; Nather, C. Weakening the interchain interactions in one dimensional cobalt (II) coordination polymers by preventing intermolecular hydrogen bonding. *Inorg. Chem.* **2023**, *62*, 10420–10430. [CrossRef] [PubMed]
33. Ma, J.; Cong, X.; Ou, K.D.; Liao, Y.G.; Yang, Y.J.; Wang, H. A luminescent sensor based on in-situ formed copper nanocluster-loading terbium coordination polymer with multicolor response for identification of antibiotics. *Sens. Actuat. B-Chem.* **2023**, *390*, 133904. [CrossRef]
34. Zhang, S.; Zhang, S.; Luo, S.Y.; Wu, D.C. Therapeutic agent-based infinite coordination polymer nanomedicines for tumor therapy. *Coordin. Chem. Rev.* **2021**, *445*, 214059. [CrossRef]
35. Kim, J.; Eygeris, Y.; Ryals, R.C.; Jozić, A.; Sahay, G. Strategies for non-viral vectors targeting organs beyond the liver. *Nat. Nanotechnol.* **2024**, *19*, 428–447. [CrossRef] [PubMed]
36. Hyldbakk, A.; Fleten, K.G.; Snipstad, S.; Åslund, A.K.; Davies, D.L.C.; Flatmark, K.; Mørch, Y. Intraperitoneal administration of cabazitaxel-loaded nanoparticles in peritoneal metastasis models. *Nanomedicine* **2023**, *48*, 102656. [CrossRef] [PubMed]
37. Xu, M.Z.; Qi, Y.M.; Liu, G.S.; Song, Y.Q.; Jiang, X.Y.; Du, B.J. Size-dependent in vivo transport of nanoparticles: Implications for delivery, targeting, and clearance. *ACS Nano* **2023**, *17*, 20825–20849. [CrossRef] [PubMed]
38. Aminu, N.; Bello, I.; Umar, N.M.; Tanko, N.; Aminu, A.; Audu, M.M. The influence of nanoparticulate drug delivery systems in drug therapy. *J. Drug Deliv. Sci. Technol.* **2020**, *60*, 101961. [CrossRef]
39. Tarry-Adkins, J.L.; Grant, I.D.; Ozanne, S.E.; Reynolds, R.M.; Aiken, C.E. Efficacy and side effect profile of different formulations of metformin: A systematic review and meta-analysis. *Diabetes. Ther.* **2021**, *12*, 1901–1914. [CrossRef]

40. Zhou, Q.Y.; Guan, Z.Q.; Liu, S.F.; Xuan, Y.J.; Han, G.; Chen, H.; Jin, X.; Tao, K.; Guan, Z. The effects of metformin and alendronate in attenuating bone loss and improving glucose metabolism in diabetes mellitus mice. *Aging* **2022**, *14*, 272–285. [CrossRef]
41. Chan, H.W.; Chow, S.; Zhang, X.Y.; Kwok, P.C.L.; Chow, S.F. Role of particle size in translational research of nanomedicines for successful drug delivery: Discrepancies and inadequacies. *J. Pharm. Sci.* **2023**, *112*, 2371–2384. [CrossRef] [PubMed]
42. McCreight, L.J.; Bailey, C.J.; Pearson, E.R. Metformin and the gastrointestinal tract. *Diabetologia* **2016**, *59*, 426–435. [CrossRef] [PubMed]
43. Li, X.W.; Zhong, H.P.; Zheng, S.J.; Mu, J.Q.; Yu, N.; Guo, S.T. Tumor-penetrating iRGD facilitates penetration of poly(floxuridine-ketal)-based nanomedicine for enhanced pancreatic cancer therapy. *J. Control. Release* **2024**, *369*, 444–457. [CrossRef]
44. Wang, D.; Jiang, Q.; Dong, Z.F.; Meng, T.T.; Hu, F.Q.; Wang, J.W.; Yuan, H. Nanocarriers transport across the gastrointestinal barriers: The contribution to oral bioavailability via blood circulation and lymphatic pathway. *Adv. Drug Deliver. Rev.* **2023**, *203*, 115130. [CrossRef] [PubMed]
45. Lee, Y.H.; Cheng, F.Y.; Chiu, H.W.; Tsai, J.C.; Fang, C.Y.; Chen, C.W.; Wang, Y.J. Cytotoxicity, oxidative stress, apoptosis and the autophagic effects of silver nanoparticles in mouse embryonic fibroblasts. *Biomaterials* **2014**, *35*, 4706–4715. [CrossRef]
46. Chen, L.L.; Chen, Z.X.; Xu, Z.Q.; Feng, W.F.; Yang, X.N.; Qi, Z.L. Polydatin protects Schwann cells from methylglyoxal induced cytotoxicity and promotes crushed sciatic nerves regeneration of diabetic rats. *Phytother. Res.* **2021**, *35*, 4592–4604. [CrossRef]
47. Fukui, M.; Song, J.H.; Choi, J.; Choi, H.J.; Zhu, B.T. Mechanism of glutamate-induced neurotoxicity in HT22 mouse hippocampal cells. *Eur. J. Pharmacol.* **2009**, *617*, 1–11. [CrossRef]
48. Khodadadi, M.; Jafari-Gharabaghlou, D.; Zarghami, N. An update on mode of action of metformin in modulation of meta-inflammation and inflammaging. *Pharmacol. Rep.* **2022**, *74*, 310–322. [CrossRef] [PubMed]
49. Shiridokht, F.; Dadashi, H.; Vandghanooni, S.; Eskandani, M.; Farajollahi, A. Metformin-loaded chitosan nanoparticles augment silver nanoparticle-induced radiosensitization in breast cancer cells during radiation therapy. *Colloid. Surface B* **2025**, *245*, 114220. [CrossRef]
50. Wasana, P.W.D.; Hasriadi; Vajragupta, O.; Rojsitthisak, P.; Towiwat, P.; Rojsitthisak, P. Metformin and curcumin co-encapsulated chitosan/alginate nanoparticles as effective oral carriers against pain-like behaviors in mice. *Int. J. Pharmaceut.* **2023**, *640*, 123037. [CrossRef] [PubMed]
51. Francoz, C.; Glotz, D.; Moreau, R.; Durand, F. The evaluation of renal function and disease in patients with cirrhosis. *J. Hepatol.* **2010**, *52*, 605–613. [CrossRef] [PubMed]
52. Pivari, F.; Mingione, A.; Brasacchio, C.; Soldati, L. Curcumin and type 2 diabetes mellitus: Prevention and treatment. *Nutrients* **2019**, *11*, 1837. [CrossRef]
53. Silamiķele, L.; Silamiķelis, I.; Ustinova, M.; Kalniņa, Z.; Elbere, I.; Petrovska, R.; Kalniņa, I.; Kloviņš, J. Metformin strongly affects gut microbiome composition in high-fat diet-induced Type 2 diabetes mouse model of both sexes. *Front. Endocrinol.* **2021**, *12*, 626359. [CrossRef]
54. Tian, J.L.; Si, X.; Shu, C.; Wang, Y.H.; Tan, H.; Zang, Z.H.; Zhang, W.J.; Xie, X.; Chen, Y.; Li, B. Synergistic effects of combined anthocyanin and metformin treatment for hyperglycemia In Vitro and In Vivo. *J. Agric. Food Chem.* **2022**, *70*, 1182–1195. [CrossRef]
55. Nahar, N.; Mohamed, S.; Mustapha, N.M.; Lau, S.F.; Ishak, N.I.M.; Umran, N.S. Metformin attenuated histopathological ocular deteriorations in a streptozotocin-induced hyperglycemic rat model. *Naunyn-Schmiedeberg's Arch. Pharmacol.* **2021**, *394*, 457–467. [CrossRef] [PubMed]
56. Han, Y.C.; Tang, S.Q.; Liu, Y.T.; Li, A.M.; Zhan, M.; Yang, M.; Song, N.; Zhang, W.; Wu, X.Q.; Peng, C.H.; et al. AMPK agonist alleviate renal tubulointerstitial fibrosis via activating mitophagy in high fat and streptozotocin induced diabetic mice. *Cell Death Dis.* **2021**, *12*, 925. [CrossRef] [PubMed]
57. Yadav, K. Nanotechnology in diabetes management: Revolutionizing treatment and diagnostics. *J. Mol. Liq.* **2024**, *414*, 126117. [CrossRef]
58. Zhou, D.Y.; Chen, L.J.; Mou, X. Acarbose ameliorates spontaneous type-2 diabetes in db/db mice by inhibiting PDX-1 methylation. *Mol. Med. Rep.* **2021**, *23*, 72. [CrossRef] [PubMed]
59. Wang, X.D.; Tian, R.; Liang, C.H.; Jia, Y.F.; Zhao, L.Y.; Xie, Q.Y.; Huang, F.L.; Yuan, H.J. Biomimetic nanoplatform with microbiome modulation and antioxidant functions ameliorating insulin resistance and pancreatic β-cell dysfunction for T2DM management. *Biomaterials* **2025**, *313*, 122804. [CrossRef]
60. Herman, R.; Kravos, N.A.; Jensterle, M.; Janež, A.; Dolžan, V. Metformin and insulin resistance: A review of the underlying mechanisms behind changes in GLUT4-mediated glucose transport. *Int. J. Mol. Sci.* **2022**, *23*, 1264. [CrossRef]
61. Kanitkar, M.; Bhonde, R.R. Curcumin treatment enhances islet recovery by induction of heat shock response proteins, Hsp70 and heme oxygenase-1, during cryopreservation. *Life Sci.* **2008**, *82*, 182–189. [CrossRef] [PubMed]
62. Moniruzzaman, M.; Min, T. Curcumin, curcumin nanoparticles and curcumin nanospheres: A review on their pharmacodynamics based on monogastric farm animal, poultry and fish nutrition. *Pharmaceutics* **2020**, *12*, 447. [CrossRef] [PubMed]
63. Lashen, H. Role of metformin in the management of polycystic ovary syndrome. *Ther. Adv. Endocrinol.* **2010**, *3*, 117–128. [CrossRef] [PubMed]
64. Vidon, N.; Chaussade, S.; Noel, M.; Franchisseur, C.; Huchet, B.; Bernier, J.J. Metformin in the digestivetract. *Diabetes. Res. Clin. Pr.* **1988**, *4*, 223–229. [CrossRef] [PubMed]
65. Zhang, D.; Fu, M.; Gao, S.H.; Liu, J.L. Curcumin and diabetes: A systematic review. *Evid.-Based Complement. Altern. Med.* **2013**, *2013*, 636053. [CrossRef] [PubMed]

66. Armour, S.L.; Frueh, A.; Chibalina, M.V.; Dou, H.Q.; Argemi-Muntadas, L.; Hamilton, A.; Katzilieris-Petras, G.; Carmeliet, P.; Davies, B.; Moritz, T.; et al. Glucose controls glucagon secretion by regulating fatty acid oxidation in pancreatic α-cells. *Diabetes* **2023**, *72*, 1446–1459. [CrossRef]
67. Soetikno, V.; Watanabe, K.; Sari, F.R.; Harima, M.; Thandavarayan, R.A.; Veeraveedu, P.T.; Arozal, W.; Sukumaran, V.; Lakshmanan, A.P.; Arumugam, S.; et al. Curcumin attenuates diabetic nephropathy by inhibiting PKC and PKC activity in streptozotocin-induced type I diabetic rats. *Mol. Nutr. Food Res.* **2011**, *55*, 1655–1665. [CrossRef] [PubMed]
68. Sawatpanich, T.; Petpiboolthai, H.; Punyarachun, B.; Anupunpisit, V. Effect of curcumin on vascular endothelial growth factor expression in diabetic mice kidney induced by streptozotocin. *J. Med. Assoc. Thail. Chotmaihet Thangphaet* **2010**, *93*, S1–S8.
69. Tikoo, K.; Meena, R.L.; Kabra, D.G.; Gaikwad, A.B. Change in post-translational modifications of histone H3, heat-shock protein-27 and MAP kinase p38 expression by curcumin in streptozotocin-induced type I diabetic nephropathy. *Brit. J. Pharmacol.* **2008**, *153*, 1225–1231. [CrossRef] [PubMed]

MDPI AG
Grosspeteranlage 5
4052 Basel
Switzerland
Tel.: +41 61 683 77 34

Journal of Functional Biomaterials Editorial Office
E-mail: jfb@mdpi.com
www.mdpi.com/journal/jfb

www.ingramcontent.com/pod-product-compliance
Lightning Source LLC
Chambersburg PA
CBHW061505210926
51850CB00008B/1827
* 9 7 8 3 7 2 5 8 4 9 5 5 0 *